The Health Care
Value Chain

Lawton R. Burns

· ·

and Wharton School Colleagues

The Health Care Value Chain

Producers, Purchasers, and Providers

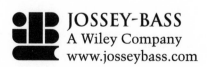

JOSSEY-BASS
A Wiley Company
www.josseybass.com

Published by

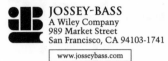 **JOSSEY-BASS**
A Wiley Company
989 Market Street
San Francisco, CA 94103-1741

www.josseybass.com

Jossey-Bass books and products are available through most bookstores. To contact Jossey-Bass directly, call (888) 378-2537, fax to (800) 605-2665, or visit our website at www.josseybass.com.

Substantial discounts on bulk quantities of Jossey-Bass books are available to corporations, professional associations, and other organizations. For details and discount information, contact the special sales department at Jossey-Bass.

We at Jossey-Bass strive to use the most environmentally sensitive paper stocks available to us. Our publications are printed on acid-free recycled stock whenever possible, and our paper always meets or exceeds minimum GPO and EPA requirements.

Library of Congress Cataloging-in-Publication Data

Burns, Lawton R.
   The health care value chain : producers, purchasers, and providers / Lawton R. Burns.
      p. cm.
   Includes bibliographical references and index.
   ISBN 0-7879-6021-7
   1. Medical care--Miscellanea. 2. Medical care--Economic aspects. 3. Organizational effectiveness. 4. Physical distribution of goods--Management. 5. Marketing channels--Management. I. Title.

RA427 .B88 2002
338.4'33621--dc21   2002016113

First Edition
HB *Printing*   10 9 8 7 6 5

Contents

. . . .

Preface

My goal in writing this book was to analyze a large segment of the health care industry that is ignored by academics and only partially understood by executives. This segment is known as *the value chain* or *the supply chain:* the trading relationships between the producers (manufacturers) of health care products, the purchasers of those products (group purchasing organizations, wholesalers/distributors), and the health care providers (hospital customers) that are the end users of those products—hence, the title of this book.

Academics have long studied the relationships between hospitals, physicians, and managed care firms. These trading relationships represent the downstream portion of the value chain. This book focuses instead on the upstream portion of the value chain. I believe there is much here for scholars to learn and mine for their research. I have elected to examine these relationships in terms of competitive strategy, market power, distinctive capabilities, and strategic alliances.

Executives in firms residing along the upstream portion of the value chain know their particular portion of the industry quite well, and perhaps some aspects of their trading partners' portions. However, I have found that some executives often have a limited view of the trading partners two steps removed from them in the chain; for example, hospitals don't really understand manufacturers, and manufacturers don't really understand hospitals. In addition, many

executives of product firms typically have a low opinion of the intermediaries who handle and contract for their products. This book
attempts to educate each side about the other and explore the
potential strategic partnerships that might develop between them.

I believe such an understanding and appreciation is essential if
the health care industry is to develop the extended trading alliances
found in other industries. Also known as *extended enterprises*, these
alliances bring together suppliers and buyers of products to improve
quality, reduce costs, and gain competitive advantage. The overall
objective of this study is to determine the potential for such
enterprises to develop in the health care industry.

The findings and conclusions reported here are based on executive interviews at a sizable sample of firms along the value chain,
background research on the firms where the interviews were
conducted, and material published in industry reports and presented
at industry conferences. This represents an enormous amount of
information on firms and their trading relationships. The general
analytic approach taken here is to immerse ourselves in the details
of these trading relationships, interpret them, and seek to draw gen-
eralizations across firms in our sample. Thus, I seek to generalize
from the bottom up, rather than impose conclusions from the top
down to try to "fit the data." The result is a lengthy report, for
which I ask the reader's indulgence. I believe that a full appreciation for the perspectives of each player along the value chain, as
well as their capabilities and weaknesses as trading partners, requires
an attention to detail.

February 2002   Lawton R. Burns
Philadelphia, Pennsylvania

Acknowledgments

• •

This book is the culmination of a three-year research initiative underwritten by an industry/university consortium—the Center for Health Management Research (CHMR)—funded by the National Science Foundation. The center's membership, a consortium of large integrated delivery networks (IDNs), asked my Wharton colleagues and me to educate them about the health care value chain. The value chain study represents one of the first efforts by health care providers to fully embrace and understand the complexities of their upstream trading relationships. This book, which serves as our final report to the center, also represents the first published book containing research findings from a center-funded project.

I thus wish to thank the Advisory Board of the Center for Health Management Research (CHMR), which selected this project for funding, financially supported it for three years, and provided ongoing feedback on our progress. I am particularly indebted to Howard Zuckerman, Ph.D., past director of the CHMR, who has had a longstanding interest in the health care supply chain and performed much of the early analyses of GPOs. Howard's unflagging support and enthusiasm helped to sustain this project. I am also grateful to Doug Conrad, Ph.D., current CHMR director, for his continuing interest in the project. I also thank the CHMR Project Advisory Committee, composed of the directors of

Materials Management from the integrated delivery networks (IDNs) that compose the CHMR. This committee helped shape the research agenda and gain access to the firms that supply products to them. Special thanks go to Larry Dickson at Sisters of Providence and Mike Rosenblatt at SSM Health Care. They also read several chapters of the manuscript.

As the final customer in the institutional supply chain, the center's IDN members helped us gain entrée to the executives of many of the country's largest product manufacturers, distributors, and group purchasing organizations. I gratefully acknowledge the assistance of the executives of these organizations that participated in the study and agreed to be interviewed. In particular, I thank John Burks at Novation, Ed Swierenga at Broadlane, Dave Pulsifer at Becton-Dickinson, Cindy Derouin at Merck, Jon Northrup at Eli Lilly, and Bob Zollars (then) at Cardinal Health. They read the case summaries that were prepared for their firms, and then labored through the chapters written on different segments of the value chain. I appreciate their candor and patience.

I also thank those colleagues and doctoral students at the Wharton School who contributed to this project: Mark Pauly, Pat Danzon, John Kimberly, Bill Kissick, and Bob DeGraaff. I also wish to thank Mark Pauly and Dean Patrick Harker for time off during the spring 2001 semester to write the bulk of this book. I also gratefully acknowledge the invaluable editorial and administrative assistance provided by Rosalie Natale, Chris Aleszczyk, and Kiersten Rogenmuser in the Health Care Systems department.

The time spent writing this book was made more pleasurable by the opportunity to take a sabbatical at the University of Cambridge (UK). I deeply thank Dr. Don Detmer for helping me to gain affiliations with both the Judge Institute of Management Studies, which served as my office, and Clare Hall, which served as the residence for my family. I value his continued friendship and collaboration. I am also grateful to Dean Sandra Dawson at the Judge Institute and Dame Gillian Beer, President of Clare Hall, for appointing me to their respective institutions.

Finally, I thank Alexandra, my wife of two decades, for her support, patience, and love while this book was written. Her companionship has enriched my life since we met.

About the Author

⬧ ⬧

Lawton R. Burns, Ph.D., MBA, is the James Joo-Jin Kim Professor, and Professor of Health Care Systems in the Wharton School at the University of Pennsylvania. He is also Director of the Wharton Center for Health Management and Economics and Visiting Professor in the Department of Preventive Medicine at the University of Wisconsin School of Medicine. Dr. Burns teaches courses on health care strategy, organization design, organizational change, managed care, and integrated delivery systems. He received his doctorate in sociology and his MBA in health administration from the University of Chicago. Dr. Burns taught previously in the Graduate School of Business at the University of Chicago and the College of Business and Public Administration at the University of Arizona. Dr. Burns has analyzed physician-organization integration over the past fifteen years. He has conducted numerous surveys of physicians at the hospital system, county, state, and national levels, and analyzed the trajectory of physician-hospital relationships over time. In recognition of this research, Dr. Burns was named the Edwin L. Crosby Memorial Fellow by the Hospital Research and Educational Trust in 1992. Dr. Burns has also published several papers on the structure and performance of the physician practice management industry, the market forces that shape the growth of group practices and investor-owned networks, and the organizational options for physicians in a consolidating industry.

In addition to this research, Dr. Burns has conducted an extensive analysis of the Allegheny Health Education & Research Foundation (AHERF) bankruptcy and is now completing a follow-up paper on its implications for hospital governance. He has also completed an analysis of the impact of ownership conversions on hospital strategy, in collaboration with Frank Sloan at Duke University. Dr. Burns has also received an Investigator Award from the Robert Wood Johnson Foundation (along with Gloria Bazzoli) to study the reasons for failure in organizational change efforts by health care providers, and to develop a conceptual model of successful and sustained change. In Spring 2001, Dr. Burns was appointed as the Arthur Andersen Distinguised Visiting Professor at the Judge Institute of Management Studies at the University of Cambridge (UK), and a Life Fellow at Clare Hall.

Dr. Burns teaches one- and two-day management seminars on behalf of the Wharton School and other organizations. These seminars are designed to prepare physicians and administrators for managing large health systems. Dr. Burns sits on the editorial boards of Health Services Research and Health Administration Press. He is a past member of the Grant Review Study Section for the Agency for Health Care Policy and Research.

The Health Care
Value Chain

· ·

To Alex and Brendan,
with All My Love

Part I

· ·

Value Chain Basics

1

The Wharton School Study of the Health Care Value Chain

Lawton R. Burns, Robert A. DeGraaff,
Patricia M. Danzon, John R. Kimberly,
William L. Kissick, and Mark V. Pauly

Focus of This Book

This book analyzes developments in the U.S. health care value chain over the past decade. Wharton School researchers spent three and one-half years (January 1998–June 2001) studying three major players at various stages of the value chain: producers (product manufacturers), purchasers (group purchasing organizations, or GPOs, and wholesalers/distributors), and health care providers (hospital systems and integrated delivery networks, or IDNs) (see Exhibit 1.1). Manufacturers make the products, GPOs purchase them in bulk on behalf of hospitals, distributors take title to them and deliver them, and providers consume them in the course of rendering patient care.

In conducting this study, the Wharton School research team had five broad aims:

1. To profile the major segments in the health care value chain and some of the key players within them, their resources and capabilities, and their recent history;

2. To document how the value chain currently operates;

3. To identify and analyze the strategic and competitive issues facing the three major players;

Exhibit 1.1   Health Care Value Chain

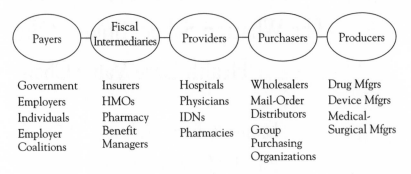

Payers	Fiscal Intermediaries	Providers	Purchasers	Producers
Government	Insurers	Hospitals	Wholesalers	Drug Mfgrs
Employers	HMOs	Physicians	Mail-Order	Device Mfgrs
Individuals	Pharmacy	IDNs	Distributors	Medical-
Employer	Benefit	Pharmacies	Group	Surgical Mfgrs
Coalitions	Managers		Purchasing	
			Organizations	

4. To assess the impact of e-commerce on the value chain; and

5. To assess future prospects for partnerships and improved efficiencies between value chain players.

We believe that an understanding of the first two topics is essential for addressing the latter three.

Our analysis is more strategic than operational. We do not provide comparative benchmarking data or measures or standards of supply chain performance, nor do we identify specific time- and cost-saving opportunities for improvements in work-flow processes. Instead, we seek to understand the bases of cooperation and competition along the value chain, the sources of efficiency in contracting between suppliers and providers, and the emerging best practices and strategic alliances along the value chain. Our overall aim is to determine whether "extended enterprise" models of supply chain collaboration found in other industries can develop in health care.

The book is addressed to both academic researchers and industry executives. We hope academics will find it a useful and comprehensive introduction to a huge segment of the health care industry that is rarely studied, as well as an analysis of the multiple problems in strategic alliance formation in health care. We hope executives will find it helpful for better understanding the motivations of their trading partners and the opportunities for working with them in cooperative endeavors.

Why Study the Health Care Value Chain?

Several major developments in the health care industry during the 1990s prompted interest in the health care value chain. These developments encompassed vertical integration, horizontal integration, managed care pressures, changes in federal reimbursement, the rise of e-commerce, and the passage of the Health Insurance Portability and Accountability Act (HIPAA) in 1996.

First, provider organizations (hospitals and hospital systems) vertically integrated into the health insurance business (for example, starting up HMOs) and the ambulatory care business (for example, acquiring physician practices), and in the process developed *integrated delivery networks*, or IDNs. Such efforts represented attempts to integrate downstream toward the patient, capture a greater portion of patient flows and insurance premiums, and develop some countervailing power vis-à-vis health maintenance organizations (HMOs). With a few notable exceptions, such efforts were spectacularly unsuccessful. Providers instead began to realize there may be opportunities to improve their financial position by partnering with upstream value chain players and, in some cases (for example wholesalers/ distributors), integrating with them.

Second, every major player along the value chain horizontally consolidated. Hospitals merged with one another or joined systems; their group purchasing organizations (GPOs) merged to form super GPOs; distributors merged to build mega warehouses and achieve economies of scale; and product manufacturers merged to gain market share, pool capital and sales forces, and deal with the other consolidated players just mentioned. By the start of the new millennium, it was unclear what were the resulting contracting dynamics within the new, consolidated chain. Was it more competitive or less competitive?

Third, provider organizations were rocked by reimbursement pressures emanating from large HMOs, which had merged to develop greater bargaining leverage with employers and to squeeze providers on payments. Providers were also rocked by reductions in both inpatient and outpatient Medicare payments resulting from the Balanced Budget Act (BBA, 1997) and the Balanced Budget Relief Act (BBRA, 1999), which included the Ambulatory Payment Classification (APC) system.

Fourth, the rise of e-commerce promised a "sea change" and "paradigm shift" in how trading partners were to transact business. Business-to-business (B2B) models using Web technology were sold as the solution to all of the industry's problems and inefficiencies. The new technology would speed up transactions; provide visibility of products and information along the entire chain; and eliminate duplication, paperwork, and processing errors.

Finally, HIPAA developed standards for providers to follow with regard to the format, use, and security of electronically stored and transmitted health care information. These standards had enormous implications for reducing overhead and administrative costs, for the development of electronic commerce, for transacting business with trading partners, and for improving the information available for decision making.

Whereas before the value chain was an unimportant side issue, the events just mentioned collectively propelled value chain issues to the forefront. The increasing importance is reflected in recent consulting firm studies of value chain improvements and efficiencies using e-commerce,[1,2] and funding for this investigation by a consortium of large IDNs known as the Center for Health Management Research (CHMR).

In addition to these developments in health care, the 1990s witnessed the formation of strategic trading alliances in the U.S. auto industry. These alliances, also known as *extended enterprise supplier networks*, brought together suppliers of component parts with large auto manufacturers to collaboratively improve quality, reduce costs, and develop competitive advantage.[3] Such strategic alliances have been held out as examples for the health care industry to follow.

What Is a Value Chain?

Michael Porter, an economist at the Harvard Business School, has popularized the term *value chain* among academic circles to mean the entire production chain from the input of raw materials to the output of final product consumed by the end user.[4,5] This chain is called a value chain because each link in the chain adds some value to the original inputs. There are really two value chains here. The first concerns the stream of productive activities *within* a given firm that allows it to manufacture a product or render a service (see Exhibit 1.2). Thus, a firm acquires inputs (for example, raw materials, labor, capital, and so on), integrates and processes them in a throughput stage, and then produces its outputs. The second value chain includes the stream of activities *across* firms, where the outputs of one set of firms become the inputs for another set of firms. Thus, a firm has input suppliers, industry competitors, distributors, and end customers. An analysis of the value created within a given firm helps to identify its contribution to the value created along the interfirm supply chain.

Exhibit 1.2   Michael Porter's Value Chain

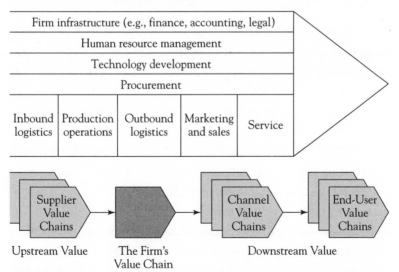

Source: Michael E. Porter. *Competitive Advantage: Creating and Sustaining Superior Performance.* Copyright © 1985, 1999. Adapted with the permission of the FREE Press, a division of Simon & Schuster, Inc.

What Is a Supply Chain?

In industry, the term *supply chain* tends to be used more frequently than *value chain*. A supply chain is a virtual (as opposed to vertically owned) network "that facilitates the movement of a product from its earliest point of production, through packaging and distribution, and ultimately to the point of consumption."[6] The supply chain is thus the path traveled by the product; each stop along that path defines a link in the supply chain.

Supply chain networks may operate to both (1) "push" manufactured products through the chain using sales forces and promotional campaigns, and (2) "pull" products through the chain to continually replenish retailers' inventories and meet customer demand.[7-9] In the former model, manufacturers promote and sell as much product as they can to customers. In the latter model, customers demand products from the preceding link in the chain; those vendors then become responsible to manage the customer's inventories.

Why Do Value and Supply Chains Exist?

Why do value and supply chains exist? There are at least two explanations, derived from industrial organization theory and organizational theory. First, supply chains exist because there is little vertical integration of manufacturers into the distribution and delivery of their products to the end customer. Vertical integration is low because manufacturers believe that the costs of transacting with the marketplace for distribution and delivery are much less than the costs of attempting to take distribution in-house and coordinating all of these exchanges using hierarchical means. That is, manufacturers believe that it is cheaper for them to "buy" distribution services from product wholesalers in the marketplace rather than "make" distribution services in-house. Consequently, manufacturers have elected not to enter the distribution business but rather let specialist firms produce these services for them.

Second, because manufacturers have left the provision of distribution services to others, they are now interdependent with external firms over whom they exercise no hierarchical or managerial control. Consequently, they need to develop contractual or strategic alliance relationships with these specialist firms in order to get their products to the end customer. Supply chains thus exist to coordinate and manage the exchanges of firms that are interdependent.

What Are the Objectives of a Value Chain?

Across firms engaged in trading relationships, a value chain is concerned with several theorized objectives:

- Optimizing the overall activities of firms working together to create bundles of goods and services

- Managing and coordinating the whole chain from raw material suppliers to end customers, rather than focusing on maximizing the interests of one player

- Developing highly competitive chains and positive outcomes for all firms involved

- Establishing a portfolio approach to working with suppliers and customers; that is, deciding which players to work with most closely and establishing the processes and information technology (IT) infrastructure to support the relationships[10]

That is, value chains are supposed to be collaborative partnerships between adjacent players engaged in economic exchange. Such collaborative activity includes coordinated planning of production and distribution to meet the customer's needs on a just-in-time basis that reduces inventory levels and delays in product availability. It is also designed to create a lowest-total-cost solution for the end customer and the manufacturer. Lowest total cost is achieved using demand planning, which relies on information gathered from the customer that "pulls products." Demand planning works backward from the customer toward the manufacturers and their suppliers and original equipment manufacturers (OEMs). This is all in contrast to traditional supply chain management, which starts with the manufacturer that "pushes product" (for example, using marketing and advertising campaigns) and works forward toward the customer. Here the manufacturer's aim is not achieving lowest total cost but increasing product sales, greatest product differentiation, and lowest delivered cost.

Value Chains and Extended Enterprises

Value chains are also supposed to develop as strategies of competitive advantage in which one set of trading partners (input supplier–product manufacturer–distributor) seeks to create more value (for example, higher quality and/or lower-cost products and services) than a rival set of trading partners. Recent research on value chain alliances in the auto industry suggests some of the essential ingredients for success.[11]

One key ingredient is dedicated asset investments in one's supply chain partners in order to increase productivity. These can include dedicated managers and account representatives who accumulate substantial understanding and know-how through long-standing relationships with trading partners. Another type of asset investment is the development of capital investments tailored and customized to a specific trading partner.

A second key ingredient is effective management of knowledge and knowledge flows among trading partners. This requires sharing of information (both explicit and tacit knowledge) rather than secrecy. This is accomplished through supplier associations, learning teams, on-site consultation, joint-study groups, problem-solving teams, and interfirm employee transfers. In this manner, suppliers provide input to product development and process improvement initiatives.

A third key ingredient is trust among trading partners. The presence of trust lowers the necessity for contract enforcement and surveillance and thus reduces transaction costs. Specific means to foster trust include selection of suppliers based on their capabilities and track record for performance (rather than competitive bidding) and previous contracting relationships, establishment of long-term contracts, stability of employment of managers involved in contracting, extensive two-way communication, financial investments in one another, and evaluation of the relationship on a broader scale than just unit price of inputs.

Research on the auto industry suggests that the presence of these three ingredients allows the formation of extended enterprises that span manufacturers and their suppliers. Such enterprises achieve competitive advantage over other manufacturers (that lack such alliances) in terms of the speed of product development, product development costs, transaction costs in procurement, product costs, quality, market share, and profitability.

Do Value Chains Exist in the U.S. Health Care Industry?

In the health care industry, this view represents more aspiration than reality. Despite all of the attention paid to the health care supply chain over the past decades, few of the elements just outlined exist today. To be sure, there are organizations operating at each stage in the supply chain (see Exhibit 1.1). Among producers (manufacturers), there are pharmaceutical companies, medical-surgical products companies, device manufacturers, and manufacturers of capital equipment and information systems. Among purchasers (intermediaries) there are group purchasing organizations, pharmaceutical wholesalers, medical-surgical distributors, independent contracted distributors, and product representatives

employed by some manufacturers. Among organized provider customers (hereafter referred to as *providers*), there are hospitals, systems of hospitals, integrated delivery networks (IDNs), and
alternate site facilities (for example, physician offices and ambulatory surgery centers). What is lacking, however, is coordinated effort
among these parties, widespread strategic alliance formation, knowledge sharing, interfirm trust, and competing value chains oriented
to delivering the greatest customer value at lowest total cost.
Indeed, some industry executives baldly state that the word *partner*
does not really exist.

Everard has recently made a similar point, claiming that supply
chain management does not exist in the health care industry. He
defines supply chain management as

> the intervention of supply chain links and players in
> determining the cost and value of exactly when and how
> a product moves, in what quantities it is moved, who
> moves it and how it is moved, who stores it and how it
> is stored, and when and how it is made available to those
> who consume or use it. Everything that happens to a
> product as it moves through the chain either adds cost
> or reduces cost. It either adds value or reduces value. The
> ultimate goal for any product moving through the chain
> is to reduce cost and add value at the same time.[12]

Within health care, information on the value or cost added at each
link is severely lacking. Indeed, the current state of knowledge on
product value/cost among producers may be so low that meaningful knowledge sharing is impossible. Moreover, there is some consensus that multiple links may perform duplicative functions or
wasteful, non–value adding functions due to this lack of information or reluctance to share information. Finally, there is some consensus that the supply chain acts more to push products down the
chain rather than pull them from the customer, due to this lack

of information at the provider level at the point of consumption. Consequently, each stage holds inventory to prevent stockouts, and providers order products based on just-in-case inventory planning. Moreover, the "product push" mentality creates distrust among providers, who believe that manufacturers are only interested in selling their products.

During the mid-1990s, several prominent supply chain participants formed a consortium called the Efficient Consumer Healthcare Response (EHCR) to combat these problems in the U.S. health care supply chain.[13] They identified an agenda of issues to be addressed, including

- Paper shuffling (manual requisitions and purchase orders, paper-based pricing information)

- Lengthy product ordering and delivery cycle times

- Multiple product handling activities

- Excessive inventory carrying costs

- Lack of information sharing among trading partners

- Little information on product location

- Little information on product utilization

- Operational (rather than customer) focus

- Pressure from managed care organizations to cut short-term costs

- Lack of trust between trading partners

- Lack of complete implementation of electronic commerce

Unfortunately, initiatives such as EHCR have yielded little fruit in terms of concrete partnerships and total-cost reduction efforts (see Chapter Two for more details on the activity of EHCR). Similarly, consolidation efforts by distributors and organized hospital buyers (GPOs) have produced some documented savings and efficiencies in portions of the supply chain without promoting systemic improvements or concerted efforts to reduce total costs. Finally, the advent of e-commerce and the rise of B2B models sparked some short-term interest in health care supply chains on Wall Street but there are few documented savings to date.

What Is Health Care's Problem?

There are several explanations for the health care industry's shortcomings as a value chain. First, unlike other industries, products are often ordered by workers on the front line of health care delivery, such as physicians, nurses, and so on. Purchasing is thus not an organizational competence, let alone a core competence, but rather the domain of non-businesspeople. Products are ordered in a way that maximizes their availability when needed, rather than minimizes the costs of holding inventory. Moreover, the end user ordering products is not typically the buyer (that is, paying for the product). Product demand is thus based heavily on the clinical preference of physicians rooted in their medical training, not on any formal cost-benefit analysis or budgetary constraint. Under the older cost-plus reimbursement environment (prior to DRGs), it did not really matter what the physician ordered or what the hospital paid for supplies. Despite the passage of the Prospective Payment System in 1983, this attitude may still be part of the culture and mentality of older generations of practitioners.

Second, the provider industry overall is largely based on nonprofit ownership. Until recently, there has been no real emphasis on budgeting, and no culture of process improvement to reduce costs. Business practices have crept into the system incrementally over time and have encountered strong resistance from professional norms of patient care and provider autonomy, as well as public goals

regarding patient access and quality of care. Thus, professional training in procurement and logistics has never been a hallmark among
providers, given the prominent role of clinicians and their preferences for branded items. Moreover, since a heavy portion of
provider revenues flow from federal and state governments, some
believe providers have developed a welfare mentality rather than a
strong profit-and-loss mindset. In this regard, the BBA is seen as
"kicking providers off the welfare rolls." Nevertheless, providers
have been buffered from this rude shock by philanthropic dona-
tions, their foundations, and the rising value of their investments
due to the surging stock market in the late 1990s.

Third, despite all of the consolidation, it is still a fragmented
industry with no real leadership at any stage. Fragmentation com-
plicates the task of connecting the thousands of parties involved at
each stage in the chain, and standardizing the formats and content
of their business transactions. Fragmentation also makes it difficult
for one large, leading firm to catalyze the rest of the industry by
changing the business model (for example, Wal-Mart). Coupled
with this fragmentation is decentralization of decision making to
front-line professional workers and moderate decentralization of
provider systems.[14] Consequently, there are lots of autonomous hospital systems and IDNs that themselves are composed of
autonomous units and professional fiefdoms within.

Fourth, providers have historically made their technological
investments in patient care rather than information systems and
infrastructure. Procurement and other functions are based in dated
legacy systems, with little direct connectivity with manufacturers.
Product master catalogs are often paper based, and their contents
(product descriptions, prices) typically differ across players in the
chain due to time lags in relaying and uploading new product and
contract information. The result is a lot of inaccurate data and thus
errors in business transactions. There are few widely accepted industry standards regarding product identifiers or communication
standards, and few decision-making support tools to assess product

spending and utilization, particularly at the point of care. All of this is deadly for an industry that is transaction intensive and facing an exploding knowledge domain.

As a consequence of these factors, the health care industry has been slow to change. Indeed, nonprofit ownership and government regulation buffer health care from market forces. The nonprofit basis has retarded flows of capital, recruitment of business-trained professionals (for example, in IT), and investments in IT needed for change to occur. The presence of third-party payment buffers physicians and patients alike from the immediate financial consequences of their decisions. The presence of professional and accrediting bodies resists the incursion of market forces and any changes that threaten professional prerogatives. And the regionally based character of health care delivery resists uniform technological solutions and standards.

Not surprisingly, analyses of the health care industry do not usually rely on Porter's value chain framework (Exhibit 1.2). Instead, they focus on Porter's "Five Forces" framework (see Exhibit 1.3),

Exhibit 1.3   Porter's Five Forces

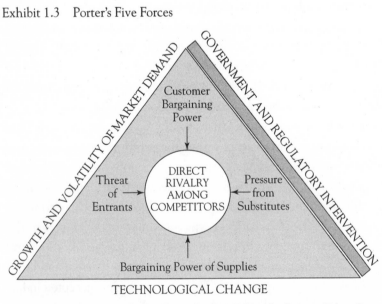

Source: George S. Day. *Market Driven Strategy: Process for Creating Value.* Copyright © 1990, 1999. Reprinted with the permission of the FREE Press, a division of Simon & Schuster, Inc.

which emphasizes competitive rivalry, supplier and customer bargaining power, and the threat of product substitutes and new entrants to the industry.

Where to Focus an Analysis of the Health Care Value Chain?

An analysis of the health care value and supply chain must consider both types of value chains described in Exhibit 1.2: the transformation of inputs into outputs at the firm level (value created by the individual firm) and the exchanges between suppliers, distributors, and customers at the interfirm level (stages of value creation as products and services are transferred from producers through intermediary purchasers toward provider customers). Such a dual focus is important for a simple reason: firms at stage X of the value chain may or may not engage in economic exchanges or strategic alliances with firms at an adjacent stage Y of the value chain, depending on their assessment of the internal capabilities of firms at stage Y to add value. Thus, to some extent, an analysis of the health care value chain requires an analysis of individual firms and their strategic capabilities.

However, a more critical requirement is the analysis of the functions performed by firms at each stage. That is, researchers must analyze what are the contributions of distributors and GPOs to the value of the products manufactured by suppliers. For example, during the past twenty years, many supply chain management functions have migrated from the product suppliers and their hospital customers to distributors.[15] Similarly, many of the purchasing functions have migrated from hospital customers to their GPOs. What value do these intermediaries add to explain their growing ascendance in the supply chain? Such an analysis is important not only for explaining their role, but also for critically assessing the possible disturbance to their role by e-commerce and the trend toward disintermediation in other industries. In the recent past, e-commerce threatened to shift functions away from GPOs to B2B firms, while disintermediation threatened to shift functions away from distributors.

In addition to functions, the analysis of the supply chain requires an analysis of the various flows within it.[16] There are three critical flows: products, money, and information. Players in the supply chain contest access to and control over these three flows. Thus, IDNs may seek to perform group purchasing and product distribution activities in-house to control product flows to the customer and capture administrative fees earned by their GPOs. Similarly, distributors may engage in forward vertical integration strategies toward the customer to gain information on customer product use and then seek to sell that information to manufacturers of the products.

Our vantage point for studying the supply chain is the IDN. The IDN perspective is adopted for several reasons. First, all supply chains are relative from the perspective of the observer. What is a supply chain to one company (an IDN) is a distribution chain to another (a pharmaceutical manufacturer). We take the perspective of IDNs as the ultimate customer because they account for the single largest portion of national health care spending ($390.9 billion, or 32 percent, of total national health expenditures in 1999), roughly 45 percent of which is nonlabor expense. Second, fifteen IDNs funded the project through the Center for Health Management Research, a consortium formed under the auspices of the National Science Foundation (NSF) to promote collaborative research between industry and academia. Industry participants (our sponsoring IDNs) include Henry Ford Health System, Intermountain Healthcare, Fairview, Baylor Healthcare, Catholic Healthcare West, Daughters of Charity, Sisters of Providence, SSM, Mercy Health Services, Northwestern Healthcare, Summa, Aurora Health Care, Catholic Health East, Samaritan Health Services, and Virginia Mason Medical Center. Third, the IDN focus allows us to delimit the boundaries of the project to manageable dimensions. We thus consider the relationships of pharmaceutical firms with institutional customers (but not with retailers) and the impact of business-to-business models (but not business-to-consumer) on the supply chain.

Study Methodology

The study relied heavily on information provided by informants from a broad sample of firms collected over a period of three and one-half years. Some detail is presented in the paragraphs that follow.

Informants

Information for the study was gathered primarily from personal interviews. Between January 1998 and June 2001, we interviewed executives at several major firms across the health care value chain (see Exhibit 1.1). Among product suppliers, we visited pharmaceutical manufacturers, medical-surgical supply manufacturers, and device manufacturers. Among intermediaries, we visited both pharmaceutical and medical-surgical wholesalers, as well as GPOs and some of their B2B technology companies. Among providers, we relied on our IDN sponsors.

Our informants spanned a wide range of functional areas, but typically included the vice presidents or directors for sales, distribution, national accounts, marketing, contracts, strategic sourcing, purchasing, global requirements planning, group planning and marketing, supply chain management, and information management. Interviews were conducted at the sites of our sample firms. Case studies were constructed from field notes for each firm we visited and were shared with those interviewed to ensure accuracy and to protect confidential information.

We conducted structured interviews using the interview protocol contained in Exhibit 1.4. Due to the protocol's length, we ascertained ahead of time which informants were best suited to answer which questions. In most cases, several informants discussed each question to ensure the reliability and comprehensiveness of our field data.

Exhibit 1.4   Specific Research Questions

Group Purchasing Organizations

1. How do suppliers differentiate between classes of GPOs:
   a) true GPOs vs. owned GPOs vs. IDNs?
   b) national GPOs vs. regional vs. local?

2. How do suppliers differentiate between specific GPOs within each class?

3. What features of GPOs are attractive to suppliers? Which GPOs possess these features?

4. What determines whether one GPO gets a better deal than another GPO?

5. Do suppliers ever use "most favored nation" contracting?

6. How big does a GPO/system have to be in order to be noticed by a supplier? How does the supplier weigh the GPO's size versus compliance rate?

7. How do suppliers view contract administration fees? What is their value?

8. What are the benefits of single vs. multi-source contracts?

9. Are GPOs tending toward restraint of trade?

10. How will the Internet (and other electronic commerce) change the role performed by GPOs?

11. How do GPOs differentiate their services to their members?

12. What is the GPO's strategic advantage? How do they maintain it?

13. How do GPOs view the manufacturers and distributors they deal with?

14. How do GPOs justify their contract administration fees (CAFs)?

Wholesalers/Distributors

1. What are the operational efficiencies for manufacturers who rely on distributors? What are the problems?

2. What are the needs and expectations of distributors? What are their views regarding number of delivery points in an IDN?

3. Are distributors willing to work through these logistical problems with GPOs/systems?

4. What other value-adding services do distributors bring to the table?

5. How do suppliers and distributors view firms like Penske Logistics which perform some of the distributors' traditional functions (transportation)?

6. What threat do drug manufacturers see in the trend by drug wholesalers to offer a source product directory?

Product Manufacturers

1. Who is the customer: GPO, system, hospital?

2. What are suppliers doing to recover their costs from discounts?

3. What reengineering have suppliers undertaken here?

4. How do suppliers view distributors' reductions in the variety and number of product lines sold to systems as part of their cost management and standardization effort?

5. What are emerging best practices in supply chain management?

6. Do suppliers believe there are higher costs of doing business with IDNs, due to the multiple parties that must come to the table?

7. What are suppliers doing to reduce turnover of national account representatives which make partnerships difficult?

8. Can account representatives speak for the entire supplier corporation and its many divisions?

9. Where does decision-making authority for contract pricing reside in the supplier firm?

10. What is the GPOs' value-added to manufacturers?

Integrated Delivery Networks (IDNs)

1. Do providers have any advantage in belonging to multiple GPOs?

2. What are emerging best practices in supply chain management?

3. How will the Internet (and other electronic commerce) change procurement?

4. What is the GPO's value added for IDNs?

We supplemented the information gathered from the interviews with a review of the literature on supply chain management (SCM) in industry as well as in health care specifically. We also attended several industry conferences on supply chain management in health care and the impact of e-commerce. Finally, we conducted case studies based on telephone interviews of provider systems that are seeking to serve as their own distributors and GPOs. Insights from these activities are incorporated into the subsequent chapters.

Project Timeline

Phase I of the project (January–December 1998) represented a pilot study of eight manufacturing and wholesaler firms along the value chain to investigate these issues. Phase II of the project (January 1999–December 2000) extended the study to six more pharmaceutical, medical-surgical, and device manufacturers and drug distributors to increase the reliability and validate the earlier findings; three GPOs and two B2B start-up firms to study new issues regarding the Internet and group purchasing; and four IDNs that had become involved in group purchasing and product distribution. Phase III of the project (January–June 2001) was devoted to preparation of the manuscript and revisions based on shakeouts in health care e-commerce and other segments. Our findings reflect the state of the health care supply chain as of early July 2001.

Sample of Firms

Exhibit 1.5 lists the firms interviewed during Phases I and II of the project (excluding the IDNs). We have attempted to collect information from a broad sample along two dimensions: type of product handled (pharmaceuticals, medical devices, and medical-surgical supplies) and role in the supply chain (manufacturer, wholesaler or distributor, and GPO). Two firms did not wish to be identified and are referred to here as *Big Pharma* and *Big Med-*

Exhibit 1.5   Sample of Firms: Phases I & II

Phase I	Phase II
Allegiance Corporation	Abbott Labs
Cardinal Health	Baxter
DePuy	Becton Dickinson
Merck	Bergen Brunswig
Medtronic	Tenet/BuyPower
3M	Eli Lilly
Big Medical-Surgical (anonymous)	Novation
Zimmer	Premier
	Big Pharma (anonymous)
	Broadlane
	Neoforma

Surg. The firms studied are arrayed along these two dimensions in Exhibit 1.6. Many of the major value chain players are represented in our sample of firms. As Exhibit 1.7 illustrates, we have included eight of the top twenty health care firms, and eleven of the top thirty, as ranked by total revenues in 1998 when the study commenced.

Organization of the Book

The book is structured into five sections. The first section, Chapters One to Three, provides an overview of our project, why value chains are important to study but underappreciated, and how the health care value chain works. A reading of Chapter Three will convey some of the enormous complexity of the health care industry in a rather mundane area such as product procurement and delivery.

The second section, Chapters Four to Six, describes the two major intermediaries (purchasers) between producers and providers

Exhibit 1.6   Product and Supply Chain Role of Firms in Sample

| Product | Location in the Chain | | |
	Manufacturer	Distributor	GPO
Drugs	Eli Lilly	Cardinal Health	Premier
	Merck	Bergen Brunswig	Novation
	Abbott		Tenet
	Big Pharma		
Med-Surg	3 M	Allegiance	Premier
	Baxter		Novation
	Big Med-Surg		Tenet
	B–D		
	Abbott		
Devices	Medtronic		
	Depuy		
	Zimmer		

Exhibit 1.7   Ranking of Sample Firms by 1998 Revenues*

Firm	1998 Rev	Rank
Merck	$ 26.9 B	1
Bergen Brunswig	$ 13.7 B	7
Cardinal Health	$ 12.9 B	12
Abbott Labs	$ 12.5 B	13
Tenet	$ 9.9 B	15
Eli Lilly	$ 9.2 B	16
Big Med-Surg (anon)		Top 20
Big Pharma (anon)		Top 20
Baxter Int'l	$ 6.6 B	22
Allegiance	$ 4.6 B	23
Becton Dickinson	$ 3.1 B	27
Medtronic	$ 2.6 B	35

*Excludes payers/HMOs

in the health care value chain: group purchasing organizations (GPOs) and distributors. GPOs buy products in bulk from producers on behalf of their hospital members, while distributors take title to the products and physically deliver them from producers to providers.

The third section, Chapters Seven to Nine, describes the perspectives and strategies of producers (manufacturers) in three product areas: pharmaceuticals, medical devices, and medical-surgical products. These chapters try to parse the different channel strategies taken by product firms and relate them to topics of interest to hospital providers, such as standardization and disease management.

The fourth section, Chapters Ten to Eleven, describes the role of e-commerce in linking up the value chain down to the provider level. Chapter Ten illustrates how e-commerce has developed in health care in the form of stand-alone dot-com firms and the technological solutions developed by GPOs, producers, and distributors. Chapter Eleven argues that all of these solutions may come to naught if providers are unwilling or unable to utilize them.

The fifth and final section represents an attempt to integrate material across the preceding chapters and draw some conclusions. Chapter Twelve discusses some of the facilitators and barriers to improved value chain operations in the health care industry, and some of the leitmotivs of the project. It also offers some forward thinking about the hospital customer of the future.

Endnotes

1. Lacy et al. *The Value of eCommerce in the Healthcare Supply Chain*. Chicago: Arthur Andersen, 2001.
2. Cap Gemini Ernst & Young. *The New Road to IDN Profitability: Realizing the Opportunity in the Health Care Supply Chain*. Chicago: Cap Gemini Ernst & Young, 2001.
3. Dyer, Jeffrey. *Collaborative Advantage*. New York: Oxford University Press, 2000.
4. Porter, Michael E. *Competitive Strategy*. New York: Free Press, 1980.
5. Ibid.

6. McFadden, Christopher D., and Timothy M. Leahy. *US Healthcare Distribution: Positioning the Healthcare Supply Chain for the 21st Century.* New York: Goldman Sachs, 2000.

7. Christopher, Martin. *Logistics and Supply Chain Management: Strategies for Reducing Cost and Improving Service.* 2d ed. London: Prentice-Hall, 1998.

8. Poirer, Charles C., and Stephen E. Reiter. *Supply Chain Optimization: Building the Strongest Total Business Network.* San Francisco: Berrett-Koehler, 1996.

9. Tyndall et al. *Supercharging Supply Chains: New Ways to Increase Value Through Global Operational Excellence.* New York: John Wiley & Sons, 1998.

10. Blackwell, Gordon. *Pharmaceutical Distribution: The Supply Chain.* Westborough, Massachusetts: D&MD Reports, 2000.

11. See Note Three.

12. Everard, Lynn J. *Blueprint for an Efficient Health Care Supply Chain.* White Paper. Norcross, Georgia: Medical Distribution Solutions, 2000, p.2.

13. EHCR. *Efficient Healthcare Consumer Response: Improving the Efficiency of the Healthcare Supply Chain.* Chicago: American Society for Healthcare Materials Management, 1996.

14. Bazzoli et al. "A Taxonomy of Health Networks and Systems: Bringing Order out of Chaos." *Health Services Research* 33(6)(1999): 1683–1717.

15. At the same time, some functions, such as the assembly of kits and trays, have migrated to suppliers.

16. Fein, Adam J. *Leaning on the Promise: Online Exchanges, Channel Evolution, and Health Care Distribution.* New York: Lehman Brothers, 2000.

2

. . . .

Importance of the Health
Care Value Chain

Lawton R. Burns and Robert A. DeGraaff

Recent Ascendance of the Purchasing
Function in Industry

While supply purchasing is a fundamental business activity, it has
historically been subordinate to other functions such as finance,
marketing, operations, and research and development (R&D). By
the early 1980s, however, global markets emerged from both a marketing and purchasing perspective. Personal computers allowed firms
to manage inventories better, automation of production allowed
firms to reduce their unit costs, and trade embargoes raised unit
prices. Input costs thus became an increasing proportion of the cost
of goods sold (COGS), ranging as high as 60 percent. By the 1990s,
purchasing costs accounted for more than 50 percent of sales in an
average manufacturer.[1] Moreover, each dollar saved in purchasing
costs translated directly into an additional dollar of profit and
increased return on investment. Executives recognized that they
could further reduce production costs by outsourcing supplies and
components to specialized manufacturers and developing trading
partnerships with them. This placed a higher premium on supply
chain management and the roles of materials managers and
purchasers within firms. The advent of electronic purchasing systems augmented the potential savings from more advanced supply
management.

One consequence has been a shift from tactical focus on supply unit prices to value-adding services in supply management. These include focus on the firm as a value chain of activities, integration of the firm's supply chain management with its overall strategy, the use of supply chain management as a strategic weapon, a shift in business competition from between firms to between supply chains, and integration of information on supplies and their utilization into the firm's management information system.[2]

Lack of Provider and Supplier Understanding

Despite these developments across industries around the world, much of the health care system was not affected. While health care product manufacturers operate global businesses, health care providers typically do not. The latter have not been exposed to global competition and sourcing of products. Moreover, due to cost-based reimbursement systems, there was little incentive historically to dwell on input prices.

In support of this view, industry observers suggest that health care supply chain characteristics and practices resemble those of industry from the 1960s and 1970s rather than 1990s and 2000s (see Exhibit 2.1). In health care, the business focus is unit cost, whereas in industry it has shifted to total supply chain cost. In health care, the supply chain is managed through budgets; in industry it is managed through measurable process and quality improvements. In health care, the supply chain is viewed as a cost center, whereas in industry it is viewed as an opportunity for innovation. In health care, the organizational structure is oriented around independent, functional department silos, whereas in industry it is oriented around an extended enterprise with trading partners; that is, both upstream (supplier) and downstream (customer) integration. In health care, the information system strategy is lacking or departmentally focused, whereas in industry it is oriented toward both internal and external visibility with one's value chain partners.

Exhibit 2.1   Industry vs. Health Care Approach to the Supply Chain

Industry	Health Care
Focus on total supply chain cost	Unit cost
Focus on quality and process improvements	Focus on managing the supply chain through budgets
Supply chain as innovation opportunity	Supply chain as cost center to be managed
Extended enterprise	Independent departments
Upstream/downstream integration	Departmental process focus
Internal/external data visibility	No information system strategy
Demand planning	Reactive planning

Finally, in health care planning capability is reactive and histori-cal, whereas in industry it is synchronized with end-user demand.[3] One result, according to EHCR, is that health care supply chain costs account for a higher percentage of the cost of goods sold (COGS) compared to other industries (38 percent in health care versus 6–8 percent in retail and 3–6 percent in gro-cery).[4] Some suggest these figures can be reduced to as little as 15–20 percent.[5]

The underlying premise of this project is that health care provider systems need a greater understanding of supply chain issues. Few health administration training programs offer courses in supply chain management; at most they offer courses in operations research. Few programs offer courses on the pharmaceutical or med-ical products and devices industries. Some exceptions are programs based in schools of business, but these programs have added these courses only recently. As a result, most executives of health care systems do not have any formal training in supply chain issues or their supply chain trading partners. The editor of *Hospitals and Health Networks* recently took health system CEOs to task for treat-ing operations as a "second-class citizen."[6] To correct this lack of understanding, the American College of Healthcare Executives (ACHE) Congress, for the first time, included two sessions on supply chain management strategies for executives.[7]

At the same time, some executives in the product manufacturing and distribution firms lack a full understanding of health care provider systems and IDNs. They are typically not trained in health administration programs and in the hospital industry. Unlike the provider side, however, this lack of understanding is not universal. Some executives of supplier or distributor organizations have prior experience in hospital materials management and thus a better understanding of IDNs. Moreover, regardless of their level of understanding, executives on the supply side have expressed a desire for a better understanding of their customer base. Some firms have sponsored their own field studies to interview such downstream trading partners as provider system and GPO executives regarding their supply chain needs.

Increasing Salience of Supply Chain Issues

Current trends in industry suggest that supply chain issues will increase in importance. First, there is a growing movement toward *disintermediation* in industry; that is, cutting out the middleman. In the health care industry, we have witnessed some nascent attempts at disintermediation in the downstream portion of the value chain in the form of provider-sponsored organizations (PSOs) that "direct contract" with the Health Care Financing Administration (HCFA) and employers. There have also been some early attempts at upstream disintermediation in the form of provider systems handling their own product distribution and/or serving as their own GPO. Moreover, there appears to be interest on both sides (provider systems and product manufacturers) to explore the potential for greater direct contracting that would phase out the role of middlemen.

Second, health care supplies (such as pharmaceuticals) account for a rising percentage of national health care expenditures

(8 percent in 1999) and of the total costs to health care systems. Overall, total contracted supply expenditures account for somewhere between 10–15 percent of a system's total budgeted expenditures, based on figures supplied by some of the nonprofit IDN members of the CHMR.[8] Of this amount,

- 15–23 percent are pharmacy costs.

- 30–50 percent are medical-surgical supply costs.

- 11–24 percent are equipment costs.

These figures resemble GPO statistics that 70–80 percent of the supplies purchased by hospitals involve pharmaceuticals, medical-surgical products, and medical devices.[9] Investor-owned hospital systems utilize a different benchmark: supply expenditures as a percentage of system net revenues. For purposes of comparison, Tenet Healthcare's $1.59 billion in supply expenditures (fiscal year 2000) equaled 14 percent of system revenues. This amount is distributed as follows:

- 29 percent are medical supplies.

- 21 percent are pharmaceuticals.

- 13 percent are implantables.

- 10 percent are nonmedical.

- 9 percent are operating room supplies.

- 5 percent are food and dietary.

- 4 percent are IVs.

In addition to direct supply costs, there are indirect supply costs due to handling and processing—what analysts refer to as "the other dollar." When these costs are factored in, the total cost of supplies

Size of the Health Care and Hospital Supply Market
Medical-Surgical and Pharmaceutical Products

Institutional Market (Hospitals and Alternate Site Facilities)

Analysts at U.S. Bancorp Piper Jaffray estimate that the institutional market for medical products, supplies, and services (that is, goods and services purchased by hospitals and alternate site facilities) in 1999 was $200 billion. Part of this amount (51 percent, or $102 billion) was spent on office supplies, food, cleaning supplies, and services. Since most estimates of hospital supply spending omit these categories, this leaves $98 billion as one estimate of supply expenditures. Of this $98 billion, $85 billion was spent on medical-surgical supplies, while $13 billion was spent on pharmaceuticals.[10] This latter figure may be too low (see the following).

The Millennium Research Group estimates the institutional market for medical supplies and equipment in 1999 to be $64 billion, exclusive of prescription pharmaceuticals.[11] Of this amount, $38 billion was spent on lower-end disposables, and $26 billion was spent on higher-end disposables and devices.[12,13] If one adds in the size of ethical drug sales to the institutional market (estimated by IMS and others to be roughly $25–30 billion), then the total market is $94 billion, close to the $98 billion figure reached by U.S. Bancorp.[14,15] Three-quarters of these purchases were made by hospitals, while the rest were made by the alternate site market.

Finally, analysts at PriceWaterhouseCoopers estimate $100 billion in supply spending in the institutional market. Of this amount, hospitals accounted for $75 billion and alternate site facilities $25 billion.[16,17]

Hospital Market Only

Hospitals are a major portion of the institutional market. Overall, analysts at PriceWaterhouseCoopers suggest that hospitals account for

$75 billion in total spending. How much of this is spent on supplies versus pharmaceuticals can be estimated in a number of ways. If, following PriceWaterhouseCoopers, one assumes that three-quarters of institutional spending is hospital based, then hospitals account for nearly $64 billion of the $85 billion in medical-surgical supplies estimated by Goldman Sachs. If one accepts the IMS data that 1999 hospital spending on drugs is $15 billion (50 percent of the institutional market), then hospital spending on medical supplies and equipment is $60 billion of the total $75 billion estimated by PriceWaterhouseCoopers. Alternatively, if one accepts the IMS figure of $15 billion and considers that CHMR hospitals spend anywhere between 15–23 percent of their supply budgets on drugs, then the remainder of their supply budget spent on supplies and equipment ranges from $52–85 billion.

The lower-bound figure is in closer accord with Muse & Associates' hospital survey data on the percentages of hospital nonlabor expenditures devoted to these supply categories. Their survey data suggest that hospital spending on medical-surgical supplies and equipment accounts for 19 percent of nonlabor costs, while pharmaceutical spending accounts for 12.25 percent. Taken together, these figures suggest aggregate expenditures of $34 billion on medical-surgical and $22 billion on pharmaceutical products, or $56 billion.

Thus, we have a range of estimates of hospital supply spending that typically range from $52–64 billion, and maybe as high as $75 billion, although the amounts for each of the two categories (medical-surgical and pharmaceuticals) vary quite a bit.[18] Finally, taking total hospital expenditures in 1999 of $370 billion, the $52–75 billion in spending on medical-surgical and pharmaceutical products accounts for 14–20 percent of hospital costs. This aligns with estimates from the CHMR hospitals.

and handling may approach as high as 25–30 percent of the hospital's budget.[19–21]

While product costs account for a sizable portion of health care system expenditures, the products themselves also represent as much as 25 percent of all system revenues.[22] This is because product costs are not reimbursed directly by payers but are captured in overall reimbursement rates.

Third, as a result of BBA cutbacks in governmental reimbursement, providers have begun to express interest in partnerships with their suppliers as means to develop new sources of revenue and competitive advantage. Academic medical centers are interested in developing closer alliances with pharmaceutical, biotechnology, and device manufacturers to serve as the sites for developing and clinical testing of new products—something they have done in the past but have recently lost market share to clinical research organizations (CROs).

Fourth, EHCR, an industry alliance of product manufacturers, distributors, GPOs, and trade associations reported that $23 billion (27 percent) of the $83 billion spent in 1995 in three supply categories (noncapital medical-surgical supplies, noncapital diagnostics, and nonretail ethical pharmaceuticals) reflected process and procurement costs rather than product costs.[23] The $83 billion represents 10.3 percent of personal health expenditures; $60 billion of these (72.3 percent of supply chain expenses, 7.4 percent of total personal health expenditures) represent product costs. The $23 billion figure was decomposed into order management costs ($8.5 billion in the areas of vendor sourcing; purchase order generation; order entry; negotiation, execution, and administration of contracts and rebates; and customer billing, returns, and credits), inventory management costs ($5.8 billion in the areas of sales and production forecasting, inventory and production planning, inventory storage), transportation costs ($5.5 billion in the areas of inbound and outbound transportation, processing payments for invoices), and physical distribution costs ($3.2 billion in the areas of receiving, putaway, and outbound distribution).[24] Of the total amount, nearly half ($11 billion) could be avoided through improved flows of product, cash, and information. This represents a savings of roughly 13 percent (of the $83 billion in supply expenditures) and an opportunity to reduce costs and improve financial performance without harming quality of care. More recently, analysts have estimated that the typical hospital spends 38 percent of the cost of goods on moving and handling supplies, versus an average of 10 percent or less for most other industries.[25]

It should be noted that the ECHR report is now five years old and has yet to be implemented. Moreover, some of the supply chain firms and trade associations that sponsored the study have departed from this coalition. Some provider organizations and GPOs have been publicly critical of the EHCR report. They question where the purported $11 billion in savings comes from and to which supply chain partners they accrue. More pointedly, they have asked, "Where is the first nickel of savings from EHCR?"[26] In support of this view, only 11 percent of pharmaceutical manufacturers responding to AT Kearney's 1999 Second Pharmaceutical Supply Chain Survey said they currently participate in the EHCR initiative. Barriers to EHCR participation include low priority status (mentioned by 67 percent), lack of knowledge regarding EHCR benefits (56 percent), and a lack of trust within the industry (33 percent).[27] The major barriers to realizing the financial benefits promised by EHCR are the failure of e-commerce to take off (see Chapters Ten and Eleven) and the failure of hospital providers to confront the inefficiencies in their own materials management and product distribution processes.[28]

Misplaced Emphasis by Providers?

Due to the rise of managed care and changes in governmental reimbursement (for example, BBA 1997), health care executives have paid relatively more attention to managing downstream supply chain relationships with payers and fiscal intermediaries than to managing upstream supply chain relationships with product manufacturers and distributors (see Exhibit 1.1). Providers have developed integrated delivery networks (IDNs), partially in an effort to leverage payers for higher reimbursement rates. With some exceptions, these efforts have experienced mixed or little success.[29,30] The HMO industry has become increasingly organized on a for-profit basis, giving plans access to the capital markets to finance mergers and acquisitions that quickly build share. Nonprofit provider systems cannot easily play catch-up by consolidating themselves using internally generated cash flows. Consequently, HMOs often enjoy much greater market share than do provider systems in local markets, thus blunting attempts at monopoly power by providers.[31] Moreover, antitrust enforcement efforts by the Department of Justice (DOJ) and the Federal Trade Commission (FTC) have been directed more at providers than at the fiscal intermediaries. This may reflect the government's interest in using managed care as a cost containment vehicle. More generally, the DOJ and FTC seem more interested in preventing monopoly power wielded by provider cartels dealing with HMOs, or by HMO cartels dealing with employers. Similar efforts are under way in state attorney general (AG) offices to combat large powerful IDNs in local markets.[32]

Providers may also have focused their attention on managed care firms due to the vast sums of money they broker and siphon away from providers. However, due to competition among health plans and the insurance underwriting cycle, profits in the managed care industry fell during the late 1990s to the low single digits. Should health care executives ever succeed in wielding greater power over managed care firms, they will not find large sums of money to reappropriate, at least in the short term.

On the other hand, the product manufacturers have been earning double-digit rates of return over the past five to eight years. Particularly noteworthy are the pharmaceutical manufacturers and the medical device manufacturers, which have been earning returns of 20–22 percent annually. Manufacturers view these returns as entirely justified, based on their rate of innovation, more efficient processes, and what they see as their "ability to take raw materials, convert them to something different, and make products that serve customer needs."[33] Providers and managed care firms alike are interested in partnering with these manufacturers in order to share in their revenue streams. The problem, at least in the eyes of the manufacturers, is that providers first need to fix their own internal systems before "looking over the fence at their neighbors' margins."

The Supply Chain as a New Source of Revenue and Cost Containment

Providers have been engaged in a series of internal cost containment efforts throughout much of the 1990s and into the new millennium. These include work restructuring, firm downsizing, and total quality management. These efforts have played themselves out and have yielded few demonstrable savings. Providers have also been engaged in efforts to boost their market power to negotiate with downstream payers and their brokers (HMOs) from more advantageous positions. These efforts have typically included horizontal integration (for example, multi–hospital system membership, hospital mergers). Antitrust limits and the lack of demonstrated economies of scale from these combination efforts limit the cost-saving potential of this set of strategies.[34,35]

Consequently, providers may be running out of places to save money and cut costs. Where might they turn next? A recent survey of health care executives indicates that providers believe the best opportunity to improve their margins lies in reducing pharmaceutical costs (27 percent of those polled) and diagnostic test utilization (20 percent). Savings on the purchase of medical-surgical supplies came in a close third (19 percent).[36] The supply chain offers an alternative, upstream approach for cost containment and revenue enhancement. One recent report targets for improvement such areas as centralized sourcing of supplies, vendor-managed inventory, and invoicing.[37] Areas to consider include product utilization and standardization, and contract utilization and compliance (see Chapter Four). A similar recommendation has recently been advanced by Cap Gemini Ernst & Young.[38] To make such an effort succeed will require greater understanding of the health care supply chain and greater executive support for pursuing this strategy. The following chapters are intended to address these needs.

Endnotes

1. Dobler, Donald W., and David N. Burt. *Purchasing and Supply Management*. New York: McGraw-Hill, 1996.
2. Porter, Michael E. *Competitive Advantage*. New York: Free Press, 1985.
3. Pandita, Vinnie. "Centralized Materials Distribution: Is It Right for Your System?" Presentation to Strategic Sourcing and E-Commerce Solutions for the Med-Surg Supply Chain Conference. Philadelphia, Pennsylvania: October 1999.
4. EHCR. *Efficient Healthcare Consumer Response: Improving the Efficiency of the Healthcare Supply Chain*. Chicago: American Society for Healthcare Materials Management, 1996.
5. See Note Three.
6. Grayson, Mary. "Second Class." *Hospitals and Health Networks* 74(1) (2000): 8.
7. Kowalski, Jamie C. "CEOs Indifferent to Operations." *Hospitals and Health Networks* 74(3) (2000): 12.
8. The Advisory Board estimates that 16 percent of hospital spending in 1998 was accounted for by supplies, with another 5 percent accounted for by equipment. Remaining hospital costs included labor (57 percent), interest expense (5 percent), business services (4 percent), repairs and maintenance (2 percent), and all other (11 percent). The Founders Council. *Online Supply Chain Management*. Washington, D.C.: Advisory Board Company (January 15, 2001).
9. Cassak, David. "Burden of Proof." *In Vivo* (June 2001): 26–40.
10. Marhula, Daren C., and Edward G. Shannon. *EHealth B2B Overview*. Minneapolis, Minnesota: U.S. Bancorp Piper Jaffray, 2000.
11. *Online Opportunities in the Medical Products Marketplace*. Stream 1, Issue 2 (October 2000). Toronto: Millennium Research Group.

12. The $64 billion figure is close to other estimates. Hambrecht & Quist suggest the total global device market to be $135 billion (excluding dental and X-ray), of which the U.S. market is 42 percent or $57 billion. (Rob Faulkner. Presentation to Wharton School. November, 2000.) According to U.S. Government figures, medical product shipments from manufacturers, including both med-surg supplies and devices, in 1999 equaled $56.5 billion. (Bureau of Economic Analysis, 2001. www.bea.doc.gov.)

13. With regard to higher-end devices, Frost and Sullivan make similar spending estimates for 1999 as follows: $19.9 billion for higher-end disposables and $7.1 billion for capital equipment. (*The Internet's Role in the U.S. Distribution of Medical Devices.* San Jose, California: Frost & Sullivan, 2000.)

14. Risinger, David, and Owen Hughes. *Healthcare Distribution.* New York: Merrill Lynch, 2001.

15. Despite their high estimate for total hospital spending, Muse & Associates (2000) suggest figures for institutional spending on medical supplies and equipment and on pharmaceuticals that are roughly comparable to those of other analysts. For 1998, they estimate total spending of $82 billion, broken out as follows: $61 billion for medical-surgical supplies and equipment, and $21 billion for pharmaceuticals. If one takes into account increased spending levels between 1998 and 1999 (for example, 10–15 percent increase in pharmaceutical costs), then 1999 spending levels begin to approximate the $94–98 billion figures cited in the text. (Muse & Associates. *The Role of Group Purchasing Organizations in the U.S. Health Care System.* Washington, D.C.: Muse & Associates, 2000.)

16. PriceWaterhouseCoopers. *HealthCast 2010: eHealth Quarterly— Procurement.* August, 2000.

17. Analysts at Goldman Sachs (GS) place a higher estimate on total institutional spending for medical-surgical supplies, pharmaceuticals, and equipment ($118 billion). Part of the difference here may reflect GS' inclusion of capital equipment. Frost and Sullivan estimate this to be roughly $7 billion (see Note Seventeen).

18. Specifically with regard to pharmaceuticals, Drug and Market Development (D&MD) estimates that institutionally based drug spending is apportioned as follows: 19 percent in the hospital channel and 9 percent in alternate sites. (Cf. Blackwell, Gordon. *Pharmaceutical Distribution: The Supply Chain.* Westborough, Massachusetts: D&MD Reports 2000.) By contrast, IMS suggests the split is 12 percent and 12 percent, respectively.

19. See Note Three.

20. See Note Four.

21. Healthcare Business. "Reinventing the Health Care Supply Chain." *Healthcare Business Special Supplement* (June 2000).

22. McFadden, Christopher D., and Timothy M. Leahy. *US Healthcare Distribution: Positioning the Healthcare Supply Chain for the 21st Century.* New York: Goldman Sachs, 2000.

23. See Note Four.

24. EHCR, Figures 2–11 and 2–12.

25. Grossman, Robert J. "The Battle to Control Online Purchasing." *Health Forum Journal* (January/February 2000): 18–21.

26. Strong, John W. "What Will Be the Impact of E-Commerce on Group Purchasing Organizations?" Presentation to Medical Equipment and Health Supplies on the Internet Conference. Chicago: May 2000.

27. Findley, Richard. "The Pharmaceutical Supply Chain." Presentation to The Global Rx Supply Chain Conference. Philadelphia: October 1999.

28. Everard, Lynn. "What $11 Billion in Savings?" *Repertoire* 9(2) (2001): 14–15.

29. Burns et al. "The Fall of the House of AHERF: The Allegheny Bankruptcy." *Health Affairs* 19(1) (2000): 7–41.

30. Burns, Lawton R., and Douglas R. Wholey. (2000). "Responding to a Consolidating Healthcare System: Options for Physician Organizations." In J. D. Blair, M. D. Fottler, and G. T. Savage (Eds.). *Advances in Health Care Management.* Volume 1, pp. 273–335. New York: Elsevier.

31. Feldman, Roger, and Douglas R. Wholey. "Do HMOs Have Monopsony Power?" Unpublished manuscript, 2000.

32. Wieffering, Eric, and Terry Fiedler. "The Health Care Shakeup: A Bold Experiment Fizzles." *Star-Tribune.* Minneapolis-St. Paul. July 22, 2001. Page A1.

33. Quotation from a medical-surgical manufacturing executive in the Wharton School study.

34. Dranove, David. "Economies of Scale in Non-Revenue Producing Cost Centers: Implications for Hospital Mergers." *Journal of Health Economics* 17 (1998): 69–83.

35. Spang, Heather, Gloria Bazzoli, and Richard Arnould. "Hospital Mergers and Savings for Consumers: Exploring New Evidence." *Health Affairs* 20(4) (2001): 150–158.

36. Health Care Advisory Board. "Advisory Board's 2000 Executive Survey." *Cost and Finance Watch.* (November 17, 2000). Washington, D.C.: Health Care Advisory Board.

37. Health Care Advisory Board. *Strategic Sourcing.* Washington, D.C.: The Advisory Board Company, 2000.

38. Cap Gemini Ernst & Young. *The New Road to IDN Profitability: Realizing the Opportunity in the Health Care Supply Chain.* Chicago: Cap Gemini Ernst & Young, 2001.

3

· ·

How the Health Care
Value Chain Operates

Lawton R. Burns

Value Chain Overview

As mentioned in Chapter One, a value chain is a virtual network designed to help move a product from the producer (manufacturer) through an intermediary purchaser (distributor), and eventually down to the provider (end user). This network may both push manufactured products through the chain using sales forces and promotional campaigns, and pull products through the chain to continually replenish retailers' inventories and meet customer demand.

Due to the advent of networking technology and global competition in the 1980s, value chains have increased in sophistication in several areas. Product manufacturers have employed inbound supply management techniques to plan their raw materials requirements, utilize just-in-time (JIT) management to reduce inventories, integrate demand management with their production processes, and develop sole-source supplier relationships. Retailers and customers have developed improvements in outbound supply chains to compete more effectively on price. These include using bar coding, point-of-sale information systems, electronic analysis of sales trends and inventory consumption rates to automate inventory management, and partnerships with suppliers and distributors to manage and track inventory.[1-4]

A value chain typically consists of two-way flows of money, products, and information between manufacturers and customers.[5] Physical goods move downward from manufacturers to distributors to customers or retailers, while information and money move upward through a back channel to the manufacturer. Chain efficiency was originally assessed in terms of the downward *velocity of inventory*; that is, the number of turns on fast- versus slow-moving items. Strategies to increase this velocity include automation of warehouses and reduction in the number of stockkeeping units (SKUs) to focus on those that turn over rapidly (and thus do not sit in inventory).

For product distributors in the chain, the critical variables are the product's brand name, the service and working capital requirements to push the product, and the margins yielded by manufacturers. Branded products that have their own promotional campaigns (manufacturer backing and thrust) and generate their own customer demand lead to higher inventory turnover, lower inventory costs, and lower marketing costs, which thus tie up less of the distributor's capital. Unbranded products, on the other hand, require the supply chain to build customer demand, and carry greater inventory costs. In such cases, manufacturers must provide higher margins to distributors. Analysts estimate that distributors earn margins two to four times higher for manufacturers of commodity and niche products than for branded products. As productivity gains from use of these strategies decrease, more attention is paid to back-channel flows as a growing source of value creation for chain participants.[6]

Why is all of this important? Product brand may not carry as much weight in patients' eyes in the health care industry as it does in consumer goods industries. With few exceptions, branded products are invisible to patients treated in health care facilities. Admittedly, some brand name items are important to clinicians who will demand them. However, for other items, product service may be more important than brand, and thus require more effort on behalf of distributors.

How Does the Health Care Supply Chain Work?

Health care systems and IDNs utilize suppliers in roughly eight different areas: pharmaceuticals, medical-surgical supplies (that is, disposables), radiology and laboratory supplies, medical devices (for example, stents or implants), capital equipment, food and dietary supplies and services, office forms and supplies, and cleaning supplies and services. Across these broad areas, providers order at least 30,000–50,000 items from their suppliers in a given year, and maybe as many as 100,000 different items for large IDNs with physician networks. Depending on the type of product, these items can be sold through one of two basic supply chains: (1) direct sale from manufacturer to hospital customer, or (2) mediated sale through wholesalers and distributors. In each instance, the sales contracts may be negotiated through a third party representing hospitals, the group purchasing organization (GPO). This yields a fourfold classification of GPO-contracted and distributor-mediated products, depicted in Exhibit 3.1.

Several observers have diagrammed the complex flows in the health care supply chain. The EHCR report provides a large

Exhibit 3.1   GPO-Contracted vs. Distributor-Mediated Products

	Suppliers Contract with GPOs	Suppliers Do Not Contract with GPOs
Suppliers' use wholesaler or distributor	Medical-surgical products of low value and high volume Generic drugs	Some branded drugs (oncology, cardiovascular) Small volume arcane items Generic drugs
Suppliers use direct delivery	Lower-end implants and medical devices Branded drugs	Higher-end implants and medical devices, specialty items of high value and low volume

flowchart of the product, information, and cash flows.[7] While comprehensive, the flowchart is somewhat dense and does not identify the major players. Wall Street industry reports offer more intelligible schematics of these flows.[8,9] Our depiction of the supply chain is even more straightforward. Exhibit 3.2 identifies the three major, incumbent players in the health care supply chain—producers (manufacturers), intermediary purchasers (GPOs and distributors), and providers (IDNs)—and the various links between them. It is along these linkages that the important flows occur. We describe the three flows of products, money, and information between these parties next.

Flow of Products

Product manufacturers represent the beginning of the flow of materials. For simplicity's sake, we do not consider the flow of raw materials to the product manufacturers from their own input suppliers and original equipment manufacturers (OEMs). Once the product is manufactured, it may be delivered to the hospital system directly by the manufacturer and its agents (for example, orthopedic implants) or indirectly using distributors (for example, gauze).

Exhibit 3.2.   Flows in Health Supply Chain

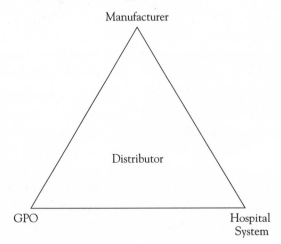

Manufacturers of devices and specialty items typically have not used large distributors for their products. There are at least three reasons for this. First, the major mission of manufacturers is to have direct contact with clinicians—contact unimpeded by intermediaries. Second, the manufacturer possesses critical knowledge about product features and product use that help to satisfy customer needs. Most distributors lack in-depth product knowledge across multiple specialty items. Third, there may be insufficient customer demand for many specialty items, deterring the use of wholesalers that, due to their low margins, rely heavily on large volume. Device manufacturers typically have delivered their products directly to providers by means of Federal Express shipments (for example, for next-day surgical procedures) or hand delivery by their field sales representatives, who serve as technical experts and after-the-sale service agents. Indeed, the latter often are present in the operating room, assisting the surgeon with the appropriate choice of device and (sometimes) with its proper use and insertion into the patient. While some device manufacturers use intermediaries, they tend to use their own franchise distributors. Thus, referring back to Exhibit 3.2, the distributors may be in the middle of the right side of the triangle that links manufacturers with hospital systems.

Manufacturers of generic pharmaceutical and medical-surgical supply products typically rely on wholesalers or distributors for delivery to institutional customers. These products, which account for the bulk of purchased goods, are typically replenishment items that lack unique specification or can be reordered based on established specifications. The distributors buy the products from the manufacturers and take ownership of the inventory, which is stored in large, regionally centralized warehouses. Distributors then use computer technology to "pick, pack, and ship" items ordered by health care provider customers—thus breaking down the boxes delivered by the manufacturer and reassembling them to fill customer orders. Distributors then ship these boxes using fleets of trucks that they either own or lease. Shipments are made either to centralized warehouses owned by the health care system or to its constituent hospitals (for example, loading docks used by the materials management department). From there, products are delivered to the appropriate areas (for example, pharmacy, central sterile supply, dietary, and so on). Product returns back up the supply chain are also handled by the distributors. The value provided by distributors here lies clearly in the logistics function of moving boxes and holding inventory for both buyers and sellers.

Depending on the estimate, the majority or near majority of products purchased by hospitals and health care systems are on national GPO contracts. Millennium states that 66.5 percent of all hospital supplies (an average of $25.1 million) are purchased through GPO contracts.[10] Supply chain executives interviewed for this study gave estimates in the 50–60 percent range; some estimated an even lower figure between 40–45 percent.[11] For these GPO contracts, large distributors tend to make delivery. The remaining percentage of products not on national GPO contracts are negotiated through local or regional purchasing contracts, and delivered through local distributors. Higher-end devices and implants (for example, hips, knees, and shoulders) and medical specialty items tend not to be included in GPO contracts but may be negotiated directly with the manufacturer. GPOs may get into the lower-end implants and devices market (for example, fracture management), especially when their member hospitals have acquired physician practices.

Flow of Money

There are several flows of money in the simple supply chain illustrated in Exhibit 3.2. One set of flows involves the manufacturers, distributors, and health care systems. The manufacturer sells the products to the distributor, which purchases the inventory at manufacturer list prices. The distributor, in turn, sells the products to the health care system at reduced contract prices negotiated by its GPO with the manufacturer. Why the divergence in prices? Distributors pay list price because they cannot anticipate all of the transactions, prices, and contracts in the market. When hospital customers place product orders through their distributors, the latter need to know the price in order to generate an invoice. Manufacturers update distributors on the prices they have negotiated with GPOs and those hospitals eligible for the discounted prices. GPOs may likewise upload contract pricing to authorized distribution agents (ADAs) for use by GPO members. ADAs are those distributors chosen and contracted by the GPO to distribute products stipulated in the manufacturer-GPO contract to the GPO's hospital members. Everard notes, "In order for the hospital to actually get the new contract price, it must be purchased through an authorized distributor. An authorized distributor is recognized both by the GPO and the manufacturer of the contracted product."[12]

This description illustrates that distributors are part of the pricing equation since they take title to the products and resell them at *cost-plus*; that is, the price negotiated between the manufacturer and GPO plus a handling fee (for example, percent of invoice) negotiated between the GPO and the distributor.[13] Once the distributor has filled the health care system's order, it issues a charge-back, or credit, to the manufacturer for the difference between the list price at which it acquired the products and the discounted price paid by the customer on all items ordered. Manufacturers pay these charge-backs on a periodic basis (monthly or quarterly) to their distributors by electronic means.[14] Distributors may also receive an additional cash discount of 1–2 percent for prompt payment (for example, within fifteen to thirty days).

Distributors receive other fees from manufacturers in addition to the rebates. For example, they receive tracing fees for documenting the volume of products sold to particular markets or providers, as well as marketing fees for distributor sales representatives who carry the manufacturer's promotional material with them on sales calls. Supply chain participants estimate each of these fees can amount to 1–2 percent of sales. Distributors may also receive rebates from vendors for a demonstrated ability to influence the manufacturer's market share within a given geographic area or customer segment.[15] The distributors' ability to move share is lessened when shipping products made by top-tier medical, surgical, and pharma manufacturers, where brand influence is important in customer selection, as well as for high-technology and physician preference items, which may be purchased directly by the customer. The distributors' ability to move share is threatened by their falling profit margins, which lowers their ability to hire good sales representatives to work with materials managers and CFOs on product utilization and standardization.[16]

Another flow of money involves the manufacturers, GPOs, and health care systems. When GPOs negotiate contracts on behalf of their hospital system members, they typically receive a contract administration fee (CAF) from the product manufacturer as part of a rebate process. One purpose of the rebate system is to demonstrate the quantity of products purchased through the GPO contract that legitimates the CAF. GPOs can receive these rebates or performance credits from manufacturers either on the front end of contracts or on the back end, as GPO members meet compliance targets (that is, committed purchases of certain products). These CAFs represent to manufacturers the cost of doing business; that is, the cost of getting access to the hospital members of the GPO. To GPOs, they represent a major portion of their revenues. CAFs typically amount to 2–3 percent of the sales contract (price × volume); some GPOs report CAFs of 3 percent for sole-source contracts (soles) and 2 percent for dual-source contracts (duals). For manufacturers that negotiate billion-dollar contracts with GPOs, these fees can be substantial. What happens to these CAFs depends on the particular GPO. While GPOs may elect to retain much of the revenue, they typically pay back to their shareholder members a sizable portion of the fees as (1) compliance rebates for adhering to the contracts signed; and (2) dividends, net of operating and other expenses. In this manner, the health care system earns back some of the membership fees it pays to belong to the GPO.

A third set of money flows involves the GPOs and the distributors. Once the GPO negotiates the product price with the manufacturer, it then negotiates delivery fees nationally and regionally with distributors. Distributors compete with one another for the GPO contracts. GPOs may play one distributor off another in order to reduce these fees or gain service concessions.

It is important to point out that the aforementioned scenario does not hold in cases where there is no GPO contract—as is true for small volume and specialty items. With small volumes, manufacturers of these products see little value in spending resources attempting to garner national GPO contracts. Hence, they typically sell their products directly to customers or to distributors and allow the latter to establish their own prices with customers.[17]

Why are these flows so complex? Wall Street analysts state that the process helps to ensure that the objectives of all parties are simultaneously achieved: compliance for the GPO, volume for the manufacturer, pricing for the provider, and margin for the distributor.[18] It still begs the question, however, as to whether this is the best means for achieving these objectives, given the amount of duplicated effort and cross-checking of orders and payments. Indeed, representatives from a coalition of distributors claim that hundreds of their employees are required to tackle and manage the rebate system.

There are other possible reasons for the existence of chargebacks and rebates, however. Some argue that they exist to benefit the manufacturer; others argue they benefit the distributor; still others claim they exist for legal reasons. First, the rebate system allows the product manufacturer to maximize its margins. A manufacturer sells products to multiple hospital customers through different GPOs. While the differences may or may not be big, GPO #1 may be able to negotiate a better (lower) price for its hospital members compared to GPO #2. But if both GPOs use the same distributor, this poses a problem for the manufacturer: at what price do you sell the inventory to the distributor, which is taking title to the goods? The manufacturer solves this problem by selling the products at list price and then allowing the distributor to apply for a charge-back after the sale that reflects the difference between the list price and the price negotiated by the GPO for a particular hospital account. The rebate system thus allows the manufacturer to sell its products to multiple GPOs at different prices through the same distributor, and maximize its margins on those products. This becomes true when hospitals are slow in paying their bills (which they are, relative to distributors). This becomes especially true when contract prices constantly change (which they do). The pharmaceutical distributor Bergen Brunswig handles four to five million contract changes per month across its various businesses. Assuming 90 percent distributor accuracy with $200 million in accounts receivables, this means there is a lot of money floating around to be correctly accounted for.

Second, the rebate system may be said to exist because it allows the distributor to take title to the manufacturer's products, and thus link itself to the product sales transaction. In this manner, the distributor insinuates itself into the flow of product information, becomes part of the pricing equation, and garners some measure of power and influence. As one executive stated, "the charge-back system is a wholesaler-originated program that enables them to participate as distributors in the contracted marketplace. Otherwise, manufacturers would be forced to sell direct and not use their distribution systems."

Third, according to Everard, "The rebate is necessary because the manufacturer will not honor the contract price unless proof exists that the hospital that bought the product on contract was in fact authorized to do so. Once such is provided, the rebate is issued."[19] Moreover, "The rebate process . . . serves to validate the quantity of products purchased by the member at the contract price. This information is forwarded to the manufacturer, who processes the 'make the distributor whole' rebate to the distributor and the administrative fee rebate to the GPO."[20]

Fourth, rebates allow manufacturers to reward distributors for helping to move market share; that is, promote their products at the expense of another competing manufacturer's products. "Rebates exist partly because of legal regulations that prohibit non-volume-based differential pricing between one distributor of the same manufacturer's products and another distributor buying the same products in the same volume."[21]

Regardless of the reason for their existence, rebates are singled out by many supply chain players as the single biggest source of inefficiency and the best area to achieve savings. Manufacturers claim, "We have more FTEs giving money back in the form of rebates than we have FTEs taking orders in." They also claim that the failure to address this area is the single biggest reason why the industry has witnessed no savings from the EHCR initiative. One reason why it has not been addressed is the presence of a strong set of large distributors whose interests are served by rebates. Another reason is that rebates and charge-backs result from communication breakdowns between manufacturers, distributors, GPOs, and hospitals regarding product prices. Such breakdowns may require the implementation and widespread adoption of Web-based ordering and purchasing before they can be resolved. A final reason, acknowledged by product manufacturers, is the lack of courage and leadership on their part to overhaul this portion of the industry and make product pricing more visible and available in real time.

Flow of Information

Just as products flow upward and downward, so does information. As mentioned earlier, information flows upward through back channels. GPOs communicate information to distributors on GPO membership changes and contract pricing. After contracts have been signed, distributors provide data to manufacturers on utilization by contract and product rebates. Manufacturers typically buy back these data from distributors (tracings) for a 1–2 percent fee to validate their sales, although some firms, such as Johnson & Johnson and 3M, are using the Internet to handle this function. This provides the manufacturer a window on its customers. Information may also flow down the chain, for example, as manufacturers coordinate product marketing campaigns with distributors, including rebates for meeting volume targets.[22]

Another important information flow is the actual ordering process. Typically, the process is initiated by the customer, who pulls products down from manufacturers. The customer (for example, physician, pharmacist, and so forth) submits product requests to the system's materials and procurement manager, who then selects the items from a product catalogue (currently paper, increasingly electronic). The order is then transmitted by telephone, fax, or Electronic Data Interchange (EDI) to the GPO and distributor for fulfillment. These orders are then bundled and transmitted to the various manufacturers for shipment. There is thus considerable manual effort involved in the ordering process, and some multiplication in product ordering and handling activities—all of which explain why product delivery may take up to seven days.[23]

Who Is the Customer?

Given the complexity of the flows described in Exhibit 3.2, it is not surprising that there are multiple customers in the value chain. Hospitals, health care systems, and nursing homes are the ultimate institutionally based customers since they pay the bill for the supplies that are manufactured and distributed. Within these institutions, however, there are multiple customers who are responsible, directly or indirectly, for ordering the products. When asked who their customer was, many manufacturing and distribution executives joked, "Whoever is on the phone" or "The person who has a P.O. [purchase order]." In a more serious vein, they stated they have to "cover all the bases" and consider each of the individuals below their customer.

Physicians are the end customer for many types of products, such as clinical preference items (for example, medical devices, surgical instruments) and brand-name drugs. Their preferences must be taken into account for several reasons. At a minimum, they may complain to senior executives if their preferences are not acknowledged; at the maximum, they may decide to take their patients and elective procedures elsewhere if they are dissatisfied. Physicians' product preferences may be tied to disease management programs. As physicians receive more information around "best practices" from manufacturers and distributors, they may be more willing to make decisions that alter the type of products they utilize. In this manner, manufacturers and distributors hope to shape customer demand for clinical preference items. Finally, physicians are key customers in both hospital-based and freestanding alternate delivery sites, such as outpatient centers and ambulatory surgical centers (ASCs). Most of the large distributors have invested in the alternate site market in terms of delivering products to ASCs and physician group practices. They anticipate this market will grow substantially in the near future, as integrated health care wanes and IDNs spin off their acquired physician practices. As stand-alone, independent sites without a hospital sponsor, they may no longer be served by the IDN's GPO contracts and ADAs.

The system's chief pharmacist is also a customer by virtue of filtering the preferences of the system's physicians and harmonizing them with any existing formularies. The system's vice presidents for materials management and purchasing represent another set of customers that actually order the products. They typically seek to standardize (as much as possible) the purchase of generic supplies in order to (1) reduce the number of stockkeeping units (SKUs) in the system's inventory and (2) increase the volume purchased in given areas in order to gain the best prices. They are currently seeking to develop standardization programs for clinical preference items. They face many barriers to their standardization efforts, not the least of which are the large number of hospital departments and customers they have to deal with (for example, physicians, nurses, respiratory therapists, operating room staff, emergency room staff, and so on), and the fact that they often each want a different brand version of the same product (see Chapter Four).

Manufacturers might also be considered customers, at least in the eyes of distributors. By virtue of the charge-back process, manufacturers constitute the source of the distributors' (thin) profit margins. Distributors are also seeking to add value for manufacturers in other ways, such as innovative product packaging (see Chapter Five).

Distributors and GPOs are not generally considered to be customers in the supply chain. They are viewed more as partners for both upstream and downstream players, as well as influencers of what the customers actually purchase. Understandably, there is some concern among other value chain participants regarding the value added from these two parties. There was also considerable speculation regarding their survival prospects with the advent of e-commerce. Any such fears quickly dissipated with the collapse of the dot-coms in the spring of 2000. These issues are explored in Chapter Ten.

To some extent, GPOs might be considered a customer of the distributors. A distributor that becomes an ADA for a GPO when it previously had no contract can experience significant revenue growth. Or, at a minimum, armed with the agreement as an ADA, the distributor can try to drive the business and focus more intensively on hospital accounts. Nevertheless, the margins allowed by the GPOs don't resemble a revenue flow. Typically, when a hospital's account with a distributor falls under a GPO contract the distributor experiences a reduction in margin. Moreover, GPOs penetrate the hospital portion of the product distribution business more than the physician and alternate site market. Thus, GPOs are not the most profitable customer for distributors. Should any favorable deals be struck, there are reportedly "no secrets" in GPO-distributor contracts. The crisscrossing pattern of distribution sales representatives in the offices of hospital clients leads to rapid aware-ness of contract prices and terms, with the result that favorable con-tract agreements have to be justified with other GPO customers. This competitive process leads to enriched distribution deals (for example, greater levels of service) for the hospital customer at lower margins for the distributor.

Endnotes

1. Bowersox, Donald J., and David J. Closs. *Logistical Management: The Integrated Supply Chain Process.* New York: McGraw-Hill, 1996.
2. Laseter, Timothy M. *Balanced Sourcing: Cooperation and Competition in Supplier Relationships.* San Francisco: Jossey-Bass, 1998.
3. Handfield, Robert B., and Ernest L. Nichols, Jr. *Introduction to Supply Chain Management.* Upper Saddle River, New Jersey: Prentice-Hall, 1999.
4. McFadden, Christopher D., and Timothy M. Leahy. *US Healthcare Distribution: Positioning the Healthcare Supply Chain for the 21st Century.* New York: Goldman Sachs, 2000.
5. Lambert, Douglas M., James R. Stock, and Lisa M. Ellram. *Fundamentals of Logistics Management.* Boston: Irwin McGraw-Hill, 1998.
6. See Note Four.
7. EHCR. *Efficient Healthcare Consumer Response: Improving the Efficiency of the Healthcare Supply Chain.* Chicago: American Society for Healthcare Materials Management Figure 2–1, 1996.
8. Marhula, Daren C., and Edward G. Shannon. *EHealth B2B Overview.* Minneapolis, Minnesota: U.S. Bancorp Piper Jaffray, 2000. Exhibits 3, 15, 17, 23.
9. McFadden and Leahy, *US Healthcare Distribution: Positioning the Healthcare Supply Chain for the 21st Century,* Figures 12, 14, 15, 16.
10. Millennium Research Group. *Hospital Online Procurement Survey.* Stream 2, Issue 1. (June 2000). Toronto: Millennium Research Group.
11. Louvierre, Michael. Presentation to Strategic Sourcing and E-Commerce Solutions for the Med-Surg Supply Chain Conference. Philadelphia, October 1999.
12. Everard, Lynn J. *Blueprint for an Efficient Health Care Supply Chain.* White Paper. Norcross, Georgia: Medical Distribution Solutions, 2000.
13. For the sake of precision, we should point out that the manner in which wholesalers earn fees differs for the distribution of medical-surgical and pharmaceutical products. Med-surg distributors resell products at cost-plus

(one source of fees) and earn additional fees on manufacturer rebates. By contrast, pharmaceutical distributors may resell products on a cost-minus basis but earn fees through speculative purchasing of drugs prior to manufacturer price hikes. This is further explored in Chapter Five.

14. Health Strategies Group. *Evolution of Integrated Systems*. Lambertville, New Jersey: Health Strategies Group, 1998.
15. See Note Four.
16. Cassak, David. "Owens and Minor: The Economics of 'Just Say No.'" *In Vivo* (July–August 1996): 42–57.
17. See Note Twelve.
18. See Note Four.
19. Everard, *Blueprint for an Efficient Health Care Supply Chain*, 11.
20. Ibid., 16.
21. Everard, Lynn J. "Rebates R. I. P.?" *Repertoire*. 8(10) (2000): 30.
22. See Note Four.
23. Marhula, Daren C., and Edward G. Shannon. *E Health B2B Overview*. Minneapolis, Minnesota: U.S. Bancorp Piper Jaffray, 2000.

Part II

· ·

The Intermediaries

4

Role of Group Purchasing
Organizations (GPOs)

Lawton R. Burns

Introduction

Perhaps the most controversial players along the health care supply chain are the group purchasing organizations (GPOs). GPOs have developed into a powerful intermediary during the past two decades, influencing both upstream manufacturers and downstream hospital buyers. This chapter describes the functions performed and services provided by GPOs, as well as distinguishes among the different types of GPOs. The chapter then provides a brief sketch of their history, their parallel growth with IDNs and some of the differences between them, and their business model (sources of revenue). The bulk of the chapter deals with their upstream relationships with manufacturers and their value added (as seen by product vendors), and then considers their strategic capabilities and competitive advantage. This discussion covers GPO efforts in the areas of clinical standardization, SKU rationalization, utilization and cost reduction, and product bundling. Finally, we address some recent issues regarding potential antitrust and restraint of trade, as well as the overall successes and failures of the GPO revolution.

What Is a GPO? What Functions and Services Does It Perform?

A GPO is an organization whose primary product or service is the development of purchasing contracts with product and nonlabor service vendors that its membership can access.[1] The GPO is a typical example of "pooling alliances," which bring together organizations that pool their resources (in this case, their purchasing dollars) to exert leverage over suppliers.[2] Joint purchasing of supplies and services offers hospitals one concrete avenue for achieving economies of scale and generating savings that may be directed toward labor services and the delivery of patient care. GPOs also offer joint purchasing programs to physician groups, nursing homes, and other alternate site providers.[3]

GPOs use their collective purchasing clout to negotiate lower unit prices with vendors of products and services in many areas. These include (but are not limited to) medical-surgical, pharmacy, laboratory, diagnostic imaging, capital equipment, dietary, office, facilities and maintenance, IT, and insurance. In addition to negotiating the contracts, the GPOs also centrally manage the contracts, update pricing changes in the contracts, and disseminate information from product vendors under contract. This is no small task, given the number of product vendors, line items, supply categories, total expenditures, and hospitals involved. Novation, for example, maintains more than 1600 agreements with leading product vendors. These agreements cover more than 890,000 line items in multiple major product categories, and total over $14 billion in purchases from over 2,100 member organizations (2000 data). Premier likewise manages $13 billion in supply and equipment purchases from its 1,829 member institutions. GPOs thus function as an efficient funnel for contracting between large numbers of product vendors and large numbers of hospital buyers. Moreover, these contracts may last as long as three to five years. Thus, GPOs also provide some form of price protection for their members.

In the past, GPOs offered their members standardized pricing, regardless of the volume purchased. In this manner, smaller members would not be disadvantaged. However, larger members felt they were subsidizing the smaller members. Vendors, too, felt they were giving away low pricing to noncompliant groups. To remedy this situation, GPOs and their vendors switched to tiered pricing, which correlates the value offered to members with the amount that members purchase. Within the GPO there are price tiers or levels occupied by hospital subgroups (GPOs within GPOs) with different levels of contract participation.[4,5]

As part of their purchasing efforts, GPOs try to increase their hospital members' adherence ("commitment") to the contracts negotiated by the GPO; that is, agreeing to use a specific contracted vendor for a contracted product across all sites within the hospital and its IDN. Committed purchasing is a strategic aim of both Premier's "Committed Compliance" program and Novation's OPPORTUNITY program. Commitment by member hospitals translates into gains for several parties along the supply chain. For the hospital, there is the promise of lower product prices, as well as cash incentives and potential financial returns from the GPO cooperative. For the GPO, there is a greater volume of GPO-mediated purchases and dollars, and thus higher contract-administration fees paid by the vendor. For the vendor, there are higher product sales and increased local market-share penetration.

To be sure, GPOs offer other services for members beyond lower contract prices. These include other cost reduction tools (for example, materials management, contract management, and operations consulting), programs to improve product standardization and reduce product utilization, programs to improve clinical operations (for example, benchmarking, clinical resource management, decision support tools, disease management, and process design), comparative data on supply chain expenditures, technology management programs (for example, technology assessment, technology life cycle management, and equipment repair or disposal), insurance services, human resource management, education, marketing—for example, the four-stage model of health care market evolution developed by the University HealthSystem Consortium (UHC)—and advocacy. In some GPOs, these functions and services may be split off from the purchasing division (the "pure GPO" that only does product buys) and reside in a broader hospital alliance.[6]

Recently, some of the largest nonprofit GPOs have invested in emerging health care technology firms and technology funds operated by themselves and outside venture capital firms. These are designed to earn profits as well as help member institutions tap into new technologies.[7,8] The GPOs may then sole-source products from the firms in which they have made such investments.

The GPOs also designate the distributors to be used for the products purchased.[9] These authorized distribution agents, or ADAs, are selected on the basis of competitive bidding; that is, lower distribution charges to members, enhanced service agreements beyond distribution, supply channel management efforts, and agreement to work with the GPOs' operating principles and new purchasing solutions (for example, e-commerce technology). The distributors help the GPOs to implement contracts through their own field sales forces, the speed and frequency of their sales contacts, and documents used by sales forces to convey GPO messages.

In addition to member services, GPOs also seek to provide services to product manufacturers.[10] For smaller manufacturers that face difficulty in getting access to large hospital and GPO accounts, a handful of GPOs offer a private label program whereby these vendors can market their products using the GPO's label (for example, Novation's NOVAPLUS program). Vendors gain incremental sales in exchange for granting hospitals lower product prices.

For larger manufacturers, some GPOs sponsor research units (for example, Premier's Innovation Institute) to evaluate new product technologies and methods for increasing their utilization among clinicians. Some manufacturers euphemistically label such efforts *value transfer tools*. "Various manufacturers have contributed money to these institutes. Now it is illegal for them to get some sort of favored contracting status in return. What the institutes do say is, We will evaluate your new product and see if it belongs on formulary. But if you don't give us the money to evaluate your product, then how do we know if it should be on formulary?" Pharmaceutical firms may balk at these institutes because they need rigorous clinical research protocols that satisfy FDA scrutiny, and the pharmaceutical firms don't believe the institutes can deliver this.

Number and Types of GPOs

The GPO industry is large. The Health Industry Group Purchasing Association (HIGPA) and SMG Marketing Group estimate there are anywhere from 600 to 700 GPOs in the U.S. health care industry, respectively.[11,12] These figures likely include regional and local distributors serving the large number of small providers in the alternate site market (for example, physician clinics).[13] The number of hospital-focused GPOs may range from 200 to 400 or more. [14,15]

The GPO industry is also concentrated. According to consultants, seven GPOs account for over 85 percent of the U.S. hospital market.[16] Data published annually in *Modern Healthcare* (see Figure 4.1) indicate there are five large nonprofit GPOs (Novation, Premier, AmeriNet, Health Services Corporation of America, and Consorta) and two large for-profit GPOs (HCA/Health Trust and Tenet/ Buypower).[17] Roughly thirty GPOs (the members of HIGPA) negotiate "sizable contracts" according to HIGPA; the remainder typically provide their members with access to the larger GPOs' contracts but also negotiate agreements with regional vendors.

As of 1999, membership in the two largest nonprofit GPOs accounted for 3,994 hospitals (medical-surgical, psychiatric, and rehabilitation).[18] This represents two-thirds of the 6,000 total hospitals in the United States. If one adds the 300 or so hospitals owned by the two largest for-profit GPOs (HCA and Tenet), the top four GPOs account for 4,300 hospitals, or roughly 72 percent of the total.

Figure 4.1   Annual GPO Revenues ($ billions)

	1996	1997	1998	1999	2000
Investor-Owned					
HCA/HealthTrust	$2.7		$ 2.9		$ 4.2
Tenet/BuyPower	$1.6	$1.8	$ 2.8		$ 3.1
Nonprofit					
Novation*	$7.1	$8.9	$11.0	$13.1	$14.4
Premier	$6.2	$8.5	$10.0	$12.0	$13.0
AmeriNet	$3.2	$3.5	$ 4.1	$ 4.4	$ 4.6
HSCA**	$2.4	$2.0	$ 2.4	$ 2.4	$ 2.6
Consorta	na	na	$ 1.4	$ 1.5	$ 2.7

*Novation is the 1998 merger of VHA and UHC. Their separate figures are combined here for 1996 and 1997.

**Health Services Corporation of America

Source: Scott Hensley. "GPOs under pressure to deliver." *Modern Healthcare*, (September 20, 1999): 38–47.

Nearly all community hospitals (98 percent) participate in some form of group purchasing, with each hospital belonging to 1.6–2.6 GPOs on average.[19–21] Typically, this includes one large national GPO and one or more smaller, regional GPOs. One of the largest hospital GPOs with the best overall pricing (using the federal government's General Services Administration) is the Veterans Administration.

GPOs differ in terms of their ownership, membership, geographic scope, and size. One basic distinction is between for-profit, nonprofit, and public GPO *ownership*. The two largest for-profit GPOs are divisions of the two largest investor-owned hospital systems: HCA (HealthTrust Purchasing Group) and Tenet (BuyPower). By contrast, the three largest nonprofit GPOs are hospital cooperatives, for example, Novation (group purchasing arm for VHA/UHC) and Premier, or strategic alliances, for example, Amerinet. The largest public GPO is the VA. Hospitals within the for-profit and VA systems are owned and operated by those systems, and thus are more directly linked and committed to their group purchasing contracts. Hospitals within the nonprofit alliances are not required to utilize their GPOs for purchasing, but voluntarily join in order to do so. Some alliances (for example, Premier) exert more influence over their members' purchasing than do others (for example, Novation).

GPOs also differ in terms of their *membership*. Some GPOs focus on the hospital market, while others focus on the alternate-site delivery market (for example, physician offices, ambulatory surgery centers, nursing homes, and so on). Due to the advent of integrated delivery networks (IDNs), many GPOs diversified their membership to include a mix of hospitals and alternate-site providers in an effort to reach both markets. Many GPOs also include both for-profit and nonprofit hospitals. For example, Tenet's GPO includes the core of Tenet's 112 hospitals but also extends its purchasing contracts to nonprofit hospital affiliates that wish to take advantage of Tenet's negotiated prices.

GPOs also differ in terms of their *geographic scope and size*. A smaller number of GPOs handle contracting on a national basis, while the majority operates on a regional scope. This latter observation reflects the fact that most GPOs developed on a regional basis. National GPOs have typically formed by consolidating regional GPOs. Premier, for example, formed by merging Sun-Health Alliance (serving North and South Carolina), American Healthcare Systems (itself a merger of GPOs based in Arizona and Missouri), and Premier Health Alliance (Illinois-based GPO). It is not surprising that the national GPOs feature the greatest number of members. Premier has 207 shareholders, which own, lease, or manage 956 hospitals; and another 871 affiliates, which utilize Premier's services (data as of May 31, 2001). Novation includes the 87 academic medical centers and 102 associates of the University HealthSystem Consortium (UHC) and the 2,200 community-based provider members of Voluntary Hospitals of America (VHA).

There are two limits to the size of GPOs. First, most GPOs include only one major hospital or IDN in a given market as a means to provide some competitive advantage. Thus, GPOs cannot amass several hospitals in a local market. Second, on a national scale, GPOs are limited by federal guidelines that create safe harbors for joint purchasing arrangements. Of relevance here is the condition that any joint purchases "account for less than 35 percent of the total sales of the purchased product or service in the relevant market."[22] That is, the total purchases by the GPO (or other joint purchasing arrangement) cannot be so high as to drive down the price of the product or service purchased below competitive levels. Here, the relevant hospital product supply market is national or regional in scope. Since each of the major nonprofit GPOs includes close to 2,000 hospitals and 35 percent of beds, they are already bordering on controlling (at least potentially through compliant contracting) one-third of the 6,000-hospital market. As they reached this ceiling, they began to level off their membership.[23]

GPOs and IDNs

It is difficult to disentangle GPOs from integrated delivery networks (IDNs) for several reasons. First, the for-profit hospital systems (for example, Columbia/HCA and Tenet) at certain times in their past have resembled IDNs by virtue of including physician divisions, insurance products, and continua of care (for example, home health agencies and ambulatory surgery centers). Second, the nonprofit GPOs often include IDNs in their membership. Indeed, one observer suggests that nearly half of GPO members are also affiliated with or owned by an IDN.[24] Third, some GPOs like AmeriNet are really strategic alliances among large IDNs such as Intermountain Healthcare.

It is nevertheless important to distinguish these two entities when discussing the health care supply chain. First, as IDNs grow in size (that is, number of hospital members, physician groups, nursing homes, and so on), they themselves develop the potential for aggregated buying clout in the local market and thus the ability to negotiate product discounts on their own. Indeed, as early as 1997,

VHA acknowledged that mergers and IDN formation among its membership lead hospitals to feel more autonomous in their supply chain management needs, to perceive less need for GPOs, and to consider direct contracting with manufacturers. At the same time, this larger size poses a management challenge for GPOs, since the IDNs lack a defined formal structure and may suffer from slower decision making that impedes cooperation with GPOs.[25] IDNs thus pose an important competitive threat (product substitute) and source of uncertainty for GPOs. The most recent data from the American Hospital Association (AHA) reveal there are roughly 455 hospital systems and networks in the United States, with an average system size of ten members and an average network size of 8 hospitals.[26] Some IDNs are much larger, of course, ranging in size from as few as 2 hospitals to as many as 300. Industry observers speculate that as many as half possess the scale necessary for group purchasing.[27]

Second, IDNs possess another feature of interest to vendors other than their size. As just noted, their composition includes not only inpatient facilities but also outpatient clinics, affiliated physician groups, nursing homes, ambulatory surgery centers, and so on. They thus provide an incentive for suppliers to (1) develop full product lines that follow the patient across different treatment settings and comprise disease management systems of care, and (2) bundle together products with services in clinical pathway programs or clinical trials.

Third, most of these systems and networks are local or regional in scope, which presents an interesting buying opportunity. For the hospitals, they may be in close enough geographic proximity to share a common warehouse and operate as their own GPO and distributor (see Chapter Six). Indeed, the local nature of IDNs may coincide with the local nature of product distribution. They may also exhibit more similar patterns of resource utilization and share enough overlap in their physician membership to standardize their purchasing around a smaller number of products and SKUs. As a result, they may develop purchasing programs with higher levels of compliance than those achieved by the national GPOs with their more diverse membership. While they do not collectively account for the same purchasing volume as do large GPOs, they offer a product vendor an alternative set of advantages including greater contract compliance, greater standardization on that vendor's products (over a rival's products), and increased market-share penetration in that local area. This situation can quickly give rise to some short-term win-win scenarios for both sides: the vendor offers the IDN a lower price than that negotiated by the IDN's GPO in exchange for increased product sales.[28] It also raises an interesting new calculus for supply chain players: would vendors prefer to have 70 percent compliance with a large GPO or 80–90 percent compliance with a smaller IDN?

Fourth, like the investor-owned GPOs and unlike the nonprofit GPOs, many IDNs have direct ownership of their hospitals. This increases the potential for higher levels of compliance and standardization.

Due to their size, IDNs are salient to all vendors.[29] However, they are particularly salient to smaller vendors that get locked out of long-term contracts with large GPOs. Partly due to the need to broadly appeal to its hospital members, large GPOs have shown a tendency to contract with large manufacturers with leading market share. Vendors that fail to win one GPO's business must compete vigorously for the others and/or compete for the IDN's purchases. Larger vendors are reluctant to grant big price concessions to gain market share, since it may hurt total profits. Smaller vendors with lower market shares are able to cede greater price discounts to win the IDN business and thereby increase the share for their products, without hurting total profits.[30] Alternatively, smaller or regional vendors may have a lower cost structure or be willing to work at lower margins in order to get the IDN's business.[31]

In sum, IDNs may thus have both the opportunity and incentive to act as their own GPOs. As further fuel to this movement, IDNs may experience growing dissatisfaction with their GPO partners as the latter grow in size. Large GPO size often leads GPOs to emphasize (1) national contracting with large vendors that can serve the majority of GPO members (for example, "one size fits all"), and (2) contract compliance over contract flexibility and the needs of local IDNs. While larger GPO alliance membership may increase purchasing volume and the potential for lower contract prices, it also makes it harder for the GPO to tailor its services to meet the needs of its hospital members.[32] As one GPO executive explained,

> There are few tailored partnerships between the manufacturer, GPO, and hospital member. Customization is coming, but unfortunately it is coming from a reactionary perspective. When the IDN calls up the GPO and says, 'I want 3M to do something differently,' that is when we react. We don't walk into the hospital with 3M and say, 'You know, we can save you X dollars if we do this differently'.

Recently one large GPO (AmeriNet) has developed its "options" program, which allows its IDN members to utilize the large GPO contracts and, at the same time, receive GPO assistance in negotiating customized, flexible contracts with individual suppliers.[33,34]

GPO Business Model and Revenues

As mentioned in Chapter Three, the primary source of GPO revenues is the contract administration fee (CAF) paid by the product vendor. This fee ranges as high as 2–3 percent of the contracted purchase price. Three percent is typically viewed as a ceiling in the industry. This stems from congressional concerns, voiced in the Omnibus Budget Reconciliation Act of 1987, over excessive GPO fees. Fees over 3 percent warrant oversight from the Department of Health and Human Services for possible abuse of Medicare Fraud and Abuse provisions. As a result of these concerns, the 3 percent figure became embodied as one of the Medicare safe harbors.[35]

To determine the size of the GPO market, one needs to estimate the dollar purchases of supplies and equipment by hospitals and the penetration of hospital spending by GPOs. With regard to the former, the Millennium Research Group estimates the size of the medical supply and equipment market to be $64–68 billion, of which hospitals purchase 76.4 percent, or $49–52 billion. With regard to the latter, Millennium estimates that two-thirds of hospital purchases are made through their GPOs and IDNs.[36] To be sure, there is a range of estimates of GPO penetration of hospital spending around this two-thirds figure. Some analysts and trade associations (for example, HIGPA) estimate the GPO penetration of hospital supply spending to be as high as 72–80 percent. Many executives in our study and elsewhere estimate a lower bound figure of 50–60 percent.[37–41] Congruent with this figure, a series of case studies of hospital purchasing suggest that GPO contracts are used only 50–60 percent of the time for medical-surgical supply orders from such departments as materials management, cardiac cath lab, laboratory, and radiology.[42,43] We adopt a middle-ground approach and estimate it at two-thirds.[44]

Taken together, these two sets of estimates suggest that GPOs mediate two-thirds of the $49–52 billion spent by hospitals on medical supplies and equipment, or $32.6–34.7 billion. In addition, they may earn 2–3 percent CAFs on the two-thirds of the $49–52 billion spend, or as much as $978 million–$1.04 billion. According to manufacturing executives, the top two GPOs each earned CAFs of $275–300 million (1998), totaling $550–600 million. At that time, they accounted for $21 billion of the total GPO volume; applying the 3 percent CAF figure to this amount would yield total revenues of $630 million. These figures suggest that the 3 percent CAF is indeed an upper bound and that, across the large GPOs, the realized CAFs may be slightly less.

The estimated revenues of GPOs do not include GPO purchases of pharmaceutical products. The percentage of hospital pharmacy purchases through GPOs may range as high as 85–90 percent, according to some case studies.[45] Nationally, prescription drug sales to the institutional market reached nearly $30 billion in 1999, of which hospitals accounted for roughly $15 billion. These figures suggest that GPOs may earn as much as 3 percent of the 85–90 percent of the $15 billion spent by hospital pharmacies, or $394 million on this $13 billion market.

Taken together, these first two sets of figures for GPO revenues on medical-surgical (over $978 million) and pharmaceutical supplies ($394 million) amount to over $1.372 billion. Total GPO-mediated purchasing dollars for medical-surgical ($32.6–34.7 billion) and pharmaceutical supplies ($13 billion), which equals $45.6–47.7 billion, approximate the combined reported volume for the top ten nonprofit GPOs in 1999 ($39 billion) and the top two investor-owned GPOs (approximately $6 billion), or $45 billion.[46,47] This figure is also close to the $45 billion in GPO purchases estimated by some GPO executives.[48,49]

GPOs have potentially three or four other sources of revenues besides CAFs.[50,51] First, nonprofit GPOs receive dues from their hospital members. These are estimated to range from nothing to $60,000.[52] Second, some GPOs may earn a slice of vendor rebates paid on order volume. Third, GPOs can charge transaction or access fees to vendors for using their e-commerce solutions (see Chapter Ten); however, these fees were waived in the past until the GPOs demonstrated that the technology worked and could deliver value to the manufacturers. Fourth, GPOs may receive a percentage of the process cost savings generated by e-commerce; these have also not yet been demonstrated. Thus, CAFs currently remain to be the major source of GPO revenues.

Upstream Relationships with Manufacturers and Distributors

GPO's relationships with upstream value chain players are controversial. There is some disjunction between the desired versus actual characteristics found in GPOs, as reported by manufacturers, as well as differences of opinion in the role that GPOs play.

Desirable Characteristics of GPOs—As Viewed
by Manufacturers and Distributors

Product manufacturers are very consistent in describing the ideal characteristics of their GPO partners. As with IDNs, they look for "clarity in governance and decision making" above all. In practice, this means the GPO can speak with one voice organizationally for its members. This trait is more commonly found in ownership-based GPOs, such as those operated by investor-owned hospital systems. Such systems have a greater ability to deliver in terms of compliance. An executive made the following comments:

> In the owned GPOs, a senior vice president signs an agreement, flicks the switch, the volume comes, and the contract terms are met. In the voluntary GPOs, on the other hand, the ability to make contracts pay out depends as much on the manufacturer's implementation plan and pull-through activities. Some of these GPOs cannot administer the agreement fully, such that the manufacturer must support the administration of the contract substantially (for example, compliance, auditability, traceability, and correct pricing).

Volume and compliance may be the two most critical points here. Manufacturers want to maximize both the breadth and penetration of their business: the number of its products the GPO contracts for, the volume within each, and its share of the hospital's purchases in that product area. As one executive explained, volume and compliance "allow you to support high levels of service, enable you to deliver committed pricing, and are the key to product velocity." Along with the GPO or IDN's efforts to standardize product purchases, volume and compliance are viewed as the key factors in the cost of doing business with the hospital industry (and thus the major source of variable pricing within a given community). Volume combined with compliance assures the vendor that the GPO negotiation will generate a predetermined level of sales. This lowers the vendor's sales risk and manufacturing costs by virtue of more accurate production forecasts. It also lowers the vendor's costs of sales, marketing, and customer relations, estimated by one GPO to be 22.7 percent of the manufacturer's total delivered costs. Savings here reflect lower costs of securing the contract, which are monetized at $418 per hospital contract. Across the GPO's 300 contracts, this amounts to a savings to vendors of $125,000 per hospital.[53] Higher levels of compliance also translate into better pricing for hospitals; indeed, the GPO membership gets segmented into price tiers based on their level of compliance with GPO contracts. By contrast, low volumes force manufacturers and distributors into a "whole different cost structure."

Several vendors remarked that Columbia/HCA was one of their most organized, disciplined, and compliant buyers. They attributed this to their purchasing control mechanisms, as well as to the presence of CEOs who "provide direction." Some nonprofit systems (for example, Henry Ford, Baylor, Baptist) are also heralded for their centralized decision making and committed volume. GPOs and IDNs that can deliver committed volume, and thus market share, are afforded good GPO contract terms up front; those that cannot are given performance-based contracts in which they receive rebates and retrospective incentives if they deliver on member compliance.

Manufacturers also mention the importance of GPO size. This encompasses several aspects: the geographic scope of the GPO (national reach), the number of members, the size of member institutions, the potential for market share (both local and national), as well as total purchased volume and compliance (committed volume). Great GPO size is reportedly a mixed blessing, according to product vendors. On the one hand, bigger GPOs "definitely get more vendor attention." As one manufacturing executive explained,

"The average large GPO has 1,000–2,000 hospitals, while the average system has ten to eleven hospitals." Another executive suggested the threshold is 200 hospitals or more. Indeed, at some large manufacturers, there are dedicated account managers for each of the large GPOs. On the other hand, manufacturers are wary of putting all of their eggs in one GPO basket. Moreover, manufacturers acknowledge that large GPOs struggle to deliver compliance and market share. They further suggest that IDNs can get the same discount offered to GPOs if they can "drive market share." Thus, vendors consider the size and relative market strength of the member hospitals of GPOs as well as systems and networks in gauging how much attention to pay these accounts. However, they state "no GPO or system gets ignored."

A third desired GPO characteristic is the ability to manage its members in a consistent way. In practice, this means that GPOs have close communication linkages with hospital members for distributing information on contracts, pricing issues, and compliance issues. Some vendors mention the importance of EDI linkages between the GPO and their larger hospitals, as well as the GPO's ability to help manufacturers with rapid introduction of new products and dissemination of new product information to their members. Such linkages help the GPO to deliver greater market share to the product vendor. Some vendors and distributors also mention the number of delivery sites in the GPO or IDN to be serviced (for example, the mix of hospital facilities and physician clinics) and the volume going to each. They state that the issues of communication and delivery points are secondary in influencing contracts and pricing, however.

Finally, manufacturers hold out the hope that GPOs and their IDN members will embrace and utilize more of the vendor's product line. Vendors view this as part of their disease management strategy. They also see this product-line approach as part of an overall strategy to look beyond unit price and focus on product bundles and services that may lower the "total cost of doing business" (see Chapters Seven to Nine).

Actual Characteristics of GPOs—As Viewed by Manufacturers and Distributors

Manufacturers view GPOs in the same way they view distributors. They help to aggregate product volume for the manufacturers, and they influence the purchasing behavior of hospital customers. Volume aggregation is viewed as especially helpful for smaller hospitals that lack EDI connections with manufacturers and distributors, and cannot afford sophisticated purchasing and materials management infrastructure. As just noted, volume aggregation is not viewed as important for larger IDNs who can potentially deal directly with manufacturers. Even though many manufacturers assign full-time corporate account directors to each of the major GPOs they negotiate with, they typically do not refer to them as customers.

Manufacturers also view GPOs as marketing aids that help to disseminate product information to hospitals, to provide members with documentation of the manufacturer's message, to have product information show up on the computer screens of materials managers when they order products, and to offer members financial incentives to comply with its contracts and "pull products through" the supply chain. GPOs also serve as an efficient communication avenue to thousands of hospitals and an efficient contracting mechanism compared to the costs of transacting with hundreds of IDNs (higher negotiation costs, higher number and greater frequency of orders, smaller shipments, and smaller base).

Beyond demand aggregation, manufacturers are reluctant to acknowledge any value-added function performed by GPOs. This stems in part from the 2–3 percent CAFs they feel they are forced to pay to get access to member hospitals. CAFs are viewed by manufacturers in several ways:

- The cost of doing business

- High margins that dwarf the margins of distributors

- Inefficiencies in the sales process that add to health care costs

- Low value added since the CAFs are not indexed to contract performance (for example, how much market share the GPO delivers)

- An entitlement that is totally unearned

- An administrative service fee offered to GPOs

- Discounts on internal P&L (profit and loss)

- An annuity (yearly fee paid in a multi-year contract)

- Access to decision makers and committed programs

- A small price to pay for the enormous cost of separately negotiating hundreds of contracts

- Something that helps get the GPO's attention, and without which the company is at a competitive disadvantage to other vendors who pay the fees and have hundreds of sales representatives competing for time

At a May 1997 Network Consulting and Information (NCI) conference, a survey of seventy-eight vendors found that 91 percent did not believe the benefits of GPO contracts were enough to make up for the CAF.[54] The contrast with distributors is quite poignant in the eyes of manufacturers: GPOs get big fees but add little value, while distributors get small fees but add greater value (see Chapter Five). Executives interviewed in this study had neither quantified the value provided by the GPO nor determined whether it was worth 3 percent, however.

This negative view of GPOs also stems in part from the reality that GPOs exist primarily to extract lower prices from the manufacturers. As the head of one GPO expressed it, "What you have is groups getting paid [CAFs] by vendors on the one hand and then trying to beat them up [on price] on the other."[55] Vendors see this as a huge opportunity cost. As one executive stated, "We do $1 billion in sales with this GPO and pay a 3 percent CAF. That translates into $30 million. That money could be used to support 350–400 sales representatives out in the field." There is widespread consensus among manufacturers (for example, especially among pharmaceutical firms) that the size of field sales forces translates immediately into greater sales volume.

Thus, while manufacturers acknowledge the position of GPOs as important intermediaries, they question whether GPOs help them to gain more market share (in exchange for the CAF), and whether they play a significant role in supply chain efficiency. Four questions manufacturers ask are

1. Can GPOs change members' purchasing behavior and thus move market share for vendors?

2. Do GPOs really improve product flow?

3. Do GPOs help their members to make wise product choices?

4. Which is more efficient—the GPO or the IDN—at driving its IT capability throughout the hospitals in a system, at coordinating its systems, at getting capabilities pushed down to its systems, at driving product protocols, and getting integrated information on product use?

Manufacturers commonly express the belief (actually *hope*) that GPOs will not survive as long as they just focus on price. They would prefer to see GPOs provide more value-adding services to both their upstream trading partners and their downstream hospital members.

Distributors also express some reservations about the committed purchasing programs of GPOs. This is largely because such programs threaten the distributor's traditional distribution patterns and value-adding services. With committed purchasing, the rewards for switching market share accrue to the GPO and its members, not the distributor. Thus, there is less emphasis on the "push" strategy of the distributor. There is also less vendor reliance on distributors to assemble product order and usage data from hospital customers.

GPOs' Views of Their Role in the Supply Chain

Needless to say, GPOs do not share the manufacturer's view regarding who is the customer. First, GPOs not only see the manufacturer as a customer but also see themselves as a customer of the manufacturer. With regard to the former role, a GPO executive remarked, "One of our customers is that business partner [manufacturer] because we play a role in making sure that they see the pull-through and the implementation strategies for their contracts." With regard to the latter role, GPOs note that manufacturers want to have a relationship with them and come calling on them.

Second, GPOs are quick to point out that their 3 percent CAFs are stipulated as a safe harbor under Medicare. Moreover, they claim to do more than just collect CAFs. An executive at one large GPO asserted they help to deliver the value inherent in the vendors' products:

> We don't collect a dime in administrative fees [CAFs]. We collect legal marketing fees. We are active, proactive marketers of the value of the products and services we put on the contract. We have a very large selling organization. We have a lot of marketing talent in the organization and not only use their knowledge and understanding of the various markets and market segments to make wise contracting decisions, but also know how to package and modify these programs to be relevant to the member alliances. So we are helping vendors to sell their products to our membership in a focused way. We're actually helping them deliver the value they create.

GPOs perceive they add value to manufacturers in terms of sales and sales support. For smaller vendors, some GPOs have private label programs that help them to reduce their sales force and marketing costs, enable them to have their products carried by the GPOs' authorized distributors, and increase their visibility in the marketplace. For larger vendors, sales may increase due to the fact their products enjoy greater visibility by being on the approved GPO contract. There are also opportunities for larger vendors to utilize their sales forces in different ways (but not necessarily to reduce them). As one GPO executive explained,

> The manufacturers don't reduce their sales force at all. In fact, some manufacturers have made the fundamental error in thinking that "Now that I have the GPO contract, I no longer have to worry about calling on those hospitals, and so I can spend time on hospitals where I don't have contracts." These manufacturers wind up potentially alienating the customer base because they don't spend the time necessarily that they should in the field. Moreover, this time should be spent differently. The time isn't necessarily spent on detailing the contract; the time is spent helping to work on process, implementation strategies, better communications with the physicians and medical team on how to better utilize the product.
>
> I stress a lot with our corporate accounts that they need to almost create a different level of sales force for our GPO hospital customers. It is not the detail folks who go "Hey, Rocky, watch me pull a rabbit out of my hat" and show them the product of the day. Rather, it's the approach of "I have the [GPO] contract, so I'm not here to wheedle with you over price or terms. I am here to show you how to effectively use this product. Who do we need to talk to within the institution to perhaps

change nurse protocols, maybe reduce your floor stock, maybe change some of your outcomes, maybe change some of your policies and procedures, maybe deal with formulary change with people on the P&T committee." So it is a different level of entry-level sales.

Despite the opportunity, GPOs do not feel that vendors are using their sales force in this manner. GPOs argue that vendors need to send out sales teams that include not only the sales representative but also specialists (for example, nurses trained in utilization management) and generalists (for example, individuals who understand a broader product portfolio and individuals who can help physicians with process improvement). By sending in only detail people (who are compensated based on commission-based sales), vendors reinforce provider suspicions that they are only interested in selling product, while providers are trying to cut costs and product use. In order to sell products, the sales representatives may also engage in counter detailing, that is, by going in "behind the scenes to try to convince a physician of the best way to do things that diverges from the way the system wants to." The result is a lack of trust between the two parties.

Maintaining and improving market share for vendors appears to be a critical performance measure for GPOs. Indeed, some GPOs have historically included the delivery of market share to their supply partners as part of their mission statement, and insist they must be able to deliver share in order to survive. One executive said

We truly believe that we must have share and show change in market share. We have these quarterly business reviews with all of our key suppliers, and the key questions we have are (1) What was the vendor's sales growth with us last year? and (2) How does that compare with how the vendor grew both nationally and with other GPOs? Unless we help them outperform the marketplace, we really have not done our job.

GPOs perceive they add value to manufacturers in terms of market share in several ways. First, committed volume programs have reportedly increased vendors' local market shares. Novation executives described the success of phase one of their OPPORTUNITY buying program, which involved seven manufacturers and thirteen product lines: "We took those manufacturers—all of them with 75 percent or higher market share in our hospitals—to over 95 percent. And for that they all contributed a small percentage in value." That is, the GPO promised and delivered over 95 percent compliance in exchange for the vendors' "maximum price tier" plus an additional set of incentives ranging from 6–8 percent. Thus, GPO executives believe they help vendors focus their resources on a segment of hospital customers in very defined and beneficial ways.

Second, outside of such programs, GPOs play a major role in maintaining the current market shares of manufacturers. GPO-manufacturer contracts often last three years with two one-year options. Over this three- to five-year period, very few contracts actually change, leading to considerable vendor stability in the product portfolios offered to member hospitals. This "sustained market share" is undoubtedly valued by manufacturers, even if they don't mention it, because it reduces their transaction costs and allows them time to convert the GPO's hospital membership to their products. During this time, incumbent vendors may see additional volume growth as the GPO (and its parent hospital alliance) adds new members and penetrates new geographic markets. GPO executives state that their greatest source of growth, however, has been encouraging existing members to switch to their committed purchasing programs.

Large GPOs also limit vendor competition for hospital business by narrowing the number of vendors who get access to GPO contracts. "They don't mind competition, but they want to have the field narrowed somewhat. If there are ten to fifteen manufacturers making the same widget, they want to make sure they are one of two or three on the GPO's portfolio." Indeed, because of the large size of GPOs and their long-term contracts with big suppliers, many small vendors have complained about the lack of competitive access to the hospital market.

Downstream Relationships with IDNs

As noted previously, the GPO has two customers: the manufacturer and the hospital member. For the former, the GPO tries to attain a certain level of volume and committed purchasing by each hospital (percentage of product purchased from that vendor); for the latter, the GPO tries to obtain a certain level of pricing. Thus, the GPO performs a basic "product for pricing" brokering role.

Basic Value Proposition: Lower Prices

The basic value for the hospital member is the GPO-negotiated pricing. GPOs recognize this as their entrée or ante into the GPO arena. As one executive explained it,

> We must have price to get into the game. It is certainly the reason we get initial support from our members. It is also the most visible element of our value added, and the one that gets benchmarked the most often.

Indeed, surveys of hospital department managers reveal that their number one expectation for group purchasing is to obtain "best price for best product." The next two most important considerations are "leverage with suppliers" and "cost analysis and cross references."[56] Cost savings are also the number one purchasing goal for hospital materials managers.[57]

IDN materials managers are convinced that GPOs have historically delivered to them lower prices than they had achieved on their own. They view the pricing practices of vendors as "opportunistic" and "irrational." As a result, they believe they never get the same price twice from vendors. They also believe the manufacturers' marketing strategy is to "keep the price as high as possible for as many customers as possible for as long as possible."[58] Of course, manufacturers feel compelled to do so in order to quickly recoup the costs of their R&D investments and increase corporate earnings. This situation has served to bind hospitals more closely to GPOs than to the vendors, increasing the perceived need for GPOs, and thus their potential bargaining power.

However, IDNs are not convinced that GPOs deliver the lowest possible prices. This is evidenced by the existence of tiered pricing and vendors' willingness to cut prices 5–10 percent below GPO-negotiated rates to win incremental business with large IDNs that are able to standardize products and rationalize vendors.[59] This may also reflect some GPOs' ambivalence toward higher prices that hurt members' budgets but increase their own CAF revenues.

As a result, IDNs tend to use their national GPO as a benchmark once they reach annual purchases of $200–250 million.[60] This benchmarking function is important for several reasons. First, it sets the new "street price" (or ceiling) for a product that other manufacturers and GPOs cannot ignore. Second, it tends to get quickly imitated in other contracts due to word of mouth among materials managers and trade journals that publicize contract terms. Third, the replication of contract terms across vendor-GPO relationships contributes to some stability (and maybe rigidity) in the marketplace. Fourth, it forms the point of departure for all subsequent contracting by IDNs shopping for a better deal.[61]

The fact that IDNs can shop their own deals and get equivalent, discounted pricing from vendors suggests that GPO savings for hospital members may be overstated. The real financial benefit may come in the GPO rebates of CAFs back to hospital members as rewards for compliance. On the other hand, some product manufacturers claim that the CAFs are built into the prices for their products, which are passed on to their hospital customers. Thus, GPOs that rebate some of the CAFs to hospital members may essentially be giving back to hospitals the original price. Manufacturers use this argument to support their belief that direct vendor-hospital contracting is the most efficient form.

What is the actual dollar value for IDNs that belong to the GPOs? There is some consensus regarding the estimated percentage savings that GPOs achieve for their members on supply contracts. Executives at Tenet/BuyPower claim they achieve a minimum of 5 percent savings for freestanding hospitals that join, with savings often as high as 15–20 percent. Consulting firms and nonprofit GPOs likewise claim that the average savings on GPO contracts are in the range of 10–16 percent, although the initial savings may be in the single digits.[62–66] Assuming a 10–15 percent savings and the total dollar volume and penetration level of GPO purchases just noted, GPOs save their members 10–15 percent of the $34.5 billion spent by hospitals on medical supplies and equipment, or $3.45–5.17 billion. If one assumes that hospitals spend $19 billion on pharmaceuticals, then GPOs save hospitals 10–15 percent or $1.9–2.85 billion. Taken together, the GPO savings estimated here of $5.35–8.02 billion are much smaller than the range suggested by Muse & Associates of $12–19 billion.

Other Sources of Economic Value

A second source of economic value for IDNs comes in the form of lower contracting costs. Novation estimates that it saves its hospitals an average of $1,367 per contract, using its group purchasing approach over the hospital's self-contracting approach. Over half of these savings lie in fewer man-hours needed to prepare bids or RFPs, to analyze bid proposals, and to implement contracts. For a hospital with 340 GPO contracts, this translates into an annual savings of roughly $465,000. However, interviews with hospital materials managers suggest they are unaware of these purchasing and contracting costs.[67]

In a similar vein, an earlier VHA-UHC study compared the total supply expense per adjusted discharge in hospitals that utilized GPOs to different degrees. For hospitals with less than 50 percent contract participation, the supply expenses ranged from $879–949 per discharge; at hospitals with more than 50 percent contract participation, the supply expenses ranged from $761–824 per discharge. This represents a savings of 7 percent per discharge.[68]

Another economic value for the GPO membership is the distribution of the revenues from CAFs. In the for-profit GPOs, CAF revenues flow first to the corporate parent, and then some percentage gets dispersed to hospital members as incentive payments for contract compliance. In the nonprofit GPOs, a percentage of CAF revenues get distributed back to IDN members and then their hospitals, after netting out the GPO's operating expenses and capitalization targets agreed to by the members. In the past, these payouts have been based on members' purchase volume due to Medicare safe harbors guidelines. In the future, they are moving toward the for-profit model of using CAFs to financially reward members for their contract participation in order to create incentive pools for purposes of promoting internal competition, or basing payouts on capitalization of the GPO. GPOs vary in terms of the percentage of CAF revenues flowing back to members, but there is a trend toward a greater share paid out to members. Many national GPOs disperse 100 percent of CAFs after expenses.

Ambivalence in GPO-Hospital Member Relationships

GPOs appear to have an ambivalent relationship with their hospital members. On the one hand, they seek to provide a wide array of services to hospitals; on the other hand, they often perceive that hospitals fail to take advantage of these services, and sometimes resist GPO change efforts.

First, they believe that many IDNs are too disorganized or decentralized to act as a coherent buyer. This problem exists at both the system level and the individual hospital level. As one executive stated,

> Four large hospitals come together to form a system, put a new name on the hospital, and still act independently. Would IBM do that? Would anybody do that on the

business side? The problem is we have had many great conversations with senior executives, but they have an inability to drive change. Many a great system has come together and fallen apart at the operations level, particularly the materials management level, because of turf issues. Obviously you don't need four materials managers in that system, but that is what happens and that is how it breaks down. They may even have created a new office of corporate materials management. But with all the integration that went on in the health care side, there are very few that have done what they needed to do to put everybody on the same materials management system.

Second, some GPO executives believe the vice president for materials management is a key customer for them but is not accorded high status within the IDN. The orientation of many GPOs toward the materials management function reflects where much of their relationship with hospital members started, where they spend a good deal of their time interfacing with members, whom they see as the gatekeepers to others in the hospital, and whom they wish to enable with programs to drive standardization and utilization reductions. These individuals are also key entry points for customer education, and "people who need to be at the table with clinicians to help us [the GPOs] with disease management and critical pathway programs." However, GPOs report that their materials management contacts lack the influence and ability to serve as effective leaders of supply chain efforts in the hospital. Part of this stems from their lack of education and preparation for their roles: "If you compare them as a peer group with their counterparts in industry, you're talking about guys who probably came out of the store room versus guys with college and post-graduate training."

Materials managers may themselves pose entry barriers—for example, by resisting incursions on their turf, by resisting change efforts that will alter their world of work, and by resisting electronic improvements (for example, CD-ROMs instead of paper-based catalogs). Some GPO executives state that the value they can provide to their hospital members is directly tied to "when we are brought into the process." When the GPO is brought in early on, there is the opportunity for transforming business processes that reduce redundant activities across supply chain partners, improve efficiencies, and benefit all parties. When the GPO is brought in late, it is typically to help with short-term problem solving on a transactional (rather than transformational) basis. This often helps to explain why GPOs are unable to develop total cost solutions for their members.

Third, GPOs generally feel that hospital members lack a sophisticated understanding of supply chain management. At a general level, there is no uniform understanding of what supply chain management means across hospitals—a problem that GPOs say they are trying to correct. Even if a shared understanding existed, there is a lack of leadership and vision for supply chain issues. As one executive stated, "There are no visionaries running IDNs the way there are visionaries running businesses such as Bob Walters at Cardinal Health or some of the executives at pharmaceutical companies. You talk about night and day!" Another executive stated, "Supply chain management is not a priority on the agenda of a hospital system CEO. It is a foreign language. They don't understand it, they don't get it, and that's what we spend a lot of our time doing." Of course, some CEOs are not used to being asked for their input in supply chain management and contracting issues.[69]

Fourth, GPOs believe that IDNs are not able or willing to push hard in the area of supply utilization. An executive explained it this way:

> This is where the real issue is, because you must get the end users (physicians and nurses) who have distinct preferences to sit down at the table and decide, Yes, I am willing to change what the custom pack looks like or give up these three products that I am very comfortable with and that I have been using since I graduated from school. This is where the disconnect is. Most IDNs have a hard

time here. Once they get the standardization piece, most
are happy with that and don't really want to do the extra
work it takes to go beyond to tackle utilization.

They can count on one hand the number of IDNs that have structured and oriented themselves to doing this detailed work. They
point to important IDN characteristics as centralized decision making, involving physicians and clinicians in the process, and involving central administration. They also note the importance of
dedicated resources to the utilization effort. These include clinical
and physician resources (personnel), both at the GPO and at the
member hospital, that work directly with clinical staff to help them
understand the importance and benefits of utilization, and who have
credibility with their peers to help them reach that point.

GPO Competitive Advantage

GPOs typically distinguish themselves from one another in terms
of their relationships with hospital members. Such relationships are
heavily influenced by the ownership model of the GPO and the
degree of organization and integration within the IDN. The content of these relationships then enables GPOs to negotiate different contracts and prices with product manufacturers, which are one
external manifestation of competitive advantage.

Contract Prices

There is some disagreement in the industry about the contract
prices that different GPOs are able to negotiate for their members.
Hospital materials management executives believe the differences
are quite small. One reason for this is price competition among different vendors for the same product. In medical-surgical supply and
portions of the pharmaceutical industry, consolidation of manufacturers has not advanced far enough to restrict competition, even
within therapeutic and specific product areas where there are clear

market leaders. Another reason is the visibility of GPO prices, which leads other GPOs and IDNs to pressure the vendor for equivalent pricing. Thus, even if there are pricing advantages for some GPOs, they tend to get quickly competed away and cannot serve as a source of any long-term advantage.

Consequently, the appearance of most favored nation (MFN) pricing in GPO contracting may be "window dressing." Manufacturers state that they resist it and "avoid it like the plague." Manufacturers also state MFN is occasionally done if the GPO demands it, but that it is (1) usually tied to contract factors such as volume, cost to serve, and hospital system composition; (2) rarely enforced and hard to enforce; and (3) useless since everyone wants it and gets it.

Some GPO executives likewise suggest that pricing differences are small:

> The manufacturers that participate in a particular marketplace essentially know where the others have priced themselves. The pricing bands have narrowed over time. The pricing highs and lows are not as great any more. The key challenge for us is to make sure we are on the low end of the band, to stay on the low end of the band, and to have effective product choices and product support.

Other GPO executives insist that pricing differences are real and substantial:

> We bring a price edge and price is important. How do I know that? Because my staff gets involved in converting other GPO contracts to our GPO's contracts. We have yet to convert somebody where we did not save them money. We actually check invoices and do all of the line item converting, and find that our price advantage beats what the consultants think it is. Most of your external

> consultants have said we have a pricing advantage of
> 1.5–2 percent, but every time we've converted somebody
> we see a 7–9 percent advantage.

Regardless of the magnitude of the differences, there are differences in how the pricing function operates for investor-owned versus nonprofit GPOs. The former typically receive up-front discounts from manufacturers (margin erosion) in exchange for mandated compliance, while the latter tend to receive back-end "rebates" for demonstrated compliance.

There are three important considerations here in interpreting these comments. First, those GPOs that reportedly have the lowest prices emphasize these pricing differences, while those GPOs that reportedly don't have lower prices emphasize other competitive advantages. Second, pricing differences among GPOs may vary by product category. Pharmaceutical pricing differences are reportedly much narrower than those for medical-surgical products. Third, the pricing differences reported by GPOs vary based on who the reference group is. Some GPOs get better prices than others on certain product items. Despite all of these differences, there are some GPOs who claim that they deliver the lowest total cost from a "total portfolio perspective—" if members implement the full portfolio rather than use it piecemeal.

Member Commitment

Executives from both invester-owned and nonprofit GPOs who claim that real pricing differences exist typically ascribe the source of these differences to the higher level of purchasing commitment and participation of their members. In practice, this means that hospital members participate in the contracts negotiated by the GPO (that is, they do less maverick, off-contract buying) and agree to purchase a minimum defined percentage of a particular supply item from a particular contracted vendor (single-source contract) or set of vendors (dual-source or multi-source contract). GPOs use the phrase *contract compliance* to empirically measure hospital members' commitment. Commitment programs not only result in better prices but can also bring additional incentives for the GPO in exchange for defined sales growth and wider sales penetration across the vendor's total line of contracted products.

By contrast, pricing differences are not necessarily tied to the overall purchasing volume of the GPO. While the investor-owned GPOs lack the dollar volume of Premier and Novation, they claim to have equivalent or better pricing. This assertion is based on an examination of the prices paid by hospitals they acquire that used to belong to the larger, nonprofit GPOs.

Compliance is variable across members and across supply item. For example, as noted previously, pharmacy departments exhibit much higher participation in GPO contracts than other departments; according to survey findings, pharmacists have more experience with formularies and thus standardization, and believe that contracting is not a good use of their time.[70] Such commitment is associated with several other efficient departmental features, including use of formulary protocols, fewer FTEs to manage materials, fewer purchase orders, higher inventory turnover, fewer vendors used and more prime vendor relationships, and more on-line procurement of supplies.[71]

Compliance is a moving target as contracts evolve, and is built into vendor contracts in the form of price tiers. Compliance is also determined to some extent by the accuracy or inaccuracy of information transmitted and maintained among trading partners after the contract has been negotiated. Thus, for example, GPOs that derive their members' purchasing from manufacturers or distributors essentially work with secondhand data that lacks timeliness, consistency (in format), and integrity. Similarly, paper-based systems, decentralized purchasing, and reliance on obsolete contract information (that is, failure to quickly access updated contract terms) lead IDNs to pay higher prices and achieve lower commitment to GPO contracts.[72]

GPOs assert that how compliance is achieved is also a source of competitive advantage. Among the nonprofit GPOs, there is a well-noted distinction between the required compliance approach of Premier and the voluntary compliance approach taken by Novation.[73] Data from one large vendor indicate that Premier's compliance level is much higher than Consorta's (55 percent), Novation's (34 percent), and AmeriNet's (5 percent). These differences are ascribed to Premier's enforcement of compliance and the lower average number of GPOs its members belong to (1.2 GPOs).[74] The hospitals that belong to these two alliances appear to largely self-select into them, based on their different purchasing philosophies. According to one executive at Premier,

> Commitment is a differentiating factor for us. We try to define for potential members what that means. We try to make them aware of the processes and procedures that we use to facilitate contract participation, the ground rules, how we make decisions—and ultimately you know what joining Premier is all about and you make that decision. This new commitment has been a learning process for people going forward. We are a committed organization, and we ask our members to commit our volume.

A different picture emerges at Novation. As explained by one executive,

> I think one unique differentiator is that we are pretty self-selecting. There is nothing mandatory about what we do. And we honestly believe that has been one of the reasons our committed "Opportunity" program has been so successful. If you want to do it, there is additional value [for the member]. If you don't, you still get to utilize the contracts agreed to and the pricing should be fair

and equitable with contracts that sit outside the committed program.

Novation takes this voluntaristic approach even farther. They
believe they allow the IDN more room for contract customization
and flexibility, that is, being willing to negotiate contracts for the
IDN outside of the GPO's portfolio, thereby achieving economic
value for both sides. One executive said

> I think the VHA side of Novation is very good at
> customizing and being flexible in their approach. That
> is why I think they win against Premier [in recruiting
> new hospital members] as many times as they have.
> Typically the way that value is structured in the
> contract—whatever the customization or flexibility
> commitment is—is in the utilization of the portfolio.
> That is where a good piece of the revenue comes from.
> So if the member can do certain things and at the same
> time get a commitment to drive business through Nova-
> tion, then financially both parties (the health care orga-
> nization and GPO alliance) come out ahead.
>
> We never want to put our manufacturer partner in the
> position of having to say to our large IDNs, "Gee, we
> would love to give you a better deal but our Novation
> contract won't let us." That is absolutely untrue. That is
> not what our contract says. In fact, our contract says that
> if you can articulate a clear business rationale as to why
> you want to offer a better deal to IDN X, we would be
> very happy to enable you to deliver that extra value and
> acknowledge that in doing so we are able to help man-
> age the market competition issue for the manufacturer.
> So we have a lot of flexibility in contract pricing. We
> understand that every IDN wants its own deal. Some

of this is "I want better price up front" and some is "I
want more services on the back end" and some of it is
"I want standardization support." Rather than forcing all
of that to be specifically articulated as a new price tier,
what we have done is maintain market competitive
pricing in between bid cycles.

Nonprofit GPOs also seek to achieve greater compliance by
reducing the number of vendors they contract with. In the past,
following its 1995 merger, some like Premier pursued a single-
source, committed-volume contracting strategy.[75] Such an
approach can work where there is a dominant supplier of a commodity item (for example, Becton Dickinson and needles and
syringes). However, this approach has been abandoned for a dual-
source strategy for several reasons. GPOs sometimes found that the
vendor selected could not handle the national sales volume for a
large alliance. Alternatively, the GPOs amassed enough size and
compliance that they could achieve comparable pricing and value
through dual-source contracts that afforded hospital members more
flexibility. Even if they could not achieve this comparable pricing,
GPOs have had to afford greater flexibility to their increasingly
large IDN members that wanted some customization. In addition,
the requirements of a single-source strategy include converting
new hospital members from their past vendor to the new vendor
under the GPO's contract. There are a lot of conversion costs and
politics (for example, persuading clinicians to change their product preferences) that must be outbalanced by the economic value
from a sole-source contract.[76] This problem increases in magnitude as GPOs merge and force a confrontation between one
GPO's portfolio choices and those of another. Finally, due to
supplier consolidation, GPOs wanted more dual-source contracts
to prevent overreliance on one large vendor. Thus, at present,
nonprofit GPOs are content to get from multi-source to dual-
source contracts.

Among the investor-owned GPOs, contract compliance is acknowledged to be roughly similar and, according to suppliers, higher than among nonprofit GPOs.[77,78] This is due in part to their common ownership, relative homogeneity, and a "culture of compliance."[79] The hospitals and GPOs are divisions owned and operated by the investor-owned chain, while the member hospitals in nonprofit purchasing alliances are often part-owners of the GPO (and thus harder to discipline).[80] Moreover, vendors cannot easily penetrate investor-owned hospitals without the GPO contract from the investor-owned system. The hospitals cannot easily order anything other than what is on the contract and what shows up on the computer screens of their materials managers. By contrast, vendors can penetrate nonprofit hospitals without a GPO contract.

Investor-owned hospitals also have more similar purchasing requirements, and common information and materials management systems. With such information, these GPOs get access to each hospital's capital budgets and can forecast capital equipment purchases over the next two years. This allows them to do "group buys," which can reduce contract costs by an estimated 20–25 percent. One executive described the process this way:

> We will analyze these capital budgets and say, "Wow, look at this. In this group of hospitals it appears that we are going to purchase thirty-two CT scanners. Why don't we get those hospitals that are purchasing CTs together, bring them in for a two-day session, and invite all of the CT manufacturers in?" We then tell the group they have to come up with a unanimous choice on who[m] they are going to purchase all of these CTs from. "OK, you have heard from every vendor. Now it is up to you. Don't worry about which manufacturer you pick, because we have got great pricing on everything. All we want you to do is focus on which manufacturer has leading technology and is going to deliver what you need

right now." We want them to pick what is clinically appropriate for their professionals, and leave the pricing to us. They make the decision right then and there, because they already have in their budgets what they are going to buy.

In this manner, the investor-owned GPOs require the participation of nursing directors and chiefs of clinical areas to assist in formulating contracting and bidding strategies for particular products. Nonprofit GPOs also pursue this approach with clinicians but more on a partnership approach. In addition, the investor-owned systems outsource responsibility and accountability for materials management to their GPOs, as well as provide them data from system-owned hospitals on their supply costs and utilization. The GPOs thus possess greater visibility of "spikes" in member utilization and the financial incentive to proactively correct these spikes in order to "deliver as corporate members and employees of the system."

In contrast to nonprofit GPOs, there appear to be only slight differences in the corporate approach to achieving these high compliance levels among the investor-owned GPOs. Some appear to be more demanding and restrictive in allowing member hospitals to utilize their contract portfolio. As an illustration, one GPO reportedly requires any hospital wishing to access the portfolio to commit to using a particular vendor and all of its contracts in the area of capital equipment. Another has developed a program called *FOCUS* (Focus On Contract and Utilization Strategies) where member hospitals are expected to comply 100 percent in fifteen to sixteen specific product categories by purchasing from one vendor. At present, many of these products are in the commodity area, where one large vendor has overwhelming market share, where there is little product differentiation, and/or where physicians and nurses have no decided preference (for example, IV pumps and sets, contrast media, imaging film, examination gloves, pulse oximeters). This makes it easier to standardize on one vendor (equivalent to single-sourcing the contract to one vendor). Full hospital compliance here is rewarded by 100 percent rebates on the CAFs earned by the GPO. These rebates sometimes enable marginally performing members to make their budgets in time for corporate performance reviews.

As a result of the different ownership structures and corporate discipline they afford, investor-owned GPOs report much higher levels of member commitment. They claim that 80 percent of the supplies purchased by their hospitals are under GPO contract. In contrast, they claim (based on prior work experience in nonprofit GPOs) that only 35–40 percent of hospital purchases in the Premier alliance are on that GPO's contracts. This figure is roughly equivalent to the 40 percent of hospital purchases that come through distributors.[81] There is a reason for this: there must be enough purchase volume for a supply item to get onto a GPO contract and to warrant a distribution agreement. The investor-owned GPOs further assert that the differences with their nonprofit counterparts may be even larger:

> That 35–40 percent [at Premier] is a percentage of what is on contract. Then you have to look at all the things a hospital has to buy. If they are 100 percent compliant with their GPO, the GPO will probably only represent 50–60 percent of their purchases. They can get up to 60 percent under a contract, and frankly I believe 60 percent is a stretch. But, in fact, they are getting only 35–40 percent, so if you do the math you come up with a very small number.

In the future, committed compliance may serve less as a means of competitive advantage. There are signs that some GPOs (for example, Consorta and AmeriNet) are willing to relax the requirement for strict contract compliance and instead support IDN efforts to do their own contracting. This trend may prove popular among IDNs in product areas (for example, implants, devices, and radiology film) where acquisition costs and thus savings are high, and where GPO influence is currently low. The technology that will enable this customization, once it is developed, is Web-based purchasing that allows IDNs and groups of IDNs to do their own group buys.

GPO Loyalty

An issue for nonprofit GPOs that is related to purchasing commitment is member loyalty. As noted earlier, community hospitals belong to an average of 2.6 GPOs. This is down slightly from 2.8 GPOs a few years earlier. This suggests a trend toward greater concentration of the hospital's organized purchasing through one or two GPOs. This growing concentration may reflect the broader product portfolios of GPOs. Alternatively, it may reflect the fact that national nonprofit GPOs expect or restrict their members to belong to only one national GPO but allow them to belong to a regional GPO for items outside the national contract portfolio. Nevertheless, three types of deviations from this expectation occur.

First, some GPOs may try to belong to more than one national GPO. The GPOs claim they police this and try to "clean this up." They also rely on their business partners (the product vendors) to identify members who show up on the lists of multiple GPOs. One executive said

> If you show up on two lists the danger is this. You are going to get the higher-priced list. So, let's just say you are on Premier's list and you might also be on AmeriNet's. If the business partner sees that and knows the price difference between the GPOs, and Premier's price is better, you are going to get stuck with AmeriNet pricing. The vendor will decide which list to choose and charge you the highest price that he can. So there is a real disincentive for hospitals to do this.

Second, and more worrisome, hospital members (perhaps more so than IDN members) frequently "cherry-pick" the GPO's contracts. Here, the hospital doesn't have to belong to another GPO. Instead, it leverages its GPO's contract prices by finding some supplier not on the national contract that is willing to discount prices on specific items by 10 percent or so. This often happens without the hospital actively seeking another contract. With long-term (three- to five-year) contracts, manufacturers excluded from the GPO's portfolio have a strong incentive to engage in "counter-detailing" to try to pick up some incremental business and market share from IDNs in the GPO. Due to just these kinds of events, manufacturers claim the word *partner* does not exist in health care.

Hospital members do not tend to share the terms of these contracts with other GPO hospitals for fear of losing that special pricing in future contract renewals. They consequently withhold pricing information from the GPO, which limits the latter's ability to measure what its members are doing, and which hurts the GPO's ability to achieve compliance targets and thereby contract for lowest possible price on behalf of all of its members. Here again, GPOs rely on their contracted manufacturers (which are losing some business) to monitor hospitals' behavior and avoid the temptation to bid on maverick hospital RFPs for better prices.

Third, some hospitals may switch their GPO affiliations either in whole or in part. This often happens among IDNs that don't fully participate in their GPO's contracts. IDNs may switch when they perceive another GPO has a better-priced portfolio or a broader product selection. They may also switch when their primary GPO displays some reluctance to tailor a more flexible, customized portfolio for their hospital members. IDNs may also transfer a portion of their portfolio purchases over to another GPO's contracts when they perceive some short-term advantage. In such cases, the IDN hopes to "fly under the radar" of its primary GPO. For their part, investor-owned GPOs may welcome IDNs and academic medical centers to join their purchasing ranks, not so much for their purchasing volume, but for "the enhanced perspective they'll provide on clinical issues" such as product utilization.[82] More frequently, members of regional GPOs may transfer some of their purchasing business to national GPOs. At present, due to the concentration of business among the national GPOs, the competition for new business is focused on the membership of "second-tier" (regional) GPOs and those freestanding hospitals that are not members of any major alliance.

However, bringing in outside members to the GPO can jeopardize the latter's high level of purchasing discipline, and thus its appeal to vendors. Thus, when they join the national GPOs, these new members are expected to reach a minimum level of participation (for example, 80 percent of purchase volume through the GPO's portfolio) and agree not to cherry-pick the contracts.

One GPO response to the cherry-picking problem is to set up a GPO for nonalliance members who only want products (not the broader set of services provided by hospital alliances) and just want to cherry-pick what they need. Such members get access to the full GPO portfolio but do not get access to the committed buying programs and their pricing. This enables the GPO to expand its market coverage, aggregate more market share for their contracted vendors, and appeal to hospitals that want to cherry-pick.

Portfolio Content, Operationalization, and Support

In addition to contract price and member commitment, GPOs claim to have competitive advantage based on their product portfolio content, the implementation of that portfolio, and the support they provide in delivering that portfolio. This means several things in practice. *Portfolio content* refers to the breadth and depth of the products offered in the GPO's contracts. The competition is not over which GPO has the contract with a given manufacturer. According to one executive at Premier,

> If you look at the product alignments between us and Novation, there are some overlaps in the products we contract for. But a lot of the differences are just the Hatfields and the McCoys. For some products, the major vendors are Baxter and Abbott. You will see that we have one and they [Novation] have the other. So how do you differentiate? Could you do well with Novation? Yes. Could you do well with Premier? You bet.

The competition lies elsewhere. As just noted, GPOs believe their advantage lies in the members' use of the total product portfolio (hence the importance of portfolio operationalization discussed next).

As noted earlier, some nonprofit GPOs seek to provide desirable product bundles from "best of breed" manufacturers to their hospital members.[83] Such GPOs offer their members greater overall (pricing) value if they "embrace the entire portfolio rather than pick it apart." At the same time, some manufacturers have engaged in mergers and acquisitions to (1) broaden their product lines and their presence in product areas that fall along the continuum of care, (2) address the bundling issue from their end, and (3) appeal to GPOs that take this approach (see Chapters Seven and Nine). Such manufacturers may enter into "corporate partnership" arrangements with GPOs that offer hospital members additional financial incentives beyond product price for "maximizing the various opportunities available in the product bundle."[84]

There are problems with this bundling approach, however. The desired bundle of products will vary across IDNs and across physicians within each IDN. This makes it hard to standardize the product. In addition, the use of bundles requires that ADAs carry all of the manufacturers' product lines, which increases their SKUs and inventory. Moreover, hospitals are fearful of getting inferior products, are thus wary of vendors and GPOs selling them bundles of products they may not want, and prefer to develop their own disease management programs in-house. One GPO solution to these problems is to dual-source contracts for products in these areas and allow multiple vendors to serve their customers' needs. Choice among vendors from which to source products is at present driven more by the vendor's market share, product pipeline, and appeal to clinicians rather than by quality outcomes.[85]

In the past few years, GPOs have taken steps to address this issue with their own version of disease management programs. Instead of offering best-of-breed bundles of products, they now offer best-of-breed bundles of manufacturers that make products to treat specific diseases (for example, cardiac rhythm problems and orthopedic injuries). The GPOs now award corporate contracts to a handful of leading vendors with the products that physicians prefer. Hospitals may choose one or more of the vendors to customize their own disease management portfolio based on their own physicians' preferences, as long as they meet an overall compliance level across vendors. Such a program allows hospital materials managers to emphasize clinical outcomes over cost issues.[86]

Finally, some GPOs also try to provide broad portfolios that appeal not only to the hospital market but also to the alternate site delivery market, either independent physicians or those affiliated with an IDN. As one executive stated,

> The physician market is not the same. It is not the same product mix. It must have a broader portfolio. Not only are you dealing with a different product mix, the scope of services also needs to be expanded. This has been one of the problems encountered by other GPOs trying to serve this market. Historically, they have just tried to take their acute care program and give it to the physicians. They were only able to capture a certain percentage of the business. What we did, which was very smart, was to

recognize that supply purchasing is the smallest piece of the physicians' expense. Physicians look for services, such as disposal or transcription, or for some other products. So what we have done through committee is really expand the portfolio of both products and services so that these physicians become truly engaged both ways.

Portfolio operationalization starts with an account manager and his or her team, which have responsibility for a certain number of alliance members. They disseminate information on contracts, programs, updates, and price changes, and "a host of other things that members could not possibly keep up with." At the same time, they try to show members the value proposition in the contracts, and what that value might look like for the member if they utilize the contract fully. They also go into the hospital, gather information, analyze it, benchmark it with other peer hospitals in the alliance, and then try to show members what the value of the contract might look like if they utilize the products appropriately or shift to alternative products. This is all in the way of customer service. These customer teams provide a unified face to the hospital customer and are cross-functional in composition, often including an RN, pharmacist, someone with a distribution background, someone with a background in the GPO's committed programs, and someone with a background in standardization and utilization. Thus, the team seeks to deliver products and services in these different functional areas to a given customer. In this manner, the GPO's functional departments at corporate headquarters have representation and input into local hospital accounts on a coordinated, multidisciplinary basis. Two problems reported by GPOs with this strategy, however, have been recruiting functional specialists in these areas who have sales expertise and background, and retaining such personnel in a labor market with low unemployment.

As another area of portfolio operationalization, some GPOs involve hospital executives and clinicians in their standing committees and task forces. Such involvement in the GPO's decision-making process is claimed to improve the credibility of and member commitment to the GPO's programs.

An important customer team activity is known as the *scrubbing session*. Here a team member seeks to validate all of the product purchases by the member hospital—what they are buying from whom—to determine if members are in compliance, if they are getting their incentive checks for being in compliance, and what they need to do to get in compliance. This monitoring is very important in committed programs, and actually becomes another program unto itself.[87] This may involve bringing in one of the other team specialists to work with the hospital in a deficient area. Such compliance monitoring is more an issue in nonprofit GPOs than in the investor-owned GPOs that have more standardized information systems and data gathering from their hospitals. In the absence of ownership, some nonprofit GPOs have had to rely on their member hospitals to tell them what they bought, and then validate this using information provided by vendors on how much product they sold and information from distributors on how much product they shipped. Sometimes large IDN members do not want to relay this information because they have "enhanced the deal" with the vendor. It is not surprising that GPOs want to provide their members with e-commerce and IT enhancements to materials management to speed up this data gathering (see Chapters Ten and Eleven). At present, however, they estimate that anywhere from 5–20 percent of their members have any such capability.

Portfolio support includes the services offered by the GPO's ADAs and, in some cases, by the GPO's pursuit of "managed distribution." As noted previously, some GPOs grade the performance of their vendors and distributors, and seek to shift contractual agreements to those that score highly. As part of portfolio support, some GPOs have larger shared-service parent organizations that claim to do things that their hospital membership values more highly over the offerings of rival shared-service organizations. These things might include performance consulting and information technology tools that enable hospitals to examine their clinical and financial data. In general, the parent offers outsourcing services that hospitals may find advantageous. Thus, some GPO executives stated that the competitive advantage lay more in the corporate parent and its service offering than in the actual GPO.

Other GPO Issues

There are several other important issues surrounding GPOs. These include their efforts to promote standardization of vendors and producers, and their consolidation into super GPOs.

Clinical Standardization and Sourcing of Contracts

Typical partnerships with vendors revolve around specific cost containment, utilization reduction, and standardization initiatives. GPOs publicize these initiatives to attract new members and improve efficiencies among their current membership. Novation, for example, publishes guidebooks on standardization and utilization each year. These volumes include case studies, written by the hospital members and product manufacturers, describing hospital efforts to (1) minimize the number of products performing the same function, or product standardization, and (2) ensure that the products selected are the most cost effective.[88-90]

In a typical case of standardization, representatives from the product vendor come into the hospital to (1) audit clinical departments' product needs and use, including practice variations; (2) develop quality specifications and/or best practices for products and packaging systems; (3) recommend and implement changes that match the appropriate product or package for the appropriate application, patient, or procedure; and (4) thus reduce waste and cost. Often, these programs consist of product and therapeutic conversions—that is, switch from one SKU or drug to another—and improved processes for utilizing them. Programmatic success is gauged by expense reductions in the specific clinical area, inventory and SKU reductions, and improved human resource utilization.

One key issue for GPOs is obtaining clinician buy-in and committed buying for their programs in clinical standardization. Such programs focus on clinical preference items in key areas (for example, cardiovascular, orthopedic, and ophthalmic) rather than commodity supply items. For example, the purchase of cardiovascular products accounts for as much as $3 billion in spending at the top nonprofit GPOs. Many of these purchase decisions are physician driven, based on direct detailing and marketing by product manufacturers. GPOs are seeking greater influence in these decisions in order to bring those products under GPO contracts and reduce their hospitals' expenditures in these high-cost areas. There is another reason for the salience of this area for GPOs. Besides relying on GPOs, the manufacturers of these products invest significant effort (selling, general and administrative costs, or SGA) in their own sales force to gain access to IDNs, "pull through" their products, and determine compliance. They thus feel they have to invest in and support GPO contracts substantially.

In some preference areas, the GPO tries to winnow down the number of vendors from double digits to single digits. In other areas, such as cardiac pacemakers, there have been three major vendors: Medtronic, Guidant, and St. Jude. Physicians develop preferences for one vendor over another based on their prior medical training or preference for particular product features. GPOs identify the major players based on their national market share and product pipeline ("You have to factor in hope for the future"), and then try to get the physicians from member hospitals to agree on using some subset of them. If physicians cannot agree but insist on having all three vendors on the contract for pacemakers, the GPO cannot drive any economic value itself, but instead must rely on market forces to drive down prices. If physicians can at least agree to go with two out of the three (dual-source the agreement), then incremental business and share directed to those two can be exchanged for lower prices.

Needless to say, vendors of physician preference and specialty items resist contracting with GPOs. They do not see any incremental market share arising from such contracts. Instead, they feel that they get the same share but at a lower price and with the added cost of CAFs. Moreover, they are not concerned about efforts to commoditize their products and reduce the effectiveness of their direct marketing campaigns.

How well does this model work? Some GPO-sponsored research suggests that hospital materials management executives view product standardization as one of their most cost-effective strategies, although certainly not as important as lower prices.[91,92] Assorted case studies of standardization programs now under way suggest savings in the range of 1–2 percent of medical supply costs.[93] Other GPO executives have acknowledged that utilization and standardization efforts have not succeeded because hospitals lacked the resources, staff, and information to do the required analysis and work. While GPO members want long-term cost reductions, fiscal stringencies orient them to short-term solutions such as contract prices.[94] It is perhaps also worth noting that utilization reduction programs may run counter to the GPO's self-interest. Any reduction in the number of supply items purchased and utilized by member institutions means lower volume flowing through the GPO, and thus lower CAF revenues.

As part of these efforts, the GPOs may commit specialized staff (for example, nurse clinicians) to work with vendor representatives and hospital members to examine the custom packs or contrast media packages that hospitals are utilizing and often wasting (for example, by throwing away certain items in the pack). The GPOs then work with the vendors to pare down the custom packs and remove SKUs in order to reduce product cost and increase hospitals' efficient use of the supplies purchased. Such partnerships are encouraged and developed as part of the bidding process. As one executive stated,

> Let me tell you what we mean by standardization and utilization. You know, you may have fourteen organizations within an IDN and some are using J&J's dressings, some are using Kendall's, and some are using 3M's. For us, working within an IDN, standardization means we would at least get all fourteen facilities to agree to purchase the product from the same vendor. And in doing that, we typically go to the vendor (supply partner) and get them to agree that they will give that system "level pricing" in exchange for volume. And most of the supply partners we work with are willing to do that. So now you have really squeezed all there is out of the product price side (about 6–12 percent). We believe there is another 8–14 percent to save if you look at the total number of line items that you are purchasing. This really gets at utilization. Utilization can mean getting the hospital to use fewer supplies, to use the supplies in a more appropriate manner, and to order fewer varieties (SKUs) of each supply item.

Some GPO executives assert that managed care has abetted their efforts here. Managed care exerts pressure on physicians not only in their practices but also on the hospitals where they admit patients. As hospitals seek to constrain physician choice and discretion, physicians respond by asking for greater involvement in the decision-making processes that limit their choice. Conversely, in markets where managed care pressure is weak, physician resistance is strongest.

This model requires that the GPO and its members know the physician practice behavior and supply utilization patterns in their hospitals. Armed with such information, the GPO can then proceed with a version of "procedure case management" that links outcomes to practice styles and resource use, and then shares this information across hospitals with clinicians. Physicians may not be fully convinced to change products based on practice variation data, however. Executives at Tenet claim the model works well when individual clinicians across hospitals in the system conduct extensive clinical trials involving competing products to gauge their effectiveness and afterward agree to use a particular vendor's product. In such cases, vendors lack direct access to any decision-making body to influence physician decision making. Moreover, individual physicians now collectively persuade vendors of their willingness to swing their business elsewhere. The model also works well when the GPO can demonstrate its own willingness to shift contracts in other product areas from a larger vendor to another, smaller vendor, that threatens supplier incumbents. The resulting benefit for the GPO is, at a minimum, physician buy-in on the basis of quality, increased physician compliance in using the products contracted for, and perhaps higher quality at a lower cost.[95]

A handful of executives at other GPOs are downright cynical regarding those who trumpet their accomplishments in this area, however,

> If you [had] talk[ed] to [this executive] at [this GPO] before he left, he would [have] be[en] the first to tell you that they got far better press for their compliance than they actually drove on the physician preference items. These accomplishments were as much public relations as anything. GPO executives have to talk this stuff up because the manufacturer will read these same reports and think "I have to give him a good deal."

More typically, GPO executives mention the challenges in working with diverse hospital members and with physicians. As GPOs increase in size, they have more diverse members and product needs. This limits their ability to do product standardization and thus their ability to rationalize the number of vendors used. This is why IDNs may be able to negotiate lower prices with vendors. For their part, vendors with large profit margins may be willing to shave a few points off these margins to maintain or increase market share. Consultants at McKinsey have flatly stated that GPOs have had little impact on either standardization or rationalization.[96]

One determinant of success in driving standardization is whether or not substitute products are available for physicians to utilize. According to one pharmaceutical executive, "There are some things for which there are good clinical substitutes. There are other things for which there are no good clinical substitutes. So, they will get resounding success in some areas, partial success in other areas, and no success in still other areas."

Success in driving standardization is also a function of the clinical nature of the disease and available therapies. As a GPO executive explained, "We had high rates of standardization on some stuff because we were not dealing with the bleeding edge of medicine that requires everything to be available; it was all routine general care." Sometimes standardization is influenced by the physician specialty involved. As one executive stated, "Interventional cardiologists are not cooperative individuals." Finally, success may depend on selection effects. For example, investor-owned systems actively select the hospitals they wish to acquire and decide which procedures they wish to do within them. In this manner, they may concentrate on general community medicine where a high rate of standardization can be achieved.

There are also several problems in working with physicians. First, as one executive stated, "I think we are three to five generations of doctors away from being able to get a doctor who will listen instead of demand." Second, when asked to express their product preferences, physicians may select higher quality, but higher cost, items. This leads to higher supply costs for the GPO's membership. Third, suppliers may factor physician preferences for higher quality into the prices they charge for their products. Fourth, physician preferences may be all over the map, leading to multi-source contracting that limits any group leverage over specific vendors. Fifth, these preferences may change quickly, especially in innovative, high-tech product areas. Such changes may prevent effective programs in product standardization. Sixth, physicians are subjected to enormous marketing messages from vendors that compete with local hospital efforts to change their behavior. On a given day, consultants estimate there are 300 detailers in an IDN trying to persuade physicians about their products.[97] Last, there is past physician resentment at not being involved in decision making, and current sentiment that physicians lack a financial incentive to get involved and/or are just not interested.[98] This is especially true for office-based physicians aligned with IDN members. In their practices, supplies are only a tiny percentage of practice expenses compared to labor; moreover, office staff (for example, head nurse or nurse manager) rather than physicians order the supplies and are "happy to let the medical sales representatives come in, inventory the examination rooms, and restock the shelves."

Several product manufacturers also question the success of standardizing efforts in clinical preference areas. First, these efforts require a lot of work for perhaps only small payoffs. According to one executive,

> Physician customers want breadth. Materials managers may prefer to have someone who can bring their physicians a large arsenal of products and services that meet the bulk of their needs and know they can depend on it. It makes their life a little easier if they can win the big wars and focus on some of the other things. As you know, the cost of the product is just a fraction of the total cost of running a health system. So it is only going to make so much of an impact to complicate the fray by having all of these other players [manufacturers] come into the bidding war. I don't know how many people

want to go and take their complicated life and com-pound it just to get those savings, versus looking at the bigger issues and getting the bigger dollars.

Moreover, standardization among a core set of physicians invited in to review and select one vendor may not sway other physicians throughout the GPO's member hospitals. Executives made these comments:

Premier is trying to do this. They have created commit-tees of surgeons and doctors to help make the choices around suppliers. With thousands of physicians across 1,700 hospitals, it's a good start to get 30 in a room, but that still doesn't cover all of the choices in selection and standardization of products that go into physician preference items. It's easy to get 30 to maybe agree with 1,700 when you're talking about a box, but when you are talking about a heart valve where there is a lot of history or experience with other products, it's going to be hard for those 30 surgeons to convince 400 others in 1,700 hospitals that they ought to use a specific valve. At the end of the day, it is still the patient's specific sur-geon or physician who makes the decision which valve to use based on an array of different decision factors.

Finally, when physicians have standardized on one vendor and the GPO switches to another vendor, oftentimes the physicians do not follow suit.

Columbia/HCA has probably done the best job with clinical preference, but even then there are some inter-esting stories. Columbia had a contract with [vendor] for central venous catheters and had pricing in place. When that pricing expired, they told Columbia they were not going to renegotiate. They walked away from the contract. So Columbia and [vendor] have been in a pretty adversarial relationship since then. And yet [vendor] continues to sell products to their member hospitals because of clinician preference.

Overall, some GPO executives believe there is much needed room for improvement in SKU rationalization.

I really do not believe we have done very well at all in basic, unit-level standardization programs. I think there is a lot more value to be had here, as evidenced by the number of codes that the manufacturers continue to offer in product lines. Moreover, we see a phenomenon that manufacturers continue to proliferate product codes as a way to continue to grow their business. If health care organizations were serious about standardization, the minute we had a new product code one would fall off the other end. And it is really not serious about standardization even at the commodity level, as evidenced by the number of exam gloves the distributor has to carry to be successful in the marketplace today. There are probably only 20 percent of our members who have had 20–30 percent success in achieving some of these goals at the commodity level.

As one illustration, some GPOs note that even for simple products like surgical sutures, there can be three SKUs for the same suture based on the length of the suture (for example, 18 inch, 24 inch, and 36 inch). Product SKUs have multiplied here as an effort by manufacturers and hospitals to meet the preferences ("whims") of surgeons. Not only do SKUs multiply, but this leads to product waste. Physicians who prefer the longer length end up using only a portion, throw the rest away, and may not even be aware they could get the same suture in a shorter version. As another illustration, GPO executives claim they can deliver only 40 percent of their members' purchases of garbage can liners to a manufacturer that guarantees the GPO 70 percent savings, regardless of what they are already paying for those liners. Here, the problem stems from multiple departments that use liners (for example, housekeeping, dietary, and OR) that have different purchasing and distribution relationships, and that are not used to working together to consolidate these purchases.

GPO Mergers and Consolidation

Another set of issues stems from the recent merger of several regional and national GPOs. These include the 1996 merger of VHA and UHC to form Novation, and the 1995 merger of Premier Health Alliance, Sun Health, and American Health Care Systems to form Premier. These issues involve the increase in GPO market power, potential to restrain trade or limit the introduction of innovative products, and the salience of GPO services to members.[99]

As just discussed, GPOs seek to use their membership size and purchasing volume to leverage manufacturers over price and service levels. Merger and acquisition is a major vehicle to augment this bargaining stance. Large manufacturers are not concerned about GPO restraint of trade for several reasons, however. First, there are Justice Department limits on GPO size. Second, the manufacturers themselves have consolidated and thereby broadened their product lines to make themselves attractive (even indispensable) trading partners. Third, manufacturers witness membership defections from GPOs, and may even encourage them by offering IDNs better deals on a spot-market basis. They also suggest that some GPOs have difficulty monitoring and policing the behavior of members who break ranks.

A greater concern over GPO market power lies in the potential exclusion of smaller, more innovative manufacturers from the marketplace. As two GPOs merge, they tend to merge their contract portfolios, which leads to the choice of the vendor used by one over the vendor used by the other. It is not surprising that informal polls of product vendors reveal that the majority has lost one or more contracts due to GPO consolidation. To be sure, GPOs may finance small, innovative firms through their "institutes." However, this represents an effort to develop sole-sourced future contracts and to "keep the big incumbents honest."

Moreover, as both GPOs and manufacturers consolidate, contracting becomes longer term in nature with large incumbent players. There is less opportunity for newer, smaller firms to get in the GPO door to discuss their products, let alone have their products supplant an established contract. In such cases, as one executive explained, "Small manufacturers have to knock on a lot of doors and build support for their product from the ground up among the GPO membership, and then hope they can get an audience with the GPO headquarters." Smaller generic drug manufacturers may also get excluded.

In the past few years, several examples of such exclusion have surfaced in the media. One manufacturer of safety syringes complained that GPO contracts with large incumbents excluded them unfairly from the hospital marketplace. For Patient's Sake, a Washington, D.C.–based lobbying group that represents small manufacturers and a patient advocacy group, argued that GPO compliance requirements ignore small manufacturers and limit patient access to medical equipment. They called for congressional hearings and the Department of Justice to investigate antitrust violations. Similarly, a consortium of 130 small device firms called the Medical Device Manufacturers Association (MDMA) complained that GPOs lock out small vendors because of the 3 percent CAFs that must be paid to win their contracts.

Finally, in June 2001, the U.S. Senate Judiciary subcommittee on antitrust, business rights, and competition announced it would hold hearings in the late fall on the competitive impact of GPOs on smaller, innovative medical device manufacturers. Some observers believe the hearings are the direct result of lobbying efforts by groups such as MDMA. Others suggest it reflects a natural interest in the GPO's rapid growth and consolidation.

The Health Industry Group Purchasing Association (HIGPA) responded to these challenges by citing studies that (1) GPOs saved hospitals and nursing homes between $14–22 billion in nonlabor costs in 1999, (2) a small hospital system saves three-quarters of a million dollars annually through its GPO participation, and (3) hospitals would have to spend an average of $353,000 annually to perform GPO functions on their own.[100]

GPOs respond to these challenges in several ways. First, they state that hospitals demand the products of larger vendors, rather than the GPOs telling them to use them. They also state that hospitals in most nonprofit GPOs can buy products off-contract if their physicians want them. Smaller vendors must therefore increase their efforts to market their products directly to clinicians who then inform materials managers of their preferences. GPOs also respond that these smaller manufacturers can get their products into hospitals using the GPO's private label programs and help them grow their market share on that basis.[101] Finally, some GPOs have initiated programs to help smaller vendors (for example, Novation's "Historically Underutilized Business Program").

There may be some benefits to this contracting situation, however. As past incumbents and smaller vendors get excluded from the large contracts, they reportedly rush to the other GPOs and to IDNs ready to execute better contracts. Moreover, smaller vendors may be able and willing to service regional, second-tier GPOs and thereby serve as a source for change in GPO contracting. Similarly, IDNs may show some willingness in the future to deal with such GPOs in order to be a bigger fish in a smaller pond. All of this is speculative, however.

Another related concern over GPO and manufacturer consolidation is the tendency for bilateral monopoly. Some executives see developing stagnation in a marketplace that brings together a handful of large GPOs contracting for products from a handful of large, diversified manufacturers. Such contracts reportedly take many weeks to negotiate on a clause-by-clause basis, leading to huge transaction costs, costs of switching, and thus inertia. As part of this stagnation, there is little change in product portfolios, little vendor switching by GPOs, and protection of incumbent suppliers due to dual-sourcing arrangements.[102]

Some analysts have characterized GPO-manufacturer bargaining as a "game of chicken" to see which party needs the other more.[103] GPOs don't want to lose a contract with a large vendor that makes products that clinicians want to use. Due to the difficulties in working with physicians, GPOs and their member IDNs may be reluctant to switch vendors and try to convert physicians to another manufacturer's products. One executive put it this way:

> You don't just switch from a Becton Dickinson syringe to a Sherwood syringe. You have to train people in doing that—the products are not the same, the packaging is different. If you switch, you have to take the old stock out, put the new stock in, and train people. Moreover, Sherwood doesn't have a 10 cc syringe; they have a 12 cc syringe. Because of these simple differences it's hard for people to switch. Hospitals don't want to go through this stuff.

Such product conversions may also result in lower compliance levels, which decrease CAF revenues flowing to the GPO. Moreover, if the GPO can get a 3 percent CAF across all of its vendor contracts, there is a clear incentive to go with long-term contracts with large vendors to minimize their transactions costs (for example, educating members about new contracts). Materials managers at IDNs may likewise be reluctant to shift contracts if these changes threaten compliance levels. Such levels are directly tied to product discounts and rebates, which directly affect their bottom lines.

Conversely, vendors don't want to lose a GPO contract because of the loss of market share (over the defined contract period), the difficulty in making that share up elsewhere in the short term, and the perceived threat to the vendor's image in the marketplace and its contracts with other buyers. As one executive stated,

We operate with a constant sense of fear of losing the contracts we already have. There is a large expense involved to re-win them. Some long-term contracts don't even have provisions for price increases. Five to seven years is a long time to go without a price increase. But we decided to go after them because it is new business. Volume is very important in this industry. Since we need a lot of volume, we keep prices down.

As a consequence of both GPO and supplier consolidation, there is a lot more at stake in losing a GPO contract. Moreover, there are some supply markets (for example, laboratory diagnostics) characterized by rapid product upgrades and revenue streams tied to products (for example, reagents) used alongside instruments already installed in hospitals. In such markets, incumbency is a major asset to be protected.[104]

Endnotes

1. Schneller, Gene. *The Value of Group Purchasing in the Healthcare Supply Chain*. Tempe, Arizona: School of Health Administration and Policy, Arizona State University, 2000.
2. Zajac, Edward, Thomas D'Aunno, and Lawton Burns. "Managing Strategic Alliances." In Stephen Shortell and Arnold Kaluzny, Eds. *Health Care Management*. 4th Ed. Albany, New York: Delmar, 2000. pp. 307–329.
3. The split between hospital and alternate site purchases at BuyPower, the GPO for Tenet, is roughly 75–25 percent.
4. Diller, Wendy. "GPOs Rethink Diagnostics." *In Vivo* (September 1999): 46–56.
5. In Vivo. "Premier Listens to Its Members." *In Vivo* (July/August 2000): 4.
6. For example, Novation is the group purchasing wing for the combined Voluntary Hospitals of America (VHA) and the University HealthSystem Consortium (UHC). Services beyond group purchasing of supplies are housed in VHA-UHC. With regard to the distinction between "pure GPOs" that only buy products versus the broader hospital alliances like VHA and UHC, executives

point out that the decision to join the former is made lower in the hospital organization by the chief financial officer or even the direc-tor of materials management, while the decision to join alliances is typically made by the CEO.

7. Jaklevic, Mary Chris. "Premier Taking New Investment Tack." *Modern Healthcare* (June 19, 2000): 36, 38.

8. Kirchheimer, Barbara. "A Technology Gambit." *Modern Healthcare* (December 11, 2000): 22–23.

9. This is a function that manufacturers have ceded over to GPOs. GPO contracts require that vendors restrict access to contracts to the GPO's ADAs.

10. For additional information, see Barlow, Rick. "Taking Stock of Business." *Repertoire* 9(4) (2001): 20–26.

11. Health Industry Group Purchasing Association, 2000. Fact Sheet. www.higpa.org.

12. SMG Marketing Group. *Multi-Hospital Systems (MHS) and Group Purchasing Organizations (GPOs): 2000 Report and Directory.* Chicago: SMG Solutions.

13. Indeed, SMG's definition of GPO is an entity consisting of (1) two or more hospitals or (2) five or more nonhospital facilities (alternate sites) that come together to offer its members access to purchasing contracts for any of the following supply categories: pharmacy, medical-surgical, laboratory, dietary, or capital equipment.

14. Swayne, Linda, and Peter Ginter. "The Premier Health Care Alliance Emerges." In Jack Duncan, Peter Ginter, and Linda Swayne, *Strategic Management of Health Care Organizations.* 3rd Ed. Malden, Massachusetts: Blackwell, 1998. pp. 825–844.

15. SMG Marketing Group states there are seven categories of GPOs. The largest of these, the multihospital system, reportedly accounts for 416 GPOs. It is not clear if these figures are correct, given that SMG estimates there are 6,970 hospitals, while figures from the American Hospital Association suggest there are only 6,000. The difference may reflect SMG's possible inclusion of specialty units like substance abuse treatment centers that the AHA does not include, or its counting of individual hospitals that have merged or consolidated (Peter Kralovec, Health Forum, personal communica-tion). SMG also estimates there are only 100 "pure" GPOs.

16. Appel, Gary. "The IDN/GPO Relationship: Its Evolution in an Era of Direct Contracting Advantages." *The Health Strategist* 6(6) (1999): 1–5.

17. Cf. Hensley, Scott. "GPOs Under Pressure to Deliver." *Modern Healthcare* (September 20, 1999): 38–47.

18. Data supplied by SMG Marketing Group, Chicago.

19. See Note Eleven.

20. This figure marks a slight decrease from the average membership in 2.8 GPOs reported in the early 1990s. Cf. Lisa Scott. "Group Purchasing Evolution." *Modern Healthcare* (September 27, 1993): 52.

21. Association for Healthcare Resource and Materials Management. *2000 National Performance Indicators for Healthcare Materials Management.* Chicago: American Hospital Association, 2001.

22. Department of Justice and Federal Trade Commission. *Statements of Enforcement Policy and Analytical Principles Relating to Health Care and Antitrust.* September 27, 1994.

23. In addition to the 35 percent of total sales threshold, group purchasing arrangements will not be challenged as long as the cost of the producers and services purchased jointly accounts for less than 20 percent of the total revenues from all products or services sold by each competing supplier in the joint purchasing arrangement.

24. See Note Sixteen.

25. Voluntary Hospitals of America. *Environmental Assessment.* Dallas, Texas: VHA, 1997.

26. Bazzoli et al. "A Taxonomy of Health Networks and Systems: Bringing Order out of Chaos." *Health Services Research* 33(6) (1999): 1683–1717.

27. See Note Sixteen.

28. The size of these contracts with IDNs can be quite large for vendors. One large medical-surgical manufacturer reported that while 45–50 percent of its sales went to hospital members of GPOs, only 38 percent of sales were for items on the GPO contracts. The difference reflected "bilateral agreements" negotiated directly between hospitals and vendors.

29. Kearney, A.T. "Redesigning the Customer Interface." Presentation to Scenario Planning Meeting. New Brunswick, New Jersey: Johnson & Johnson. January 26–27, 1999.

30. Appel, Gary. "Integrated Delivery Systems Purchase More Competitively." The Health Care News Service. *The Business Word.* January 8th, 1998.

31. See Note Twenty-Nine.

32. See Note Fourteen.

33. Cf. Howard Larkin "Alliances: Changing Focus for Changing Times." *Hospitals* 63 (December 20, 1989): 34–35.
34. Cassak, David. IDNs and GPOs: "Changing the Leopard's Spots." *In Vivo* (July/August 2001): 32–44.
35. House Conference Report 1012, 99th Congress, 2nd Session, pp. 310–311 (1986): October 17th. "Providing for Reconciliation Pursuant to Section 2 of the Concurrent Resolution on the Budget for Fiscal Year 1987." Also see www.hhs.gov/progorg/oig.
36. Millennium Research Group. *Online Opportunities in the Medical Products Marketplace.* Stream 1, Issue 2 (October 2000). Toronto: Millennium Research Group.
37. Frost & Sullivan. *The Internet's Role in the U.S. Distribution of Medical Devices.* San Jose, California: Frost & Sullivan, 2000.
38. Muse & Associates. *The Role of Group Purchasing Organizations in the U.S. Health Care System.* Washington, D.C.: Muse & Associates, 2000.
39. See Note One.
40. Murawski, Ken. "Jump In. The GPO Water's Fine." *Repertoire* (April 2000): 54, 57.
41. Cassak, David. "Novation's E-Commerce Play." *In Vivo* (July/August 2000): 66–77.
42. Novation. *Value of Commitment Study.* Dallas, Texas: Novation, 1995.
43. In line with this figure, executives at Tenet/BuyPower estimate that 40 percent of their purchases are traditional GPO-contracted products, another 40 percent are small volume arcane items that are typically not on contract, and another 20 percent are high-technology physician preference items for which they may or may not have a GPO contract but might like to (Cassak, David. 1998). These lower figures may reflect the fact that the GPO's share of hospital spending varies widely across hospital departments. A mid-1990s study of hospital participation in GPO contracts found that use rates vary from a high of 87 percent (pharmacy) to a low of 28 percent (facilities). Across the twelve hospital areas studied, the average contract participation rate was 71 percent (Novation. 2000. *Value of Group Purchasing Case Studies.* Referenced in Schneller, Gene. 2000. Cf. Table 1).
44. The salient fact here is that hospitals procure only a percentage of their products through their GPOs. Not only are merely two-thirds

of products covered by GPO contracts, but also the level of hospital compliance with these contracts may be only 80 percent or so (covered next). Thus, hospital acquisition of supplies through GPOs is the product of these two terms, or 80 percent of two-thirds (53 percent). This leaves a lot of room for off-contract buying.

45. See Note Forty-Two.
46. Becker, Cinda. "For GPOs, E-Commerce is All Show." *Modern Healthcare* (October 9, 2000): 26–38.
47. Appel (1999) suggests that the top seven GPOs account for 85 percent of the hospital market. Applying his figures suggests that the total GPO market is closer to $48 billion.
48. Becker, Cinda. "GPO Maverick." *Modern Healthcare* (May 21, 2001): 28.
49. These calculations also do not include GPO purchases for the alternate site market. This market is estimated to be $16–25 billion, depending on what products are included. The estimated savings from GPOs are estimated to be 20–40 percent here, due to high product markups by distributors, but may not be realized in the short term due to the fragmentation of buyers in this market and the GPOs' historic lack of presence here. Alternate site spending is estimated at roughly one-quarter of all purchasing, but is expected to grow for several reasons: (1) the aging of the population, which increases demand for long-term care; (2) increasing managed care penetration and shorter lengths of hospital stay, which decrease hospital utilization; (3) declines in the number of hospitals and hospital beds; and (4) changes in Medicare such as the Balanced Budget Act, which reduce inpatient reimbursement. Indeed, some drug distributors (for example, AmeriSource) that have moved into this market have reported 50 percent growth in sales during 1998–99 and suggest 20 percent growth rates into the future. (Alan Clock, personal communication).
50. Hensley. "GPOs Under Pressure to Deliver." *Modern Healthcare* (September 20, 1999): 38–47.
51. Everard, Lynn. *Blueprint for an Efficient Health Care Supply Chain.* White Paper. Norcross, Georgia: Medical Distribution Solutions, 2000.
52. See Note Twelve.
53. See Note Forty-Two.

54. Smith, Charlie R. "Determining When Integrated Delivery Systems Should Belong to GPOs." *Healthcare Financial Management* 52(9) (1998): 38.
55. Cassak, David. "Tenet Shakes Things Up." *In Vivo* (July/August 1998): 41–53.
56. See Note One.
57. Gillett et al. *Hospitals' New Supply Chain.* Forrester Research. www. forrester.com, 2000.
58. See Note Thirty.
59. See Note Four.
60. See Note Twenty-Nine.
61. See Note Thirty.
62. Chapman, Timothy, Ajay Gupta, and Paul Mango. "Group Purchasing is not a Panacea for U.S. Hospitals." *McKinsey Quarterly* 1 (1998): 160–165.
63. See Note Thirty-Eight.
64. See Note Forty-Two.
65. In a 1996 survey of 131 GPOs (primarily outside of health care) conducted by Arizona State University, the average GPO achieved an annual dollar savings of 13.43 percent. Cf. Schneller. 2000.
66. Frost, Scott. "Buying In: IDN Reaps GPO Benefits." *Hospital Materials Management* 26(7) (2001): 11–13.
67. See Note Forty-Two.
68. See Note One.
69. See Note Fifty-Five.
70. See Note One.
71. See Note Forty-Two.
72. Accordus. *Contract Price Management in the Healthcare Industry.* White Paper. Accordus. www.Accordus.com, 2001.
73. Plummer, Patrick M. "The Future of Group Purchasing." *The Health Strategist* 5(1) (1998): 1, 2, 5.
74. See Note Twenty-Nine.
75. Premier also wanted aggressive price discounts from vendors under threat of being dropped.
76. Despite the politics of persuading physicians to change to products under committed contracts, there may not be much economic fallout. A survey of physicians found that 72 percent said the risk of losing physicians when implementing committed contracts in the facility was low or none. Eighty-four percent said their institution

had experienced no physician turnover due to compliance or commitment initiatives.

77. See Note Twenty-Nine.

78. This statement applies to the hospitals owned by the investor-owned systems, but not necessarily to the nonprofit hospitals that contract with the investor-owned GPO for buying.

79. Lutz, Sandy, and Preston Gee. *Columbia/HCA: Healthcare on Overdrive*. New York: McGraw-Hill, 1998.

80. See Note Four.

81. The figure of 40 percent is from Tenet's GPO, BuyPower.

82. Volunteer Hospitals of America. *Environmental Assessment*, 47.

83. Investor-owned GPOs, by contrast, take the position that "every product category must stand on its own," and that "pricing must be competitive in that particular [product] marketplace." Moreover, they feel that their nonprofit GPO counterparts never really know whether they are getting good prices across products in the bundles for which they contract. According to one executive, the nonprofits "take bids from five manufacturers and the lowest bid wins. But they don't know if that lowest bid is the best bid or the best price in the market. That is because they don't have access to the data on prices that their member IDNs are paying for these products. The big IDNs are not going to tell Premier or Novation what they are paying because they likely have enhanced the deal with the manufacturer to some degree [on their own]."

84. For IDNs these incentives consist of some portion of the CAFs that flow back to the hospitals. For freestanding hospitals, the incentives are a bonus discount.

85. Investor-owned GPOs tend to avoid the product bundling approach. They are concerned over what happens when you contract for five products and one product category fails. If you seek to disengage from that contractual relationship, the other product categories suffer. Instead, these GPOs state that each product category must stand on its own in terms of both price and quality.

86. DeJohn, Paula. "Disease-Based Contracts Reflect Clinical Realities." *Hospital Materials Management* 26(7) (2001): 1, 9–11.

87. See Note Twenty-Five.

88. Novation. *Standardization: A Guide to Reducing Variations to Improve Outcomes*. 3rd Ed. Dallas, Texas: Novation, 1999.

89. Novation. *Utilization: A Guide to Reducing Variations to Improve Outcomes*. 3rd Ed. Dallas, Texas: Novation, 1999.

90. Novation. *1998 Standardization and Utilization Poster Book*. Dallas, Texas: Novation, 1998.

91. See Note One.

92. See Note Fifty-Seven.

93. DeJohn, Paula. "GPO Deals Still Golden: Compliance Is the Key." *Hospital Materials Management* 25(10) (2000): 1, 9–11.

94. Cassak, David. "Novation's E-Commerce Play." *In Vivo* (July/August, 2000): 66–77.

95. See Note Fifty-Five.

96. See Note Sixty-Two.

97. See Note Sixty-Two.

98. See Note Fifty-Five.

99. There are other issues beyond these. One is the need to integrate different cultures of GPOs. This issue surfaced in the formation of Novation, which combined the customer relationships and purchasing patterns for private nonprofit hospitals in VHA (customized contracts for IDNs) with the academic medical centers (potentially more physician preference) and publicly owned hospitals (public bidding process) in UHC. Both here as well as in the formation of Premier the GPO needs to develop one standard portfolio of products for the larger, more diverse membership. Another is the need to develop one consistent face for the hospital member that can service that account.

100. DeJohn, Paula. "Senate Subcommittee to Probe GPO Influence." *Hospital Materials Management* 26(8) (2001): 1, 10–11.

101. Some innovative products such as skin staplers have entered the market in this manner.

102. See Note Fifty-Five.

103. See Note Fifty-Five.

104. See Note Four.

5

Role of Wholesalers and Distributors

Lawton R. Burns and Robert A. DeGraaff

Wholesalers are independently owned and operated intermediaries in the distribution channel. As noted in Chapter
Three, they are to be distinguished from the manufacturer's sales
force (a captive wholesaling operation) and from independent
agents and brokers (who do not take title to the goods they buy and
sell). As independent intermediaries, they also operate their own
warehouses for product inventories.[1]

It is appropriate to clearly define two terms that tend to be used
interchangeably: wholesaling and distribution. *Wholesalers* are firms
that resell products to another intermediary; thus a pharmaceutical
wholesaler may purchase drugs from the manufacturer and then resell
them to a pharmacy, which in turn sells them to the end customer.
Distributors are firms that resell the product to the end customer
directly; thus, a pharmaceutical distributor purchases drugs from the
manufacturer and then resells them to a hospital, which dispenses
them in-house.[2] Pharmaceutical intermediaries typically serve both
functions and thus are correctly labeled wholesalers/distributors.
Medical-surgical product intermediaries typically resell directly
to the end customer and thus are accurately labeled as distributors.
For the sake of simplicity, we will refer to both sets of intermediaries
as distributors.[3]

What Functions Do Distributors Perform?

The two basic functions performed by distributors are (1) to satisfy customer needs and (2) to match supply and demand. More specifically, distributors serve to

- Aggregate demand across many small buyers.

- Allow manufacturers to produce steady quantities of product.

- Mediate customer wants (desire small quantities of many different products) and manufacturer needs (produce large quantities of a few products).

- Simplify product, payment, and information flows between manufacturer and customer (for example, reduce the number of purchase orders and shipments that manufacturers have to process, and provide product availability and use information to the customer).

- Simplify credit issues for manufacturers in dealing with small and local customers.

- Allow manufacturers to ship products in large batches by "breaking lots."

- Permit regional distribution networks to service the majority of locations to which products are shipped.

- Hold inventory (rather than manufacturer or customer).

- Protect the quality and integrity of the product through proper storage and handling.

- Provide an off-site customer service department for the manufacturer.

- Serve as part of the manufacturer's push strategy to move products to customers.[4]

Distributors in the United States typically act as multichannel distributors, which sell products from a wide range of manufacturers rather than serve as the exclusive agent for one product vendor. Health care distributors state they prefer to handle single-source contracts—that is, handle a given product from only one manufacturer—for two reasons: processing a large volume from one supplier drives the best prices and service levels, and high compliance levels on the part of the customer within a single-source contract is "the lowest-cost scenario." At the same time, single-source contracting is difficult for health care distributors for several reasons. First, distributors may not have sufficient capacity to service a nationwide GPO contract. Second, they may be unable to service a national GPO that seeks to drive committed purchasing due to shortcomings in manufacturer or distributor "fill rates." Third, the hospitals serviced by the distributor may be on different contracts for different brands and manufacturers of the same product.

Distributors and Electronic Data Interchange (EDI)

Distributors have been instrumental in the diffusion of electronic data interchange. The following paragraphs describe what EDI is, its prevalence across value chain players, and its benefits.

What is Electronic Data Interchange (EDI)?

One of the most significant contributions of distributors to the health care supply chain was the deployment of electronic order-entry systems to their customer base. The first entrant here was Analytic Systems Automatic Purchasing (ASAP), a computerized system for ordering, tracking, and managing hospital supplies developed back in the late 1950s by American Hospital Supply Corporation (AHSC), a medical-surgical distributor.

In 1985, AHSC was acquired by Baxter Travenol. When Baxter's chief products competitors, Abbott Laboratories and Johnson & Johnson, saw that one of their main distribution channels (ASHC) was acquired, they developed their own electronic order systems (COACT and QuikLink). What followed was a proliferation of order-entry and materials management systems, each of which originally sought to be a proprietary marketing channel. Competition among them, however, forced them to develop multivendor systems where hospitals could order products from a large number of different manufacturers. Hospital customers in fact demanded open access in order to derive value from their linkages. Baxter's own product here, which rolled out in 1988, was ASAP Express. In this manner, the distribution industry began to migrate away from a dedicated system with proprietary protocols toward an open system with a common electronic data interchange (EDI) platform. In 1995, Baxter spun off its distribution business into a separate firm known as Allegiance, the largest distributor of medical-surgical products.

As a consequence of these efforts to link with providers, EDI is now the major electronic form of communication used by distributors. By virtue of their large volume, distributors could afford the expensive investment in and deployment of EDI systems to their hospital customers. Formally defined,

> EDI is the direct electronic transmission, computer to computer, of standard business forms, such as purchase orders, shipping notices, invoices, and the like, between two organizations. In a purchasing environment, documents are transmitted "over the wire," eliminating the need to generate hard copies and to distribute them manually. By utilizing EDI, a buyer and a supplier are operating in a near real-time environment, which can reduce material delays by shortening procurement lead times.[5]

EDI relies upon commonly accepted message formats, or transaction sets, that contain the information to be exchanged among trading partners. EDI messages can be transmitted using value-added networks (VANs) or point-to-point dedicated systems.

Prevalence of EDI

EDI is found to varying degrees among value chain players. Distributors have a much greater EDI capability compared to providers and manufacturers.

Distributor EDI Capability

Analysts estimate that more than three-quarters of distributors exchange data electronically with customers and generate three-quarters of their business using EDI systems.[6,7] The volume of EDI-based business may vary by distributor. Large distributors like Allegiance report that 80–90 percent of their incoming orders are received computer-to-computer via EDI. Smaller local and regional distributors may do less. A survey of national and regional distributors (covering medical-surgical, pharmaceutical, and medical equipment products) revealed that 70 percent of distributors overall take customer orders using EDI, but only glean 22 percent of revenues in this manner. Ninety percent of distributors still take orders via fax or telephone. Eighty percent have a salesperson doing order entry, 59 percent take orders via e-mail, 33 percent use proprietary order-entry technology, and only 41 percent take orders over the Internet (the latter accounting for only 2 percent of revenues).[8]

As a result of the development of open (rather than proprietary) systems, distributors no longer enjoy exclusive marketing channels in dealing with hospital customers. Instead, they have focused on providing customer benefits.[9] Based on their large volume and their focus on customer service, distributors have developed strong customer relationships focused on improving supply chain management.

Hospital EDI Capability

Distributors report that their customers vary widely in their EDI capabilities, which are described as "relatively weak" at present. Hospital capabilities appear to be among the strongest. EDI is now the major way in which hospitals do electronic procurement. Data from the early 1990s indicated that 80 percent of acute care hospitals handled their 15,000 annual purchase orders using electronic order-entry systems (EDI); 15 percent used manual systems while the remaining 5 percent used standardized EDI interfaces.[10] More recent published survey evidence suggests little advance here. Two surveys of hospitals and IDNs reveal that 80 percent or more use EDI for purchasing.[11,12] However, the figures appear to be lower for smaller hospitals, which lack the dedicated linkages to large distributors. According to these surveys, the prevalence of electronic capability in hospital procurement varies by procurement function: placing orders (67 percent of hospitals), issuing purchase orders (59 percent), tracking orders (44 percent), and billing (30 percent). More recent data from Arthur Andersen reveal that less than 31 percent of all EDI transaction sets are actually used. Outbound purchase orders have the highest level of EDI use (90 percent), followed at a distance by invoicing (31 percent), catalog and uniform pricing (12 percent), purchase order confirmation (11 percent), and advance ship notice (0 percent).[13]

Alternate Sites and EDI Capability

EDI may be less common in the rest of the health care industry. EDI capability in the alternate site market clearly lags behind hospitals. Data on physician office supply orders reveal that 69.7 percent are made by phone, 34.2 percent involve an in-person sales call, 18.8 percent involve faxes, 5.4 percent are EDI based, and only 1.7 percent are made on the Internet.[14] The Millennium Research Group cites industry estimates of only 20–30 percent of total medical supply purchases using EDI, primarily limited to large manufacturers able to use the technology.[15]

Manufacturers' EDI Capability

A survey of forty-six global health care firms indicated that EDI transactions account for 36 percent of their revenue, while the majority of revenues (61 percent) are through nonelectronic means (phone, fax, or external order entry). Only a small fraction (3 percent) of revenues come through Internet commerce.[16] Indeed, pharmaceutical manufacturers spend only 5.5 percent of total company external expenditures on proprietary EDI (versus 27.4 percent in sixteen nonpharmaceutical industries) and 13.3 percent of total company external expenditures on Internet EDI (versus 23.6 percent in other industries).[17]

One reason why product vendors have not directly linked to hospital customers using EDI is that their products are sold through a large number of distributors, which "limits the ability of the EDI system to process critical information all the way back to the manufacturing stage so that manufacturers can tailor production schedules to customer ordering and distributor inventory levels."[18] Another reason is that it is inefficient for a large number of manufacturers to have dedicated EDI linkages with thousands of hospital customers. Indeed, compared to others, distributors appear to be most electronically linked to the other supply chain players; more than 80 percent are linked to manufacturers, more than 75 percent are linked to customers, and more than 40 percent are linked to GPOs.[19] However, while the few large distributors are linked to major manufacturers, it is not the case that the thousands of manufacturers are linked to distributors. Manufacturer-distributor EDI linkages are not as prevalent, due to the excessive number of one-to-one connections (and the cost of multiple integrations) that have to be made.[20]

EDI Benefits and Barriers

The implementation of EDI across the health care value chain requires use of common data sets that facilitate standardized electronic communication. At present, there are multiple versions of

EDI in the market. WEDI estimated one-time implementation costs for providers to establish or upgrade existing operations to a standardized EDI capability at $3.8–11.2 billion.[21] While providers would bear the bulk of the implementation costs, they would also reap the bulk of the savings (estimated at $9.0–15.5 billion). This would yield operational savings of $0.64–1.07 per transaction for hospitals and $1.01–1.96 for physicians. It would also reduce the cost of processing a purchase order as follows:

	Manual Processing	Proprietary Order-Entry System	Standardized EDI Interface
Provider Cost	$40–150	$28	$11.20
Supplier Cost	$30–150	$24	$3.20
Total Cost	$70–300	$52	$14.40

The benefits of the standardized EDI approach to business communication include the elimination of data reentry by provider or supplier, increased efficiency in repetitive business processes, reduced errors in rekeying data input in high-volume transactions, faster submission and quicker turnaround of orders, the elimination of paperwork, reduced personnel time devoted to manual tasks, the facilitation of just-in-time inventory, and "full-cycle data integrity" across the value-chain transactions.[22]

To implement a standard requires the presence of a standard-setting body, however. In other industries, the development of universal EDI formats and networks has taken many years (for example, the spread of ATMs with standard formats required almost two decades). These industries have frequently created "action groups" to fulfill the need for EDI development, coordination, and education to foster data standards and their quick implementation. WEDI was a public-private task force formed after a Department of Health and Human Services (DHHS) forum in 1991 on ways to reduce administrative costs. Their solution called for tax credits and small business loans as incentives to adopt a standardized EDI approach.

More recently, the Health Insurance and Portability Accountability Act (HIPAA) encouraged but did not mandate the use of EDI by health care organizations. Those organizations using EDI, however, are required to abide by HIPAA transaction and security standards developed by DHHS. The lack of uniform standards (as well as disparate databases) has been one major obstacle to the widespread diffusion of EDI. In the future, the costs of compliance with the HIPAA standards (estimated at $4 billion) will be another.[23]

Distribution Industry Dynamics

There are several important trends shaping the distribution industry. These include outsourcing by other value chain players, rise of generics, horizontal consolidation, vertical integration, and product diversification.

Outsourcing

The distribution business in health care is characterized by several dynamics. With the exception of medical devices, capital equipment, and some medical-surgical products (made by Allegiance Healthcare), manufacturers outsource the distribution of much of their products to wholesalers (rather than engage in direct customer delivery). Some suppliers talk of their capabilities (whether real or potential) in product distribution, but they have nevertheless allowed wholesalers to perform this function. Goldman Sachs analysts estimate that only 16 percent of medical-surgical supplies (over $5 billion) are shipped directly by manufacturers.[24] Exhibit 5.1 illustrates the heavy reliance of drug manufacturers on drug wholesalers for the distribution of their drugs, particularly for independent drug stores (96.0 percent) and health care providers (79.8 percent for hospitals, 89.2 percent for nursing homes).

Exhibit 5.1   Manufacturers' Sales of Drugs Through Distributors (1998)

Class of Trade	Mfgr Direct (Percent)	Chain Wholesaler and Mail Order (Percent)	Wholesaler (Percent)
Indep Drug Store	3.7	0.3	96.0
Chain Drug Store	3.3	73.6	23.2
Mass Merchants	0.2	60.0	39.8
Hospitals	20.2	0.0	79.8
Clinics	39.9	0.2	59.9
LTC/Home Health	10.6	0.2	89.2
Health Plans	46.8	0.1	53.2
TOTAL	12.6	32.6	54.8

Source: National Wholesale Druggists' Association. *1999 NWDA Industry Profile and Healthcare Factbook.* Reston, Virginia: NWDA, 1999.

Wholesalers handled 54.8 percent of the product flow across all classes of trade; only 12.6 percent of sales were direct from the manufacturer to either the dispenser, or the hospital or retailer that acted as its own warehouser.[25] Of the $122 billion sales in the U.S. pharmaceuticals market in 1999, distributors handled $106 billion, or 87 percent. The vast majority was distributed to the retail market, while roughly $30 billion was distributed to hospitals and alternate site facilities (where the hospital portion is estimated at $15 billion).[26] Drug manufacturers are also outsourcing more noncore functions in 1999 compared to 1997, such as information systems (33 percent outsourced), distribution (50 percent) and transportation (56 percent).[27]

Further fuel to the outsourcing trend is the rise in the number of delivery sites from which products are dispensed. IMS Health reports that pharmaceuticals are now dispensed from 135,000 sites in 1998, an increase from 90,000 sites ten years ago. For drugs alone, there are 20,000 independent pharmacies, 19,000 chain pharmacy outlets, 60,000 clinics, 7,000 hospitals, and 12,000 mass merchandisers and food stores.[28] With over 1,000 drug suppliers, the volume of potential transactions is enormous. Drug distributors reduce the overall number of transactions between manufacturers and pharmacies from 439 million to 40 million.[29] In 1998, the median number of vendors per drug distributor was 650; the median number of shipping points served per distributor was 525.[30] Sixty-seven percent of distributors made deliveries five times a week; another 31 percent made deliveries six days a week.

For medical-surgical supplies, the logistics are even more daunting. The number of product manufacturers are estimated to be anywhere from 10,000 to 22,000.[31–33] According to the Medical Device Register, there are 12,000 medical device manufacturers. Most of these manufacturers are small. Eight hundred members of the Health Industry Manufacturers Association (HIMA) reportedly generate 90 percent of the revenues.

Just as manufacturers have increasingly outsourced product delivery to distributors, so too have customers increasingly outsourced procurement functions to distributors. Exhibit 5.2 shows the increasing percentage of drug purchases made by hospitals and health systems that are mediated by drug wholesalers. Much

Exhibit 5.2   Pharmaceutical Distributors' Customer/Revenue Mix

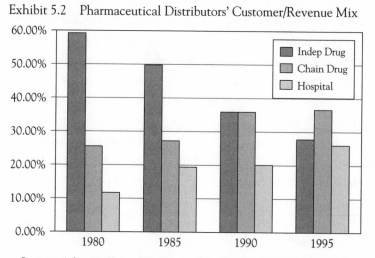

Source: Adam J. Fein. "Understanding Evolutionary Processes in Non-Manufacturing Industries: Empirical Insights from the Shakeout in Pharmaceutical Wholesaling." Journal of Evolutionary Economics, 8 (1998): 231–270.

of this shift occurred during the 1980s when wholesalers began to manage hospital pharmacy inventories using superior asset management, logistics, and on-line ordering systems.[34] Distributors thus assumed purchasing and warehousing functions, and developed a valuable window into the inventory of an important downstream customer. Given all of these outsourced functions, hospitals became an engine of growth for the pharmaceutical distribution industry. By 1998, 79.8 percent of hospital sales were mediated by distributors; among nursing homes and home health units, distributors handled 89.2 percent share; among clinics, distributors handled 59.9 percent share.[35] To be sure, some large drug chains do warehouse their own products to benefit from price increases. Analysts estimate that these chains may purchase up to 2,000 items in speculative buying for products where they can earn the greatest profit. They nevertheless rely on distributors for the other 20,000 or more items, or 80–90 percent of their total SKUs.[36,37]

Emphasis on Generics and Commodities

In contrast to branded products and advanced medical equipment and devices—which are more direct-ship and distributed through fragmented channels—generic drugs, commodity supplies, and low-tech, nonphysician preference items have traditionally been handled by large distributors. There are several reasons for this pattern. One reason is that it is easier to achieve product standardization on such items. Distributors can pursue "line rationalization" on commodity items (that is, carry a small variety of widely used products) and thereby reduce the number of SKUs they carry. In this manner, they pursue the Pareto principle: promote and distribute the 20 percent of product items that account for 80 percent of the product volume (and allow hospitals to directly source the less frequently ordered items). Conversely, it is harder to achieve line rationalization on branded drugs because the priorities in product selection are often efficacy, safety, and then cost. Nevertheless, in the pharmaceutical area, distributors carry a handful of the leading brands and their generic equivalents in each therapeutic area. In the medical-surgical area, distributors carry more brands (reflecting different customer choices) since it is harder to standardize.

One vehicle to achieve this line rationalization is to develop "source programs" whereby the distributor grants a price discount to hospital customers that select generic items from a select list of manufacturers. This may generate price wars among generic product vendors and allows distributors to move share from one vendor to another. Consequently, distributors have become less brand neutral in trying to use their logistical leverage as distributors to offset the lack of brand leverage among the generics they are handling. Another vehicle to achieve line rationalization is for the distributor to adopt an integrated strategy that seeks to influence both the hospital's formulary (especially with regard to generics) and product selection.

Another reason why distributors carry generic or commodity items is that manufacturers do not want distributors to have the ability to influence or switch branded product purchases by customers. Manufacturers prefer direct sales for branded items in order to retain control over supply chain channels and hedge against commoditization of their products. Manufacturers also want to inhibit cross-referencing of their products and comparison shopping with competitors' offerings by customers. This is likely one reason why manufacturers (in some product categories) have resisted placing Universal Product Numbers (UPNs) on these items.

The spread of UPNs has also been inhibited by a chicken-and-egg problem: manufacturers will not assign bar codes unless hospital customers use them, and hospitals will not use them unless all products are labeled with them.

Universal Product Numbers (UPNs)

UPNs are eight to twenty character numbers derived from either the HIBCC-LIC or UCC-EAN bar code labeling data structures (manufacturers choose which one they will use). The former is published by the Health Industry Business Communications Council (HIBCC), while the latter is published by the Uniform Code Council (UCC). UPNs uniquely assign a number to each medical-surgical product at all levels of packaging (shipping cases; shelf packs; and unit of use packages, or "eaches"). The UPN number includes a code for the manufacturer, the item number, and the level of packaging.[38]

Bar code technology has many advantages:

- Permits fast and relatively error-free data entry

- Provides immediate data capture

- Automates the flow of information into business practices

- Integrates product flow with the flow of information

- Permits efficient tracking of purchasing, price information, and supply utilization

- Contributes to cost accounting

- Reduces the amount of time distributor sales representatives spend in order taking, product pushing, and customer calling

- Obviates the need to cross-reference numbers on different product lines or conduct extensive catalog search to identify or order items

After the advent of barcode technology for drugs in the 1970s, McKesson's sales jumped from $1 billion supported by 1,000 representatives to $6 billion supported by only 500 representatives.[39]

Some hospitals have been pushing vendors to place UPNs or bar codes on their products at the unit level. Several GPOs and IDNs (for example, BJC, Columbia/HCA, Tenet, and Amerinet) had stated as early as 1996 that they were making bar-coding capability a major consideration in contract awards to help them improve their materials management ordering, receiving, and invoicing. Indeed, UPNs facilitate the use of EDI. Two bills were introduced in Congress to tie reimbursement to a requirement that hospitals report the UPN on products used by government-insured patients (neither bill was enacted). The Department of Defense (DOD) mandated that all manufacturers providing medical products to DOD facilities must have purchase unit of measure packages identified by UPNs. More recently, in February 1998, twenty major health care groups (orchestrated by the Healthcare EDI Coalition, or HEDIC) endorsed a joint communiqué establishing a target date of July 1999 for industry-wide implementation of (1) UPN standard identifiers as the industry accepted key reference to product information; (2) UPN standard compliant bar-code labels on all products at each unit of inventory; and (3) automatic data capture technology, software functionality to process UPN product information, and EDI connectivity throughout the supply chain.[40]

Finally, during 2001 the Centers for Medicare and Medicaid Services (CMMS, formerly the Health Care Financing Administration) considered a request to require the use of UPNs as a means of reporting all new medical devices qualifying as new technologies. Such UPNs would be incorporated into the existing ICD-9-CM coding system for inpatient hospital care. CMMS demurred at the time, citing the lengthy process of public discussion and rule making needed to designate national standards for medical coding.

At the same time, the Senate Commerce Subcommittee on Science, Technology, and Space held hearings on e-commerce. GPO executives testified about the benefit of UPNs, and urged Congress to enact federal regulations for a standardized identification system covering medical-surgical supplies. Such a system would not only

(Continued on next page)

Universal Product Numbers (UPNs) (*Continued*)

improve hospital efficiency but would also help serve to reduce medical errors and improve quality (for example, through reduced drug administration errors).

Despite these efforts, UPNs are unevenly found across product areas. Some of the aforementioned coalitional efforts collided with the Y2K initiatives of supply chain participants and got derailed. According to the Health Industry Distributors Association (HIDA), only slightly more than 40 percent of medical-surgical supplies carry UPNs. In a 1996 report, HIDA cited statistics on the prevalence of bar codes: 39.8 percent of all packages, 38.6 percent of all cases (shipping cartons), 55.1 percent of all boxes (shelf packs), and 27.7 percent of each unit of issue.[41] Similarly, a 1997 HIDA audit indicated that 77 percent of shelf-quantity boxes of medical-surgical supplies carry the bar codes, while only 26 percent of product units that can be scanned on nursing floors bear UPNs.

The HIDA statistics must be viewed with caution, however, since they are based only on products going through distributors (HIDA's membership). To the extent that products that get shipped directly from manufacturers to providers have bar codes, HIDA may understate the prevalence of bar codes. Indeed, recent survey data collected by HEDIC suggests manufacturers are progressing toward the adoption of UPNs, at least on medical-surgical product cases. Among 269 manufacturers and distributors surveyed, 150 reported 100 percent compliance with putting UPNs on cases. Over 70 percent placed UPNs on individual units. These vendors accounted for 65 percent of the 96,442 products reported in the survey. Conversely, only sixty-seven respondents reported zero compliance with UPNs, but represented only 7,225 (7 percent) of products.[42]

The pharmaceutical area is a bit different. There is a unique numbering system using National Drug Codes (NDCs)—which have a UCC/EAN data structure—that is recognized universally and mandated by the Food and Drug Administration (FDA). A 1996 study by the National Wholesale Druggists' Association (NWDA) found that virtually all over-the-counter drugs are bar coded with either an NDC number or a U.P.C. code, and 95 percent of consumer products contain a U.P.C. code in bar-code format on their label. Nevertheless, uniform product codes may also be a problem here. Only half of the pharmaceutical products utilize bar codes on a case or unit-dose level.[43] A recent survey revealed that drug manufacturers place less importance on the use of bar codes on both cases and individual product packages, compared to distributors.[44] They are also less likely to use bar codes for most applications.

A consortium of GPOs (Novation, Premier, Consorta, and HealthTrust Purchasing Group) and B2B firms (Medibuy and Neoforma) formed in June 2000 to jointly demand that product manufacturers and distributors adopt standard product codes to facilitate supply purchasing over the Internet. The consortium, known originally as the "e-standards work group" and since renamed the Coalition for Healthcare Electronic Standards (CHeS), has worked to adopt UPNs and health care identification numbers (HINs)—often supporting the efforts of other organizations, such as HEDIC—and to develop a taxonomy and hierarchy for product names (that is, to standardize what products are called by materials managers, GPOs, vendors, and clinicians).[45,46] CHeS' taxonomic efforts focus primarily on commodity items ordered by GPOs.

Despite their effort, GPOs have not consistently enforced their policy requiring vendors to use bar codes on products. Some industry representatives have suggested this lax enforcement has prevented the Defense Department from fully implementing its own policy (noted previously). GPOs have been asked by their IDN members why they have not demanded that vendors place bar codes on all items they sell. GPOs respond in several ways. First, they state that vendors often

(Continued on next page)

Universal Product Numbers (UPNs) (Continued)

place UPNs on cases of products but not on each unit of use that can
be scanned on the nursing floor. Vendors would have to redesign their
packaging to place bar codes on each unit. Second, they state that
IDNs are equally or more responsible for demanding UPNs on products purchased from vendors. While hospitals lack the clout of GPOs
to force vendors to adopt UPNs, there are preliminary case reports of
IDNs succeeding in these demands.[47] The director of HEDIC stated
that UPNs will not be adopted until industry giants take the leadership
here as they have in retailing (for example, Wal-Mart).[48,49]

Finally, distributors earn higher margins on generic items due to
the "push" nature of product demand (versus the "pull" of branded
items). The difference in margins is anywhere from three to five
times that for branded items (that is, 12–20 percent versus 4 percent). It is important to note that these higher margins are earned
in a growing market. Generic and commodity items compose roughly
half of the U.S. medical supplies market according to analysts at
Goldman Sachs, but only 19–20 percent of the prescription drug
market.[50] However, over the next three years $10 billion in branded
prescription patents are tracking to expire; over the next five years,
the figure is $35 billion. As one interesting side note, the drug dis-
tribution industry and generic drug industry posted the first and second largest increases in share price (66.7 percent and 43.7 percent,
respectively) during 1998 across all health care segments.[51]

Increase Value for Upstream and Downstream Partners

Distributors recognize the precarious nature of their middleman role
and foresee an end to wholesaler consolidation.[52] They have thus
sought to become more important to both their upstream and downstream trading partners. Looking upstream toward manufacturers,
distributors have tried to develop large scale and field forces to provide "product push." They have also sought to broaden their chan-

nels to reach additional customers (for example, ability to reach new markets and alternate sites) and provide an information window to manufacturers on their customers. Looking downstream, distributors have used consolidation and automation of warehouses to pursue operating efficiencies, which are then passed on to customers. They have also sought to streamline and automate the ordering process by their customers, provide software support for their customers' materials management functions, reduce customer inventory management expenses, and reduce the cost per delivered item—all of which enables the health care system to cut supply costs, improve internal efficiencies, and better deal with managed care pressures. In this manner, distributors have shifted from sellers of products to hospitals to managers of the hospitals' assets. Most recently, they have acquired several new product and service businesses to add value for their hospital customers (see the following for an illustration).

In general, the distributors seek continued integration and strategic partnering with their downstream customers.[53] Potential benefits include increased coordination of activities, competitive advantage over rival distributors, improved adaptability to market changes, and increased salience in the eyes of product manufacturers. More specific distributor benefits vary by customer segment. In the hospital market, where GPOs drive a lot of the product contracting and selection, distributors generally provide logistics support; in the alternate site market where GPOs are less active, distributors provide logistics support, contracting, sales and marketing, and information.

Horizontal Consolidation

As in most wholesale distribution industries, health care distributors have pursued efficiencies through consolidation.[54–56] Exhibit 5.3 lists the top drug distributors and their acquisition activity during the period 1978–1995. Exhibit 5.4 lists their 2001 revenues and market share. The top three firms now have a combined share exceeding three-quarters of industry demand. Near the end of 2000, Cardinal Health (the number-two player) announced its acquisition of Bindley Western (number-five player), a deal which would make

Exhibit 5.3   Mergers of Drug Distributors

Firm	1978–1995 Acquisitions	1995 Dollars Target Revenues*
Alco-Standard/ AmeriSource	17	$1,024
Bergen Brunswig	11	$3,019
FoxMeyer	11	$2,125
Cardinal Health	11	$5,214
McKesson	3	$926

*Sum of acquired companies annual revenues in year prior to acquisition. Revenues inflated to constant 1995 dollars using Producer Price Index for prescription drugs.

Source: Adam J. Fein. "Understanding Evolutionary Processes in Non-Manufacturing Industries: Empirical Insights from the Shakeout in Pharmaceutical Wholesaling." *Journal of Evolutionary Economics*, 8 (1998): 231–270.

Exhibit 5.4   Leading U.S. Drug Distributors Market Share Analysis, Calendar 2001 (EST)

	Percent Share
McKesson Corp. / HBOC	27
Cardinal Health/Bindley Western	29
AmeriSource/Bergen Brunswig	32
Other	12

Note: Calendarized Stock Sales

Source: David Risinger and Owen Hughes. *Healthcare Distribution.* Merrill Lynch, Table 11, January 8, 2001.

Cardinal the largest drug distributor. However, in August 2001, Bergen Brunswig and AmeriSource completed their own merger, making them the largest distributor.

Unlike other firms upstream and downstream in the health care value chain, distributors have physically consolidated capacity into megawarehouses and utilized automation to drive greater volume through these warehouses at faster speed. Business historian Alfred Chandler argues that these are the necessary conditions for achieving engineering-based economies of scale.[57] McKesson, for example, has reduced the number of its warehouses from forty to five, using megawarehouses. In the Cardinal-Bindley Western deal, analysts expect the two firms to combine their warehouses (twenty-four Cardinal facilities and seventeen Bindley facilities) into twenty-eight sites, further enhancing "Cardinal's capacity to use scale as a competitive advantage and leveraging its well-capitalized infrastructure."[58,59.]

One measure of the greater volume is the level of sales going through a reduced number of megawarehouses. According to NWDA, the average pharmaceutical distribution center has increased annual sales almost fourfold during the 1990s, from $117 million in 1990 to $452 million in 1998.[60] Sales per warehouse square foot more than doubled from $1.7 to $3.6 million. One metric of the faster speed is the number of invoice lines picked per hour off of warehouse shelves. From 1970 to 1998, this rate of speed increased from twenty-six to fifty lines.

Consolidation and automation allow distributors to efficiently handle large amounts of product. Pharmaceutical wholesalers, for example, carry up to 25,000 items in a warehouse and as many as 60,000–70,000 items across their divisions.[61] This requires huge investments in information technology to communicate with manufacturers and customers; to manage the inventory in-house; and manage the ordering, tracking, and delivery of products. These investments have enabled distributors to substitute labor for capital. Between 1970 and 1998, total compensation as a percentage of gross profit declined from 49.4 percent to 30.7 percent.[62]

Consolidation offers benefits beyond operational efficiency. Consolidation results in higher product volume, which helps to smooth out demand patterns (that is, lower volatility of demand) and allow distributors to provide better service. Consolidation also allows the acquisition of assets that may be complementary. For example, according to analysts, Cardinal's strong hospital relationships may help it to leverage Bindley's specialty nuclear pharmacy operation

(Central Pharmacy Services), which offers unit-dose radio-pharmaceuticals for use in imaging centers.

Exhibit 5.5 shows the decline in the number of drug distributors and their distribution centers.[63] The result of drug distributor consolidation and automation has been a decline in the overall operating expenses of distributors as a percentage of their net sales from 11.5 percent (1975) to 3.5 percent (1996). The expense ratio is even lower among the larger distributors. This consolidation and greater efficiency in operations has also raised the entry barriers into the drug distribution industry. There were no new market entries between 1981 and 1996.

The growing oligopolization of drug distribution has not threatened competition, however. While distributors have consolidated, so have their customers (hospitals and nursing homes). Consolidated customers have pressured distributors (and manufacturers) for better prices and service. Surviving firms in this industry have vigorously competed with one another by lowering their margins and

Exhibit 5.5   Number of Drug Distributors and Distribution Centers

Year	# NWDA Firms	# NWDA Distribution Centers
1970	144	372
1975	145	395
1980	139	347
1985	104	327
1990	84	263
1995	63	224
1996	55	233
1997	54	222
1998	70	220
1999	70	235

Sources: National Wholesale Druggists' Association. 1999 NWDA Industry Profile and Healthcare Factbook. Reston, Virginia: NWDA. 1999; Adam J. Fein. "Understanding Evolutionary Processes in Non-Manufacturing Industries: Empirical Insights from the Shakeout in Pharmaceutical Wholesaling." Journal of Evolutionary Economics, 8 (1998): 231–270.

offering new services to maintain and increase market share. These increasingly lower profit margins are evident in Exhibit 5.6.

Nevertheless, while pharmaceutical distributors have low returns on their sales, they have a good return on their equity. A pharmaceutical manufacturer explained it this way:

> Since they are using other people's money, they are getting a pretty good return. They just don't want to admit that. They love to come in and bemoan their 2 percent returns on sales versus our 20 percent in pharma. But this does not take into account our asset turnover. Our asset turnover is horrible because we have so many assets invested in the future [R&D] and not in the current sales period. All of their assets are invested in the current sales period. Another issue is what is their leverage position? They are leveraged to the hilt, because it is all

Exhibit 5.6   Financial Trends in the Wholesale Drug Industry

	Gross Profit Margin (Percent)	Operating Expense (Percent)	Operating Profit Margin (Percent)	Net Profit Before Taxes (Percent)	Net Profit After Taxes (Percent)
1989	7.3	4.9	2.5	2.0	1.4
1990	7.4	4.7	2.6	2.0	1.4
1991	6.8	4.4	2.4	1.9	1.3
1992	6.5	4.2	2.3	1.9	1.3
1993	5.8	4.1	1.8	1.6	1.0
1994	5.4	3.7	1.7	1.8	1.2
1995	5.1	3.6	1.5	1.4	0.5
1996	5.4	3.7	1.7	1.3	0.8
1997	4.5	3.0	1.5	1.2	0.8
1998	4.5	2.9	1.6	0.8	0.6

Note: All calculations on a FIFO basis

Source: National Wholesale Druggists' Association. 1999 NWDA Industry Profile and Healthcare Factbook. Reston, Virginia: NWDA.

hard assets, inventory, buildings, and stuff. We can leverage some parts of our business, but nobody will loan you
money to put into research. So they have strong asset
turnover and are leveraged to the hilt. So at the end of
the day, their return on equity doesn't look too bad compared to the pharmaceutical industry, when you adjust
for the amount of risk they take on.

How do distributors make money under these conditions? One
means is increasing volume (available through consolidation). On
the sell side, distributors earn small margins on large volumes. The
margin on pharmaceutical products is usually less than fifty basis
points above wholesale acquisition cost.[64] Distributors may also earn
a premium for delivery to multiple sites for a customer (for example, physician offices affiliated with a health care system and retail
sites of a pharmacy chain).

A second method is asset management (that is, management of
working capital). Pharmaceutical distributors receive incentives
from manufacturers for prompt payment for the products they
receive (usually 2 percent discount for thirty-day payment).
Manufacturers make these incentives available to increase their
cash flow and maximize their investments in new product development. Since distributors' customers usually pay within twenty days,
the distributors enjoy a ten-day float, which allows them to finance
inventories without tying up as much capital as other types of
distributors.

Third, distributors can earn fees from drug manufacturers by
moving market share (that is, inducing their customers to switch
brands). However, there are several difficulties with the pursuit of
this approach. As noted previously, manufacturers don't want distributors to influence the brand choices of their customers, and thus
don't abandon their role in brand positioning. At the same time,
hospital and physician customers tend to favor the top brands and
may not easily switch. In addition, with falling profit margins,

distributors may be increasingly unable to hire good sales representatives who can work with hospital materials managers on standardization and utilization initiatives. Consequently, distributors may be able to move share for smaller manufacturers or for generic drug manufacturers, but not for branded drugs.[65]

A fourth, more controversial, method is to arbitrage manufacturers' price increases; that is, anticipate the increase, buy in bulk ahead of time, and then sell the products at the higher price to customers.[66] This practice is known variously as "forward buy gain" and "speculative buying." Speculative buying requires price forecasting capability (for example, in-house economists), large warehouses to store the inventory purchased in bulk, strong financing capability, and good inventory management. These conditions favor large distributors over their smaller competitors.

Abetting this speculative buying tactic is the fact that pharmaceutical prices have been rising over time. As a result, drug inventories appreciate rather than decline in value. To be sure, the cost of carrying inventory rises at the same time. However, inventory costs are only one of three cost components for distributors; the other two—product handling and delivery—are activity-based costs that don't vary much by product. Since distributors get paid a percentage of the product's value, and since the product's value is rising, they are getting paid more to do tasks for which their costs are not rising quickly.

It is also evident that a growing percentage of the distributors' gross profit margin (sales minus cost of goods sold) comes from the manufacturer rather than the customer. In the late 1980s, roughly half of the distributors' margins came from sell margins (upcharges to customers of roughly 400 basis points) and half came from buy-side margins granted by manufacturers. By the late 1990s, upcharges to customers amounted to only thirty-five basis points (.35 percent). The bulk of the distributors' gross margins came from manufacturers in the form of cash discounts for prompt payment for products received, manufacturer incentives to promote certain products and move its own inventory and market share, and inventory profits based on both speculative and nonspeculative buying.[67] This suggests that manufacturers are indeed a major customer of the distributors and that the distributors are somewhat the "captive agents" of the manufacturers.[68]

To be sure, many manufacturers are not thrilled with the idea of speculative buying by their wholesaler intermediaries. Such buying behavior costs them lost sales revenues. It also leads to peaks and valleys in the manufacturers' production and packaging schedules, which are accompanied by inefficiencies in labor and plant operation (for example, overtime, downtime, and excess inventory). They would prefer to have more even, predictable flow to their product and sales revenues. One set of remedies they take is to tell distributors to hold off on speculative buys, ask distributors to justify the large volumes ordered, modify their orders, ship them less than what they ordered, or elect not to fill their orders. One possible solution, reportedly being considered or implemented, is for the manufacturers to give distributors the monies they would have made off of speculative buying up front, in exchange for greater predictability in product flow.

According to an AT Kearney survey, 56 percent of pharmaceutical firms have adopted a "VMI fee" to deal with the problem of distributor stockpiling and demand variability.[69] VMI (vendor managed inventory) is an agreement between the manufacturer and wholesaler where the former manages the inventory of the latter. It is an electronic communication where orders are created on demand based on off-take of the wholesaler. VMI customers are under contract not to speculate.

On the other hand, speculative buying may actually be encouraged as well as discouraged. Some manufacturers "game the system" by discounting prices and filling the supply chain channel with enough volume to meet quarterly sales targets. In this manner, they give away earnings to time their earnings.

Much of the same consolidation has occurred among distributors of medical-surgical supplies. Unlike drug distribution, the market here is more fragmented. One reason is that there are four distinct market segments: acute hospital care (40 percent of business), extended care and home health care (24 percent), imaging supplies (16 percent), and physician offices (13 percent) (see Exhibit 5.7). The largest player in the industry has only 10 percent share overall. However, within market segments, there may be significant concentration. For example, Allegiance Corporation, Owens and Minor, and General Medical control over 90 percent of the hospital market. On the other hand, the top three players in the physician office segment (Physician Sales and Service, General Medical, Henry Schein) control 45 percent share, while the top three players in the extended care market (General Medical/Redline, Gulf South, and Medline) control only 44 percent share. As a result, much of the consolidation here is large national players acquiring smaller, regionally based distributors. Often, these acquisitions are made to fill in regional gaps in distribution coverage (for example, Owens & Minor acquired Medix because it lacked a presence in the State of Wisconsin). Moreover, as noted earlier, the medical-surgical distributors operate under a different economic model compared to drug distribution: they enjoy cost-plus margins (rather than cost-minus) but do not participate in speculative buying.

There are some downsides to the consolidation movement. One is the potential for antitrust violations. On July 31, 1998, U.S. District Court Judge Stanley Sporkin granted the Federal Trade Commission's request to block two proposed megamergers on the grounds that (1) the resulting two firms would have nearly 80 percent market share, (2) a large segment of their customers (especially hospitals) would have no reasonable substitutes to using the two resulting firms, and (3) the two firms would have a greater ability to engage in anticompetitive behavior.

Exhibit 5.7   Selected Medical Products Distribution Channels List
of Major Company Participants (2001E Market Share)

Participants	Revenues	Mkt. Share (Percent)
Hospital Market Channel Participants		
Allegiance/BBMC	$5,700	48
Owens & Minor	$3,700	30
General Medical	$1,600	14
Bergen Med'l	$ 475	4
Burrows	$ 240	2
Henry Schein	$ 150	1
Total Market Size	$ 12 B	
MD Office Channel Participants		
Henry Schein	$ 805	16
General Medical	$ 750	15
PSS	$ 720	14
PHCC	$ 480	10
AEH/BBMC	$ 450	9
Total Market Size	$ 5 B	
Long-Term Care Channel Participant		
Gen Medical/Redline	$ 580	19
Gulf South/Gateway	$ 380	13
Medline	$ 350	12
AEH/BBMC	$ 200	7
Total Market Size	$ 3 B	

Source: David Risinger and Owen Hughes. *Healthcare Distribution.* Merrill
Lynch, 2001.

Another possible downside to consolidation is the threat posed
to smaller product manufacturers. The latter claim that distributor
consolidation reduces distribution channels and limits their customer
access. Larger-sized distributors means greater time and effort
required by the manufacturer to gain the distributor's support, greater
distributor bureaucracy and slower response, greater scrutiny of any

additional products and SKUs, and greater distributor efforts to rationalize SKUs and eliminate redundant or duplicative products. Moreover, consolidated distributors engage in less effort to "detail products" and more effort to provide services to customers and manage customer assets. Finally, consolidated distributors now have cost-plus agreements with hospital customers, which leave the distributor with little financial incentive, time, and interest in selling new products or promoting new innovative technologies.

Vertical Integration

Distributors have pursued avenues other than horizontal consolidation in an effort to drive greater volumes over their fixed-cost infrastructure. These new strategies, while in place for some time, received new impetus following Judge Sporkin's decision to block the proposed Cardinal Health-Bergen Brunswig and McKesson-AmeriSource mergers. Two avenues have been vertical integration (value-adding services) and product diversification (channel breadth).

Vertical Integration at Cardinal Health

Vertical integration has been quite evident at Cardinal Health. Over the past several years, Cardinal Health has been actively acquiring several businesses. Businesses oriented toward its upstream trading partners include

Business	Year	Functions Performed
PCI Services	1996	Pharmaceutical packaging to manufacturer specifications and/or improve patient compliance, clinical trials packaging, printed components (inserts, labels, promotional packaging)
R.P. Scherer	1998	New drug delivery systems (for example, soft gel capsules)

Automatic Liquid Packaging	1999	Aseptic liquid packaging
Cord Logistics		Warehousing, distribution, transportation, inventory for biotechnology firms
Comprehensive Reimbursement Consultants		Strategic reimbursement planning, product advocacy with payers
SP Pharmaceuticals	2001	Contract manufacturing and development for pharmaceutical and biotech products
Rexam Healthcare Packaging	2000	Manufacturing of cartons used to package prescription and OTC medicines

Businesses oriented toward downstream partners include

Business	Year	Functions Performed
Pyxis Corporation	1996	ATM dispensing of drugs on hospital units
Owen Healthcare	1997	Hospital pharmacy and materials management
Allied Pharmacy Service		Hospital pharmacy management
Medicine Shoppes	1995	Retail pharmacy franchising
Cardinal Information		Information integration via MediQual and Jericho systems (for example, outcome studies, and clinical data capture)
National PharmPak Services		Drug repackaging for retail drug chains

National Specialty Services		Distribution of pharmaceuticals and med-surg supplies to oncology practices
HelpMate Robotics	1999	Advanced mobile robotic systems used in hospitals and laboratories

Cardinal's strategic intent here has been to more deeply integrate with the customer (for example, the manufacturer, hospital, or pharmacy) and be a more critical trading partner (see Exhibit 5.8). For example, Cardinal is seeking to gather data on its downstream customers and the products they are using (for example, via the Pyxis machines). This is an effort to take advantage of the small percentage (18 percent) of health systems with automated dispensing systems.[70] Cardinal hopes to integrate the various strands of data it is collecting into knowledge that both its downstream and upstream customers will find useful. Much of the data it is assembling are patient specific concerning drug use and compliance. Cardinal sees these data as the beginning of its disease management infrastructure. It also sees a potential to use these data to help influence product selection by downstream customers, and thus offer upstream manufacturers the ability to increase channel penetration. Some observers also believe that Cardinal is seeking to move further down the supply chain to more closely resemble the end user.

In addition, these acquisitions have helped Cardinal to diversify away from its core business of drug distribution. While drug distribution has been a cash-cow business, the margins have been falling steadily over time. The operating margin for Cardinal drug distribution was only 2.6 percent, and for Allegiance med-surg distribution was only 4.2 percent; by contrast, operating margins for Medicine Shoppes and Pyxis were 52 percent and 30 percent, respectively.[71] In the first half of fiscal year 2000, drug distribution accounted for 71 percent of revenues and but only 38 percent of earnings; conversely, services provided to manufacturers and providers accounted for only 9 percent of revenues but 32 percent

Exhibit 5.8   Vertical Integration at Cardinal Health

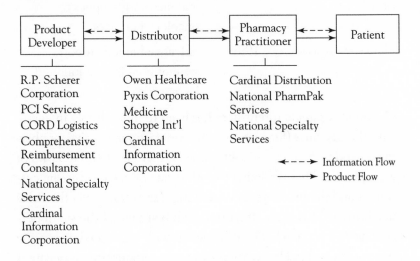

of operating earnings. The last component of Cardinal's financial results derive from its recent acquisition of Allegiance, a medical-surgical products manufacturer and distributor, which accounted for 20 percent of revenues and 30 percent of earnings.[72] As a result of this vertical integration, Cardinal now enjoys a more diverse earnings platform than its competitors. Moreover, Cardinal developed the Cardinal Health Capital Corporation in 1999 to perform a central financial services function for all of its businesses including capital assets financing, real estate portfolio management, and receipts and payments processing. In this manner, Cardinal can use all of the dollars flowing through the distributor as a float.

Some pharmaceutical executives believe that vertical integration efforts may augment the power of these intermediary organizations:

> Because you see them getting into repackaging, manu-
> facturing, customized delivery, I think we are going to
> see more power shift to the big four or five wholesalers
> faster than we realize as an industry. I think they are

extremely savvy at managing their businesses very efficiently because they operate on basis points.

Other supply chain participants are not entirely convinced of the wisdom of Cardinal's strategy. At a general level, some question what is the overall vision behind the acquisitions, or the fit between the new information-based businesses with the core business of distribution. For example, do the new businesses make product movement more efficient? Is there synergistic sharing of information across the different lines of businesses (for example, drug distribution and dispensing)? Can Cardinal really integrate all of these capabilities to determine drug efficacy and safety, and thereby recommend one product over another? Are GPOs better positioned than drug distributors to exploit the information gathered and use it to provide better service for hospital customers? Do Cardinal's customers want an integrated and customized package of services?

In response to this question, Cardinal executives claim that 65 percent of its hospital and health system customers utilize services from two or more of these new affiliate businesses listed previously, suggesting their complementary nature with Cardinal's core business. Nevertheless, manufacturers believe all of these projects are very complicated and difficult to properly implement—even when it is the core of someone's business. Can Cardinal be expert at each of the stages it has entered? Others note that the new businesses may now compete with Cardinal's current customers.

Specific questions regarding Cardinal's strategy revolve around the uses to which it might put its new information. One pharmaceutical executive stated, "Drug distributors have the information engines to put all the data together for pharmaceutical therapeutic choices and act like a PBM [pharmacy benefits manager]. This is scary because it will focus more on the cost than the evidence base." However, most pharmaceutical executives do not believe that Cardinal's data will be that valuable. First, it is just one company that cannot offer a global view of drug information like IMS. Even though IMS's data are not entirely accurate or complete, IMS performs algorithms to fill the holes and provide accurate "deltas," or rates of change in usage and market share. To get a similar product, pharmaceutical firms would have to buy data not only from Cardinal but also Wal-Mart and PCS, combine it, standardize it, scrub and clean it, and perform the algorithms to fill in missing data. Second, executives question whether Cardinal's sample of patients in a hospital is large enough and representative enough to fairly capture all of the patients with that condition. Similarly, is their sample of hospitals where they have Pyxis machines large enough and representative of patients with a given condition. Third, executives characterize distributors' data as too fragmented (lack of data integration across distributors) and too disconnected (lack of data integration with other meaningful information) to be helpful to drug companies. Cardinal's data is not national data but just data on where it ships product. It thus cannot help drug firms to measure market share or to pay their sales representatives. Finally, executives question whether Cardinal's efforts to influence product choice at the hospital level will extend beyond generic drugs into branded products. "Cardinal does not have a say as to whether a pharmacy gets [brand A]; it is the doctor who wires the prescription." Still others do not believe that the data collected by distributors have in fact been fed back to pharmaceutical manufacturers.

Product Diversification

Diversification has been another common strategy pursued by distributors. Pharmaceutical distributors have diversifed into medical-surgical products and vice versa, and both firms have diversified into the alternate site market.

Pharmaceutical and Medical-Surgical Distribution

In addition to vertical integration, distributors have also pursued a strategy of product diversification. Cardinal Health has actively adopted this approach in its acquisition of (first) Cardinal Daly and (later) Allegiance Corporation (1998), the largest distributor of medical-surgical products. In a similar vein, McKesson has acquired General Medical (1997), a leading medical-surgical distributor to several channels, and Redline Healthcare Corporation (1998), a distributor of medical products and services to the long-term care industry. Earlier, Bergen Brunswig acquired Durr-Fillauer Medical (1992) and subsequently developed its "IntePlex" program. The general strategy here was to build a larger volume of goods and product expertise across multiple market segments, supported by a common corporate infrastructure (for example, purchasing, information technology, human resources, capital management), and service the continuum of care developed by IDNs (for example, hospitals, physician offices, and nursing homes).

The product diversification strategy occurs in the distribution industry roughly every ten to fifteen years. Past efforts in the 1980s to marry these two businesses together resulted in failure (for example, McKesson and Gentec, Bergen Brunswig and a hospital supplier, and Owen & Minor and a drug supplier). In the 1990s, this diversification strategy has resurfaced to replace horizontal consolidation (where acquisition opportunities are drying up on the pharmaceutical side) and to take advantage of provider integration efforts (see the following).

What are the rationales for pursuing both pharmaceutical and medical-surgical product distribution? One obvious goal is to enable pharmaceutical distributors, which are faced with fewer acquisition opportunities on the drug side, to grow on the medical-surgical side. Compared to drugs, the medical-surgical distribution industry is fairly large ($33 billion) and fragmented. A second goal is to use combined drug and medical-surgical distribution as a platform for disease management. Thus, the distributor can offer hospitals the drugs and medical supplies that might be jointly used in targeted disease efforts. A third, related goal is to use one business as a lead-in to the other—that is, cross-selling. Thus, the sales representative for one set of products can identify customer needs or opportunities to use other product lines, and then develop an integrated customized offering. A related benefit here is the development of a one-stop shopping capability that increases customer convenience and offers one face to the customer. For the distributor's suppliers, this means a senior procurement officer responsible for the purchases made on behalf of the distributor's different businesses. For the distributor's provider customers, this means a single account executive to handle all purchases across product categories. For all of these reasons, the combination of the two businesses is believed to allow distributors to offer hospital customers "true partnering" from an efficiency standpoint.

Other rationales include sustain company growth and earnings, expand market and customer account penetration on both sides of the business, increase potential for technology transfer from pharmaceutical to medical-surgical distribution, help customers improve their technological capabilities in the medical products area (for example, using information systems), counterbalance low pharmaceutical margins with higher medical-surgical margins, increase the procurement clout of hospitals as suppliers consolidate, and combine the financial resources of the two firms. For example, in the case of the Cardinal Health-Allegiance transaction, there may have been an effort to combine Cardinal's capital assets and information technology investments with Allegiance's cash assets.

Critics of the strategy are quick to point out, however, the numerous mismatches between the two businesses (see Exhibit 5.9): different physical logistics (small drug packages versus large medical-surgical supply boxes), different returns (high value but low average gross margin of 4 percent on drug shipments versus low value but high average gross margins of 10 percent on hospital med-surg shipments and 26 percent on alternate site supplies), different economic bases (for example, lower selling, general, and administrative costs of 3 percent for drugs, versus higher SGA costs of 7–10 percent for hospital medical-surgical supplies and even higher costs of 25–35 percent for alternate sites), different degrees of automation (higher for pharmaceutical products), different product variety (more SKUs among medical-surgical products), different levels of information and electronic capability (greater product numbering, information, and electronic ordering for drugs), different technological proficiency (technology-proficient drug distributors versus backward technology in many medical-surgical distributors), different customers (pharmacists versus materials managers), different growth rates (12–14 percent CAGR for pharmaceutical products versus 3–5 percent for hospital supplies and 6–8 percent for alternate site medical supplies), different growth patterns (rising volume and prices for drugs versus flat prices but rising volume for medical-surgical),

Exhibit 5.9 Pharmaceutical vs. Medical-surgical Distribution

	Pharmaceutical	Medical-Surgical
Physical Logistics	Small packages	Large boxes
Shipment Value	High value	Low value
Avg Gross Margins	Low margin	High margin
Economic Bases	Lower SGA costs	Higher SGA costs
Level of Automation	High	Low
Product Variety	Fewer SKUs	More SKUs
Product Information	More product numbering	Less product numbering
Electronic Capability	More electronic ordering	Less electronic ordering
Customers	Pharmacy directors	Materials Management
Purchase Patterns	Formularies	No formularies
Growth Patterns	Rising prices & volume	Flat prices & rising volume
Cumulative Avg Growth Rates	12-14% CAGR	3–5% CAGR

Sources: David Cassak. "Do Drugs and Hospital Supplies Mix?" *In Vivo* (June 1997): 39–50; Christopher D. McFadden and Timothy M. Leahy. "U.S. Healthcare Distribution Overview Comments" Presentation to the Wharton School, Dec. 7, 2000.

different sales strategies, and different purchase patterns (formulary versus non-formulary).[73]

On top of this, the two industry sectors diverge quite widely. Drug distribution has undergone greater consolidation into fewer vendors compared to med-surg distribution. This allows a drug distributor greater ability to perform one-stop shopping. In med-surg, by contrast, with the larger number of vendors, more fragmentation, and more products, customers have to access several distributors to get the full breadth of products they need. There is less potential for one-stop shopping. Moreover, there is greater customer expertise on the pharma side (training and knowledge of hospital pharmacists) compared to the med-surg side (training and expertise of materials managers). Finally, there is greater ease of standardization on pharma due to higher levels of bar coding than there is on med-surg, and lower levels of hospital spending on pharma than on med-surg products.

The simple fact that there are separate customers or buyers for the two sets of products may make success with the diversification strategy difficult, at least until hospital systems centralize all purchasing in one individual. Moreover, it has never been fully demonstrated that customers desire a combined approach, or want cross-sales of pharma and med-surg products that are not *both* "best-in-class." More recently, a Goldman Sachs survey of 361 hospital executives in pharmacy and materials management revealed that bundled product offerings are not important in either driving their contracting decisions with distributors or shaping their perceptions of distributor reputations.[74] Indeed, two of the top three ranked distributors by hospital customers are "pure plays"—that is, operate solely in one product area.

It is also unclear whether a large pharmaceutical distributor that acquires a smaller medical-surgical distributor will experience any real improvement in its overall returns. Unlike the horizontal consolidation strategy, there is no opportunity here to consolidate operations and warehouses across the two businesses. Indeed, distributors may need to erect a firewall between the two sets of supplies for security reasons. Thus, the supplies may physically reside in the same building, but the distributor must handle them separately (except for some combined shipments). Thus, there appears to be no potential for scale economies.[75]

Diversification into the Alternate Site Market

Instead of (or in addition to) joint pharmaceutical and medical-surgical distribution, wholesalers are now pursuing diversification out of the hospital market into the alternate site market (ASM). The main goal here is to diversify out of the relatively stagnant growth in the medical-surgical supply business for hospitals into the faster-growing market for physician offices and extended care sites. Another oft-stated goal here is to follow the patient before and after hospitalization by building a technology business (for example, using the Internet or telesales force).

The ASM is defined in various ways but typically includes physician offices, ambulatory surgery centers (ASCs), long-term care and nursing homes, and "other" (for example, home infusion therapists). The size of the alternate site market has been estimated at $14 billion in med-surg products, $11 billion in pharmaceutical products, and $5 billion in lab products.[76]

Medical-surgical manufacturers have viewed this as a desirable market for their products, given that GPOs have historically not operated here. With no GPOs, there are no rebates and CAFs, and vendors can enjoy higher prices and margins. Distributors are important for manufacturers in the ASM, since manufacturers often lack sales representatives who can go in and restock thousands of physician offices. The manufacturer's price and thus the distributor's product acquisition cost is the same for both the hospital market and ASM. However, some estimate the markups in ASM to be as high as 35–50 percent. This partly reflects the higher cost of distributing products to lots of small offices; it also partly reflects the lack of group buying.

Several large distributors and GPOs are now pursuing this market. One point that is rarely emphasized is that the ASM is a series of fragmented markets that have failed in their 1990s' consolidation effort. The physician market was unsuccessfully consolidated by the physician practice management companies (PPMCs) that went bankrupt; a similar fate befell the nursing home chains (for example, Genesis Health Ventures) and home infusion companies (for example, Coram). A customer market of fragmented buyers typically translates into higher margins for the product manufacturers and their distributors, since GPOs are only recent entrants here.

The ASM strategy faces several challenges. First, can distributors generate enough sales volume out of these small practices to make the accounts profitable? The logistical challenge here is servicing a large number of geographically dispersed and smaller-sized physician practices, as compared to the large physician groups and networks affiliated with IDNs. Are distributors willing to support and service this dispersed market with its attendant higher costs? As part of this support and service, distributors may need to offer many of these accounts hands-on help in ordering products, as well as education regarding products and product use. A related challenge here is that physician offices are typically not tied to the distributor by EDI linkages. Without EDI, it will be more difficult for both sides to sort out ordering problems, such as getting the right product at the right price. With an estimated 30,000 office products, this problem can be enormous.

Second, there is great heterogeneity among office physicians that may require even more customization. For example, oncologists have different supply needs than do surgeons in ASCs and respiratory therapists—all of whose supplies differ in size and type from those used in hospitals. Thus, in contrast to IDNs and large physician groups, smaller sites may require more customized, frequent, and smaller deliveries (for example, including low unit of measure, or LUM) across a wider geographic area. This may require distributors to utilize a different sales force or sales strategy for these accounts. Distributors may also need to set up smaller, satellite distribution facilities to serve a specific geography and thereby balance the need to deliver products within a day, provide faster service, and serve more customers out of fewer facilities.

Third, there is the more general issue of the integrity of the class of trade. Given its heterogeneity, it is unclear what constitutes an alternate site market. The manufacturer and distributor may have difficulty classifying the customer; that is, is this particular physician or ASC covered under the manufacturer's contract with a GPO and thus authorized to access the product? Such confusion leads to chargeback rejections for the distributor and thus delays in payment. One manufacturer's solution to this problem, noted earlier, is to eschew GPO contracting for products sold to this market and let distributors set their own prices with customers.

Another issue raised by the strategy of diversification is whether consolidated, diversified distributors can assume the contracting and service functions now performed by GPOs? These combinations allow distributors to develop large groups of customers who tend to themselves develop some loyalty with their distributors. Consolidation and diversification has the potential effect of limiting the distribution options for health care providers and raising the stakes of switching from one distributor to another.[77]

Finally, can manufacturers and distributors build brand name for medical-surgical products in the ASM? Do physicians care about brand names for such products?

How Do Supply Chain Participants View Distributors?

Product manufacturers and GPOs generally have complimentary things to say about their distributor partners. Distributors are recognized for their basic contributions in the areas of aggregating customers, simplifying sales to final customers, stocking and distributing contract items at contract prices, and gathering and sharing purchasing compliance and sales data. Distributors are also credited with removing FTEs from the supply chain by virtue of their automation and inventory management efforts, as well as with bearing financial risk by taking title to the products and providing quicker payment than do hospitals.

A survey of manufacturers highlighted three valued traits in distributors: responsiveness from sales and customer service, order turnaround time, and order "fill rate" (that is, the percentage of orders accurately filled). The problem for distributors here is that the distributors' fill rate to hospitals is estimated at 90–95 percent while the manufacturers' fill rate to distributors is only 60–70 percent.[78]

Our site visit interviews provided a variety of insights into the perceived value of distributors. Pharmaceutical executives often emphasized the efficiencies with the following comments:

> In our eyes, the distributors add market efficiency. They have efficiency of ability to deliver. They have extreme expertise in delivering just-in-time inventory. They are so good at it that it makes little sense for others to try to duplicate them at best, let alone try to outperform them.

> I think that distributors are a highly efficient and cost-effective means to distribute products in the business. Their capability is far greater than individual manufacturers could ever attempt to be.

> I think we get tremendous savings in terms of bulk shipments—that is, to ship truckloads and pallets for them to break down and redistribute rather than sending thousands of FedEx's out of here. I think we get further efficiencies in inventory and buffer management. Having back-up systems is also very important because there are so many drugstores, pharmacies, and wholesalers out there going through all the Y2K planning.

The main efficiency that distributors offer us is credit management. The wholesaler essentially takes the credit risk of our customer, because we do all of our billing and shipping through a wholesaler. We do have fewer points to ship to also, so that adds a lot of simplicity to our distribution operation and helps us keep our costs down. But from my standpoint it is the credit function of not having to manage accounts receivable with thousands of places.

I don't see them as distributors. I see them as asset managers. They manage that inventory and accounts receivables.

Manufacturers of medical-surgical products mention some of the same advantages of using distributors:

Distributors get inventories closer to the customer. That is value. It is something that we couldn't really do efficiently ourselves with the current infrastructure. It's not that we couldn't do it, but why duplicate the infrastructure that is out there.

The distributor's value is the ability to get that single shipment to a hospital or to a floor that increases the breadth of product offering so that everyone can make it easier for the customer to order more frequently and still meet some minimum quantity orders so they don't lose the price points that they need to be at.

The distributor helps to reduce inventories and manage our inventory as well. They also manage the transfer of the product, leveling out sales volume.

Distributors now focus more on the total picture—lowest cost, asset productivity, waste elimination in the supply chain—in response to supplier and hospital interest, and are dropping their prices and tacking on value-adding services.

Distributors have infrastructure that enhances efficiency in the supply chain: volume going to one place, frequency of going to that one place, business transactions (EDI, continuous replenishment, efficient shipments). IDNs cannot replicate this without critical mass. So for now distributors are valued partners.

We are more efficient shipping to a distributor. Our distributors break large shipments into smaller quantities, assemble orders, manage all of the individual transactions with specific customers, and implement what we have negotiated with the GPOs.

Distributors also help manufacturers to execute their strategy in a number of ways. They can facilitate rapid distribution of a new product that maximizes sales as well as articulates with marketing campaigns. They can deliver committed customer groups and foster generic alliance partnerships. As the number and size of manufacturers grow, and thus as the number and scope of their products grow, distributors would seem to be well positioned to add value. They can help manufacturers to better understand the demographics of their broadening market and the buying behavior of their customers, and provide feedback from customers on products and product features.

Distributors can also develop compliance packaging to increase the product's therapeutic benefit and tie customer drug use to packaging (develop packs of 14, not 100 pills), as well as develop private-label programs. Some pharmaceutical manufacturers report compliance packaging happens on a small scale with a handful of nursing homes. But for this practice to take off it must come from the customer who demands packaging convenience and congruence with how they use the product. Other pharmaceutical manufacturers view compliance packaging as a potential area for future partnership with distributors, but first they need to create compliance factors that adhere to FDA guidelines on packaging. The problem here is that this effort takes time. Moreover, pharmacy chains are less interested in these types of services and more interested in the number of inventory turns for prescription drugs.

However, such value-adding programs are recognized as more valuable on the retail than on the institutional side. With regard to the latter, some pharmaceutical and medical-surgical executives are skeptical of the compliance and other value-adding programs offered by distributors. With regard to compliance, drug firms want to see persistency in refilling prescriptions, compliance in taking prescriptions, and even filling the prescription that the physician wrote. These take primacy over compliance packaging. Other executives offered the following criticisms of distributor efforts to add value:

> Other than their volume, we don't really regard their [compliance] programs as adding much value. They talk about being able to drive compliance, but their compliance programs do not exist to a level that is acceptable to us. [Pharmaceutical executive]

> They may try to provide other value-adding services, but the pick, pack, and ship operation of distributors is the valued portion of the wholesaler to me. When they ask me what else they can do, my answer is nothing. [Pharmaceutical executive]

> For us their main value is getting product closer to the end user and doing the pick and pack. That is their business. All the other things they do that supposedly creates [sic] value for those end users, you'll have to ask them about that. They each have programs and are supposed to add value to the end customer, but I'm not quite sure what that value is. [Medical-surgical executive]

> Distributors don't make a lot of money right now and are
> always looking to the manufacturer for 'margin funding'
> (for example, put a best-value program on top of the deal
> and get an additional 3 percent margin over and above
> the original 4 percent upcharge to the hospital cus-
> tomer). They have a hard time recouping the cost of all
> the services they provide. [Medical-surgical executive]

> Distributors have played around with consulting, just-in-
> time delivery, taking title to the hospital's warehouse or
> central sterile supply. But these are shell games. [Medical-
> surgical executive]

Part of this skepticism over value-added programs appears to be
based in fear of distributors usurping some of the manufacturers'
control over the supply chain. Some executives commented

> They deliver value to customers but want to deliver more
> value and move up the food chain and gain more control
> over what goes into the end-user customer. This is not in
> our interest. We just want them to distribute. We don't
> want them to direct product choice and steer it towards
> someone else willing to give them another 4 percent. But
> this is what the distributors are trying to do—'line ratio-
> nalization'—push the fraction of items they carry in their
> warehouse that account for 80 percent of their volume.

> Distributors are trying to arbitrage the manufacturer's
> price, provide the services that the manufacturers do,
> and become a 'selector of products.'

Distributors are also recognized for their information capabilities.
They are developing "information engines" regarding (1) IDN purchases to help identify potential cost savings—for example, through
generic substitution, reducing off-contract purchasing, changes in pur-

chase quantity, and so on; (2) IDN purchases by department or site; and (3) drug therapeutic choices that confer some ability to act as a pharmacy benefits manager (PBM).[79] They also provide an "information window" on customers and product shipments. In addition, they are building electronic bridges at contracting points, assisting IDNs with inventory management via EDI, JIT, and robotics systems; and developing e-commerce capabilities in the areas of invoicing and payment. According to one medical-surgical executive, "Distributors bring critical mass to the hospital customer from an EDI and IS [information system] perspective. Since one distributor may bring in 85 percent of the business, and since the distributor may give the EDI software to the hospital customer, the distributor can automate the customer's link to the distributor and reduce costs for both sides. The distributor can also assist with the system's integration. Our operating companies can only do this piecemeal."

According to GPOs, all of this information capability may help them to drive process improvements, standardization, utilization management, and demand-based delivery among their hospital members.

A handful of manufacturers commented on strategic initiatives with their distributors. Such initiatives included direct shipping from the factory, shipping on a scheduled basis, and preplanning product pallets. However, most product manufacturers do not rely on or develop strategic alliances with a single distributor. According to some pharmaceutical executives,

> We have scores of wholesale companies operating hundreds of distribution centers across the country and we use all of them equally.

> They aggregate customers that suppliers cannot sell directly to. But we don't have much else to do with them, other than good relationships with all of them.

> We don't exclusively market to some wholesalers rather than others. We go through all available wholesalers. I

view dealing with wholesalers as a pretty nondescript part of the business. I would say we have a very dedicated group of people who deal with wholesalers, but from a brand standpoint we deal very little with the wholesalers hands-on. However, when dealing with a wholesaler, size certainly does matter, especially if we get into product shortages and that kind of thing.

There also appears to be little joint research and programming between the two parties. "In some instances we do collaborative research studies with them, but not as much as we would like—simply because of their restriction on expenses."

Similarly, most GPOs do not have a single preferred distributor for a given class of products (for example, pharmaceuticals and medical-surgical supplies). They typically contract with multiple distributors in a given class ("open distribution"), mainly because no one distributor is large or national enough in scope to service all of the members of a large GPO. Moreover, different distributors offer different kinds and breadth of service to hospitals. These multiple distributors represent the authorized distribution agents (ADAs) for the manufacturer's products under contract with the GPO. GPOs try to get their hospital members to support these ADAs since they have mechanisms in place to help them obtain slightly more favorable pricing and better information and product tracking. However, hospitals are free to go off-contract and obtain supplies from other distributors. In the past, a few GPOs adopted the approach of "managed distribution," in which hospital members are asked to select one distributor based on service differentiation. The rationale here is that the GPO considers itself the supply chain manager and, in that role, believes that it must contract with a preferred distributor in order to effectively manage the total delivery cost for the hospital. In support of this approach, the GPO may conduct hospital customer satisfaction surveys regarding distribution. During the 1990s, the top issues reportedly have been fill rates (percentage of line items ordered that are delivered on the first truck) and pricing accuracy. Consolidation among distributors, however, has resulted in most distributors being "preferred" and thus on contract with the GPO.[80]

In a similar vein, some GPOs state that they often avoid using a single wholesaler (unless approached by a regional group of member hospitals) to allow customers more voice and leverage in negotiations. IDNs similarly prefer multiple wholesalers to avoid being overly dependent on one distributor and its prices and service levels. They also state that the source product directories (that is, generic formularies) that distributors developed in the 1990s pose a competitive threat to suppliers, and indeed have already driven several smaller generics suppliers out of the market.

How do IDN's view distributors? One might expect IDNs to appreciate all of the services that distributors provide. Hospitals have long benefited from the software and electronic information linkages provided by their distributors. Other valued distributor services include cost management and the provision of information for standardization programs. Some distributors send a full-time account team and clinician or product expert into hospital clients to identify cost-saving opportunities and areas to reduce ordering and practice variations (for example, drug dispensing). Standardization efforts can be furthered by "custom procedure packs" for certain surgical procedures (for example, cesarean sections and appendectomies) that are standardized across all physicians in the hospital. Other valued services include fee-for-service consulting.

Unfortunately, IDNs may not always recognize distributors' efforts in all of these service areas. One reason is the ubiquitous focus on product cost and markup in the health care supply chain. The value add of distributors may be lost on customers because the cost of their services is melded with the price of the products they distribute. Another reason is that distributors charge lower cost-plus pricing on contracted (high-volume items) and compensate with higher cost-plus pricing on noncontracted (lower volume) items. Customers may resent two-tiered pricing that doesn't reflect the actual value of the service provided.[81]

A similar view is presented in a Goldman Sachs survey of hospital executives in pharmacy and materials management. According to these data, hospitals select their distributors based primarily on price and GPO affiliation (that is, with whom does the GPO contract). Secondary issues include contract terms, service reputation and guarantee of the distributor, relationship and incumbency; tertiary issues include bundled offerings.[82] According to product manufacturers, IDNs want to be able to get everything they need from one source; the use of distributors fulfills this need. Nevertheless, IDNs appear to draw limits on the types of services they want from distributors. Several IDNs foresee their distributor in the future delivering products closer to the site of use in the hospital as well as off-site, providing separate packaging for satellite clinics and pharmacies, and more automated dispensing at alternate sites. They also would like distributors to combine hospital benchmark data (for example, patient days and case-mix index) with product consumption data to permit better evaluation of their purchases, and offer consultant pharmacists and pharmacy newsletters to help with pharmacotherapy management activities.[83] However, IDNs see little role for distributors in coordinating market share programs for manufacturers, or for conducting health data management functions using clinical outcomes information (since such information is not widely available).

Endnotes

1. Fein, Adam J. "Wholesale Distribution." *U.S. Industry and Trade Outlook*. New York: McGraw-Hill, 2000. Chapter 41.

2. Ibid.

3. Another distinction is between the pure distribution model and the agency model. In the former, the distributor buys the product and takes title to it; in the latter, the distributor holds and distributes the product, but the manufacturer owns the inventory and holds the receivables.

4. For more detail on the functions performed by distributors in the supply chain for medical-surgical products, see Arthur Andersen, *The Value of Distribution in the Medical Products Supply Chain*. Alexandria, Virginia: HIDA Educational Foundation, 1996.

5. Monczka, Robert M., and Joseph R. Carter. "Implementing Electronic Data Interchange." *Journal of Purchasing and Materials Management* (Summer 1988): 242

6. McFadden, Christopher D. *E-Distribution Update and Survey Results*. New York: Goldman Sachs, March 10, 2000.

7. Grossman, Robert J. "The Battle to Control Online Purchasing." *Health Forum Journal* (January/February 2000): 18–21.

8. See Note Six.

9. Cassak, David. "The New Internet Supply Chain: Issues for Device and Supply Companies." *Start Up* 5(3) (2000): 16–26.

10. WEDI. *The 1993 WEDI Report*. Workgroup for Electronic Data Interchange (October 1993).

11. Gillett et al. *Hospitals' New Supply Chain*. www.forrester.com, 2000.

12. Millennium Research Group. *Hospital Online Procurement Survey*. Stream 2, Issue 2. (September 2000). Toronto: Millennium Research Group.

13. Lacy et al. *The Value of eCommerce in the Healthcare Supply Chain*. Chicago: Arthur Andersen, 2001.

14. Thill, Mark. "Face-to-Face Still Sells." *Repertoire* 8(9) (2000): 28–36.

15. Millennium Research Group. *Online Opportunities in the Medical Products Marketplace*. Stream 1, Issue 1 (July 2000). Toronto: Millennium Research Group.

16. Boehm et al. *Sizing Healthcare eCommerce*. www.Forrester.com, 1999.

17. Findley, Richard. "The Pharmaceutical Supply Chain." Presentation to the Global Rx Supply Chain Conference. Philadelphia: October 1999.

18. Cassak, David. "E-Health's Second Mover Advantage." *In Vivo* (March 2000): 26–42.

19. See Note Six.

20 For the distributors that lack EDI linkages to manufacturers, a new Internet Web site has developed that allows them to place and track orders. It has contracted with National Distribution and Contracting (NDC) to help its 230 non–EDI-enabled distributors order products from suppliers.

21. See Note Ten.

22. See Note Ten.

23. Lee, Richard D., Conley, Dierdre A., and Andy Preikschat. *eHealth 2000: Healthcare and the Internet in the New Millennium*. Wit Capital Research, www.witcapital.com, 2000.

24. McFadden, Christopher D., and Timothy M. Leahy. *U.S. Healthcare Distribution: Positioning the Healthcare Supply Chain for the 21st Century*. New York: Goldman Sachs, 2000.

25. National Wholesale Druggists' Association. *1999 NWDA Industry Profile and Healthcare Factbook*. Reston, Virginia: NWDA, 1999.

26. The $122 billion figure derives from IMS Health. This amount includes not only prescription drugs but also over-the-counter (OTC) drugs and diagnostics, and health and beauty care products. Distributors handle $106 billion of this total. Of this $106 billion, $87 billion are direct deliveries, while $19 billion are chain and warehouse sales. Of the $87 billion in direct deliveries, $78 billion are prescription drugs. At first glance, the IMS data do not resemble data from the Health Care Financing Administration (HCFA). HCFA data reveal $99.6 billion in national health expenditures on retail prescription drugs in 1999. These data do not include prescription drug sales to hospitals and alternate sites. When these figures are added to the HCFA statistics, total sales resemble the IMS data. Cf. David Risinger and Owen Hughes. *Healthcare Distribution*. New York: Merrill Lynch, 2001.

27. See Note Seventeen.

28. See Note Twenty-Four.

29. Oswald, Sharon L., and William R. Boulton "Obtaining Industry Control: The Case of the Pharmaceutical Distribution Industry." *California Management Review* 38(1) (1995): 138–162.

30. See Note Twenty-Five.

31. Frost and Sullivan. *The Internet's Role in the U.S. Distribution of Medical Devices*. San Jose: Frost and Sullivan, 2000.

32. PriceWaterhouseCoopers. *HealthCast 2010: eHealth Quarterly—Procurement*. August 2000.

33. Millennium Research Group. *Online Opportunities in the Medical Products Marketplace*. Steam 1, Issue 1, 2000.

34. Fein, Adam J. *Macro Shock: How Wholesale Distribution Industries Are Being Revolutionized*. New York: Lehman Brothers, 1999.

35. See Note Twenty-Five.

36. Dunn, Homer. "Pharmacy Distribution Trends: Expert Perspectives in a Turbulent Market." In Marsh, Feinstein, and Raskin. *Health Care Supply Management Distribution/Outsourcing Guidebook*. New York: Lehman Brothers, 1999.

37. Marsh, Lawrence C., Feinstein, Adam T., and Joshua R Raskin. *Health Care Supply Management Distribution/Outsourcing Guidebook*. New York: Lehman Brothers, 1999.

38. HIDA. *UPN Bar Coding of Medical/Surgical Products in Distribution and Patient Care*. Washington, D.C.: Health Industry Distributors Association, 1999.

39. Repertoire. "Distributors Remain the Low-Cost Solution." *Repertoire* 8(4) (2000): 36–37.

40. Healthcare EDI Coalition. Joint Communique (February 19, 1998). www.hedic.org.

41. HIDA. *Toward the Year 2000: A Status Report on the Implementation and Use of Bar Codes in the Medical-Surgical Industry.* Alexandria, Virginia: Health Industry Distributors Association, 1996.

42. Becker, Cinda. "Using Bar Codes Could Lower Costs." *Modern Healthcare* (June 4, 2001): 16.

43. National Wholesale Druggists Association. *Bar Coding Practices in the Wholesale Drug Industry.* Reston, Virginia: NWDA, 1996.

44. See Note Twenty-Five.

45. Hensley, Scott. "Hospital Co-Ops Seek to Ease Purchases on Web." *Wall Street Journal* (June 13, 2000).

46. Hospital Materials Management. "CHeS Seeks Industry-wide Set of Standards." *Hospital Materials Management* 26(6) (2001): 2, 10–11.

47. Becker, Cinda. "Singing the Bar Code Blues." *Modern Healthcare* (June 25, 2001): 34.

48. DeJohn, Paula. "Hospitals Awaiting Arrival of E-Commerce Standards." *Hospital Materials Management* 26(6) (2001): 1, 9–10.

49. In July 2001, the National Coordinating Council for Medical Error Reporting and Prevention (nccmerp.org) issued a set of recommendations that called on the FDA to collaborate with pharmaceutical manufacturers to establish and implement uniform bar code standards, including standards for unit-of-use packages. Here the push for bar codes is linked to a parallel effort to reduce medical errors through information technology.

50. In 1998 generic drugs accounted for 45 percent of dispensed prescriptions but only 19–20 percent of prescription drug sales.

51. *Jenks Healthcare Business Report.* Volume 9(7): 1–2. January 9, 1999.

52. Doucette, William R., and Thani Jambulingam. *Drug Wholesalers and Their Customers: Attitudes and Expectations on Current and Future Services and Integration.* National Wholesale Druggists' Association, 1999.

53. Ibid.

54. See Note One.

55. Fein, Adam J. "The Triggers of Consolidation in Drug Wholesaling." *Healthcare Distribution* (November 1997).

56. Fein, Adam J. "Understanding Evolutionary Processes in Non-Manufacturing Industries: Empirical Insights from the Shakeout in

Pharmaceutical Wholesaling." *Journal of Evolutionary Economics* 8 (1998): 231–270.

57. Chandler, Alfred D. Jr. *Scale and Scope: The Dynamics of Industrial Capitalism*. Cambridge, Massachusetts: Belknap Press of the Harvard University Press, 1990.

58. McFadden, Christopher D., Savas, Stephen, and Timothy Leahy. *Cardinal Health Inc.* New York: Goldman Sachs, December 18, 2000.

59. On the medical-surgical side, Allegiance has similarly automated and consolidated its warehouses.

60. See Note Twenty-Five.

61. See Note Thirty-Six.

62. See Note Twenty-Five.

63. See Note Twenty-Five.

64. Marhula, Daren C., and Edward G. Shannon. *EHealth B2B Overview*. Minneapolis, Minnesota: U.S. Bancorp Piper Jaffray, 2000.

65. Movement of market share for generic manufacturers may be easier because distributors can pick from any generic bin in the warehouse where the product margins are higher.

66. Speculative buying characterizes drug distribution but not med-surg distribution. In the latter arena, manufacturers often notify distributors about price increases ahead of time.

67. Lehman Brothers decomposes the components of these gross profit margins as follows: 41 percent based on cash discounts, 20 percent based on owned inventory profits, 16 percent based on speculative inventory profit, and 6 percent based on program incentives. Lawrence Marsh, Adam Feinstein, and Joshua Raskin. *Healthcare Information Technology and Outsourcing/ Distribution Guidebook*. New York: Lehman Brothers, 2000.

68. See Note Thirty-Seven.

69. See Note Seventeen.

70. See Note Sixty-Seven.

71. Ibid.

72. McFadden, Christopher D., and Timothy M. Leahy. *Cardinal Health Inc.* New York: Goldman Sachs, 2000.

73. Cassak, David. "Do Drugs and Hospital Supplies Mix?" *In Vivo* (June 1997): 39–50.

74. McFadden et al. *Hospital Executive Survey*. New York: Goldman Sachs, 2000.

75. See Note Seventy-Three.

76. Phillips, Perry. Allegiance Healthcare Corporation Presentation to the Healthcare Manufacturers Marketing Council Spring Conference. Key Biscayne, 2001.

77. See Note Seventy-Three.
78. Repertoire. "Who Moves the Market Share—The Rep or the Company?" *Repertoire* 8(4) (2000): 42–43.
79. See Note Fifty-Two.
80. Some manufacturer reports of problems using distributors reflect the nature of the product. Very lightweight products like heart valves are susceptible to damage during shipping; in such instances, there is little perceived value in using distributors. Nevertheless, manufacturers may still use distributors to handle these products because "the customers want it that way." In general, manufacturers may continue with certain distributors just because of customer preference.
81. Everard, Lynn J. *Blueprint for an Efficient Health Care Supply Chain.* White Paper. Norcross, Georgia: Medical Distribution Solutions, 2000.
82. See Note Seventy-Four.
83. See Note Fifty-Two.

6

....

Threats of Disintermediation
Facing Distributors

Robert A. DeGraaff and Lawton R. Burns

The threat of *direct* contracting between buyer and seller (disintermediation) continually confronts any wholesaler/distributor. Today, these threats might be analyzed in terms of (1) the capabilities of third-party logistics firms to supplant distributors, (2) the emerging capabilities of e-commerce firms to supplant distributors, and (3) the willingness of some IDNs to serve as their own distributors and GPOs. These three threats are discussed next.

Capabilities of Third-Party Logistics Firms (3PLs)

There are third-party logistics firms (3PLs) such as Penske, UPS, CSC, TNT, Livingston, and Caliber Logistics that have entered the market to deliver small parcels when the customer is outside the service area of the manufacturer's or distributor's private fleet. Distributors sometimes use 3PLs for drop shipping, since firms like UPS have a distribution network with small distribution centers. They may also take over the distribution functions that health systems might consider performing on their own.

3PLs offer potential value to IDNs. According to one analyst, a medium-sized IDN can spend $500,000 a year in both inbound and outbound small package delivery. Manufacturers estimate that a twelve-hospital IDN can spend up to $800,000 a year in FedEx shipping. These are individual shipments (typically by 3PLs) that are not bulk or palletized delivery from a distributor. Moreover, there is a savings opportunity of anywhere between 7–25 percent by consolidating and committing all package freight to one contracted vendor. 3PLs might be able to do this consolidation.[1] In addition to this, 3PLs may be able to help hospitals manage "the last 100 yards of the health care supply chain" that spans from the hospital's loading dock to the patient floors by picking up products from manufacturers and delivering them directly to the point of use. In this manner, no one in the hospital moves or hoards products.

3PLs offer potential value to manufacturers in terms of pricing and the charge-back problem. Unlike large distributors, 3PLs move boxes without charging for what is in the box. According to one manufacturer, "Right now, if we ship a 6-inch by 6-inch box that has a value of $1,000, we pay 4 percent of that to have it moved by a distributor." By using 3PLs, manufacturers also solve the charge-back problem. Penske Logistics has set up "turnkey operations" in certain metropolitan markets where it builds a warehouse, contracts directly with manufacturers, moves their products in and out, and serves local IDNs. Some manufacturers believe 3PLs are the future of the industry. As one executive stated, "They are on the goal line; they have the money; they just need to invest more in IT and billing systems."

One concern about 3PLs expressed by manufacturing executives is how they will affect the vendors' traditional relationships with large distributors. Manufacturers may have strong relationships with distributors that help to promote their products to clinicians.[2]

3PLs may also offer value to the alternate site market (ASM). This is a fragmented market with thousands of delivery sites where physician offices have become accustomed to receiving daily UPS shipments. It is also a market where manufacturers of medical-surgical products have fewer sales representatives and thus have a potential to capture sales. Big med-surg distributors have been somewhat late in entering this market. Compared to distributors, 3PLs offer a stripped-down delivery vehicle that "just takes orders and fills them," rather than try to provide value-adding services, operate a field sales force, and help manufacturers sell their products.

The 3PLs firms tend to specialize in one of three functional areas: trucking (for example, Penske and UPS), warehousing (for example, TNT, Livingston, and Caliber), and information systems (for example, CSC). One challenge for these firms is developing capabilities in all three areas—something that distributors now do for the provider community. Logistics supply chain managers suggest that a good 3PL offer most or all of the following services, which cut across the three areas previously mentioned: purchase and brokering of transportation, distribution, warehousing, demand planning, order management, inventory management and optimization, information technology, modeling design and strategy, and integration of logistics.[3]

Another challenge for third-party logistics firms is handling "nonconformance" in the medical-surgical supply chain; that is, finding a product for an emergency operation when it is not available, handling product recalls, and placing products in a pyxis machine. Manufacturers that have vested relationships with distributors question whether these third-party firms can buffer both vendors and their customers from unpredictable demand and uneven product flow rates.

Moreover, it is unclear how the 3PLs are going to remove cost from the distribution process. On the pharmaceutical side, distributors are operating with low operating margins and low expenses. Many supply chain participants wonder where the 3PL savings are, other than offering a lower price to manufacturers, and are skeptical that manufacturers will offer the 3PLs additional margins ("behind-the-line incentives") elsewhere. Of course, the 3PLs might argue that their approach serves to rid the current supply chain of one of its biggest inefficiencies—the administrative cost of managing the rebate program between manufacturers and distributors. As argued previously, manufacturers benefit from the rebate program and may not be willing to alter it. On both the pharmaceutical and medical-surgical side, 3PLs do not take title to the products they carry and thus do not function as wholesalers. As noted previously, pharmaceuticals have been subject to some price inflation (facilitating speculative buying) while medical-surgical products carry relatively high margins. Thus, 3PLs are foreclosed from the areas in which traditional distributors make some of their profits.

A final challenge facing 3PLs is the lack of their widespread use by IDNs for the delivery of medical-surgical products.[4] 3PLs represent a risky proposition for IDNs, which have come to be dependent on the many services distributors provide, and which may be unsure whether 3PLs possess the same level of product knowledge, industry knowledge, customer service, and capability in handling contract pricing. As one distributor executive stated, "3PLs just deliver a box from point X to point Y. But the distribution of medical products is more than this. 3PLs are attractive to those who do not understand all of the stuff behind the scenes that gets a product to a customer priced correctly and invoiced." Moreover, if the 3PLs succeed in handling the high volume A items, then the mainstream distributors are left handling the lower volume B items. This will raise the distributors' costs, which then get passed on to the IDNs, who do not save any money.

Capabilities of E-Commerce Firms to Supplant Distributors

Like other industries, health care is witnessing the emergence of Web-based firms that threaten to disturb trading relationships in both retailing and wholesaling. The former are known as business-to-consumer (B2C) models; the latter are known as business-to-business (B2B). B2B firms are also known as e-commerce and e-procurement providers. Chapters Ten and Eleven provide a thorough introduction to e-commerce and its broader role in the health care supply chain. Here we focus on its role in product distribution.

With regard to product distribution, e-commerce firms confront a series of functions currently performed by wholesalers. These include

- warehousing and delivery logistics

- contract management and adjudication

- sales and marketing support

- receivables financing

- returns processing

- inventory management

- IT support

- generic purchasing

- speculative purchasing and forward buying

These functions are often distinguished in terms of being front end and back end (see Exhibit 6.1). Over the past decade, distributors have moved away from traditional back-end distribution where the core business is providing and detailing products, focusing on prices, and serving as an extension of each manufacturer whose lines the distributor carried (manufacturer/distributor convergence model),

Exhibit 6.1   B2B Medical Products Supply Chain

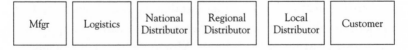

Back-end functions:
logistics, fulfillment, shipping, fulfillment tracking,
financial processing, order management,
customer service, data warehousing

Front-end functions:
sourcing, purchasing,
procurement, data capture
financial processing, order
management, fulfillment
tracking

and instead moved toward the provision of more value-adding, front-end services, designed to lower costs for their hospital customers (hospital/distributor convergence model).[5]

Distributors now typically perform multiple functions for their customers and offer a bundled pricing model, which captures their costs in the upcharge to customers or is embedded in the products' list price.[6] E-commerce firms, by contrast, focus on a discrete subset of these functions and offer customers a plug-and-play solution. That is, the customer is offered the option to purchase one or more of these functions from the B2B firm rather than the distributor, which is then left with the potential problem of pricing its once-bundled package of services one by one. These functional areas differ in terms of their barriers to entry, value added for customers, strategic importance, and potential for returns.

For example, the logistics function—the core business of distributors—has high entry barriers due to the need to develop warehousing and automation infrastructure and the scale economies enjoyed by the top firms in each product market segment. Logistics is strategically important for health care providers to minimize their costs and maintain quality, but adds little value and features small economic returns. For example, the large pharmaceutical distributors have already squeezed out most of the savings here, and have left themselves with margins of roughly 0.2–0.5 percent (twenty to fifty basis points). It is not surprising that this function is not targeted by e-commerce firms. Indeed, the leading e-retailers in industry (for example, Amazon.com) utilize a drop-ship model that relies on existing distributors for order fulfillment. Deliveries using this model typically take two days, whereas some health care provider customers want next-day delivery. Moreover, these customers do not want hundreds of small shipments from hundreds of suppliers showing up every day on their loading dock, but rather prefer the large shipments from distributors. Consequently, the emergence of e-retailers has led to a growth in wholesale distribution, not a decline.[7] Instead, as just discussed, the threat to distributors here comes from 3PLs that might serve as alternative partners to e-commerce firms that target other functional areas.

Threat of Process Improvements by Internet Firms

What are the emerging e-commerce threats to distributors? The real savings may be in process improvements, not in product logistics. These improvements are likely to take place using one of two business models: a catalogue model and an auction model. The former brings together buyers and sellers to purchase goods from an on-line catalogue, typically for more standardized items. This catalogue can be interposed between manufacturers and distributors, and between distributors and providers. The auction model brings together buyers and sellers to set their own prices for specific products (for example, capital equipment and specialty purchases).[8] While auctions may serve to lower sales prices for vendors, they allow them to reduce some of their costs (for example, field sales force salaries and travel expenses) as well as reach new customers.

In the functional area of *contract management and adjudication*, e-procurement companies automate the buying process spanning from creating requisitions, having them approved, processing purchasing orders, sending purchasing orders to suppliers, receiving back invoices, and creating a matching voucher to accounts payable system to pay the invoice.[9] This is a particularly important area since errors here are common and require expensive rework for everyone involved. Invoice errors, for example, are measured by distributors in terms of the number of pricing credits per thousand lines. Such errors are often due to either the manufacturer being late in getting the price to the distributor or the hospital customer being late in getting the updated price (outdated customer price files).

In the area of *sales and marketing support*, e-sellers (e-retailers) offer on-line catalogues in several product markets including wholesale drugs, retail drugs, medical equipment, medical supplies, scientific products, laboratory and scientific supplies and instruments, and medical devices. In the area of *purchasing*, e-market and e-auction firms bring buyers and sellers together in several product markets and collect a commission of consummated transactions.

Threat to Distributors' Product Bundling Approach

One threat these firms pose is the potential unbundling of the distributors' functions, using the plug-and-play approach.[10] In this model, channel specialists emerge to focus on doing one or two functions well to achieve economies of scale. Thus, UPS would specialize in materials handling and shipping, CSC would specialize in information integration and exchange, Caliber would specialize in warehousing, and a new firm ("the distribution assembler") would emerge to link and optimize the networks of burgeoning specialist firms. Some of the principles behind this hypothesized shift are (1) customers focus on the price and efficiency of each service that heretofore was bundled, (2) inefficient services get jettisoned, (3) buyers and customers drive the structure of distribution channels by demanding customized bundles of distribution solutions, and (4) the key competence is the ability to interconnect.

This potential threat is real for distributors that have sought to develop bundles of value-adding services beyond logistics. One issue they face is the need to cost and price each function offered within their bundled package, and thereby demonstrate its value added. Distributors such as Owens & Minor (O&M) responded by applying activity-based costing (ABC) techniques to analyze their internal costs and then price their external contracts using activity-based pricing (ABP). In the traditional method of cost-plus pricing (in med-surg), the distributor's fee is based on the product cost plus a percentage markup, rather than the actual cost of product delivery. Under the new method, O&M tied its product distribution fees to the activity levels demanded by customers (for example, number of deliveries per week, bulk versus low-unit-of-measure delivery, number of purchase orders generated per month, and number of lines per purchase order). The advantage here is threefold. First, it allows the distributor to justify its contract pricing and avoid cost shifting or subsidization across functions. Second, it allows the distributor to partner with customers in economizing their transactions and lowering customer costs. Third, it allows customers to separately consider the product decision from the distribution decision. By the end of 1999, O&M derived nearly 15 percent of its total revenues from ABP contracts.[11]

More recent data provided by O&M executives tout the advantages of its ABC and ABP systems for itself and its trading partners. Under the traditional distribution model, the cost to the provider might include $0.94 in product cost (supplies); $0.06 for the distributor's fee; and $0.40 in internal (distribution) costs such as ordering, receiving, breaking down, and distributing inside—for a total of $1.40. Under its new "CostTrack" model, O&M attacks the $0.40 spent by the hospital internally by consolidating the number of orders per day, decreasing the number of deliveries per week, reducing the number of departments placing orders and reducing the number of vendors used. According to O&M executives, "It's all about changing behavior."[12] Using CostTrack, supply costs drop slightly ($0.90), distributor fees rise ($0.10), and distribution costs fall sharply ($0.20)—for a total of $1.20. Overall, the provider saves 14 percent in costs, while the distributor realizes a 66 percent gain in fees.

Still, the plug-and-play threat of e-commerce may be more imagined than real. As Adam Fein has emphasized, e-commerce firms do not address the warehousing, logistics, and fulfillment functions performed by distributors and do not take title to the products they carry.[13] They instead insert themselves into the value chain at that point where hospital customers make decisions regarding the vendor source, quantity, and amount of their supply purchases; and hope to detach the presales information and order processing functions from the distributors. The problems here are multiple:

First, the distributor is well-ensconced in a complex web of existing relationships where it has sought to make itself indispensable to hospital customers via its hand in inventory management, electronic linkages, and so on.

Second, the distributor is already an efficient supply chain channel. Assuming a gross margin of 5 percent, taxes and expenses incurred in operating the fixed cost infrastructure of trucks, warehouses, and so on to handle logistics and fulfillment functions consume nearly four-fifths of this margin, especially in pure-play distributors. This leaves roughly 1 percent available for e-commerce firms to vie for, unless they can take costs out of the remaining channel functions.

Third, e-commerce firms hope to earn revenues by charging transaction fees of 1–2 percent of sales to sellers of products. However, this sales commission represents over 50 percent of the distributor's net margin, and rewards the e-commerce firm for transmitting larger invoices, even though the cost of transmitting a large invoice is equivalent to that of transmitting a small invoice. Not only are manufacturers unlikely to want to pay these graduated fees, but the transaction fees are likely to get bid down due to competition, leaving less than e-commerce firms expect.

Fourth, it is not clear that manufacturers will disintermediate their own distributors by utilizing e-commerce firms. As indicated in Chapter Five, manufacturers recognize that distributors represent the lowest-total-cost solution for the delivery of their products. They also believe that if they begin to utilize e-commerce firms to handle their high-volume products, their former distributor partners may start pushing the product lines of their competitors.[14,15]

Nevertheless, manufacturers may use e-commerce firms to "lend cyber-visibility" to the 50 percent or so of their products that constitute only a fraction of their sales and that distributors either don't stock or don't sell.[16] Manufacturers may also allow e-commerce firms to handle product sales when customers use their Web sites for information and then decide they want to purchase products. In such cases, the manufacturer may seek to "re-intermediate" the distributor with a "virtual reseller commission" in order to keep the distributor from pushing a competitor's products, elicit future cooperation, and to give them an incentive to help hospital customers shop for niche items through their own Web sites.

Threat of Internet Substitution for EDI

Another threat is the substitution of the Internet and B2B transactions for the more traditional EDI linkages between distributors and customers. In Chapter Five we discussed the advantages of EDI over manual, paper-based systems. Here, we discuss the advantages of the Internet over EDI.

EDI vendors perform two basic functions: provide a format translation (for example, format invoices, orders, and claims) and perform electronic routing.[17] Distributors and health care systems process roughly 75–80 percent of their supply transactions using EDI. However, EDI runs on expensive networks that are installed from scratch for each pair of buyer and seller computer systems. EDI thus facilitates only one-to-one connectivity. EDI is also expensive to run and maintain, requiring significant manpower costs. Given the high cost of installing and maintaining these networks, EDI is also typically available only to larger organizations. Moreover, it does not permit easy integration with providers' materials management or accounting systems, and fails to simplify the need to consult multiple catalogues, prices lists, and discount schedules.[18] Finally, EDI networks are more proprietary than standardized, are nonscalable and inflexible, and are slower than Internet-based communication.

EDI-based transactions are threatened by the Internet and its improved accessibility and connectivity to multiple users. Larger customer firms no longer face high exit barriers to shifting to another distributor or vendor, since the communication formats (using XML) are more standardized than customized.[19] Smaller customer firms that could not previously afford EDI linkages will be able to access their supplier and buyer trading partners using the nonproprietary linkages afforded by the Internet. Moreover, the Internet serves to accelerate the procurement process, automate it, and integrate it into financial and materials management systems.

Moreover, as the Health Insurance Portability and Accountability Act (HIPAA) standards (for example, use of X12 standard format for data) penetrate the EDI market, there will be less need for an EDI intermediary. As a result, according to analysts, EDI revenues in health care are expected to peak by 2005.[20] Internet trade as a percentage of total sales revenues will grow from 3 percent to 32 percent between 1999 and 2002, while traditional EDI will shrink from 36 percent to 21 percent, and non-e-commerce revenue will fall from 61 percent to 47 percent.[21]

According to industry estimates, the cost of processing an electronic invoice is anywhere from one-fifth to one-twentieth of the cost of processing a paper invoice, which can range $40–150 on the buyer's side and $30–150 on the supplier's side.[22–24] Some observers have further speculated that the cost of Web-based transactions are one-eighth to one-tenth the cost of EDI-based transactions. If so, then the Web constitutes a major cost saving over EDI. In a recent survey, 63 percent of national, regional, and local distributors reported that e-commerce was less expensive than EDI; 58 percent said it was more flexible, but only 33 percent said it was easier to operate.[25]

However, there is some early evidence (albeit from a potentially biased source) that there are no major cost savings from transitioning from EDI to Internet linkages, since both are electronic processes. The vice president for distribution at Allegiance (the largest medical-surgical distributor) reports that EDI is very efficient for order processing. A phone or fax order costs $.63 per line to enter, while an EDI-based order costs $.03 per line. The Internet drops the cost even further to less than $.01 per line, but the real savings are in automating the manual order-entry process, a task that EDI already does.[26] Interviews with major GPOs indicate further limits to Internet savings: the difficulty in getting customers to use it. One of the largest medical-surgical suppliers reportedly discovered that over 40 percent of the hospitals with a direct electronic link to the firm do not use it; instead, they continue to phone and fax in their product orders.

The savings to be expected from the Internet may depend on one's perspective. If one adopts a narrow view of a hospital that purchases its supplies from one distributor, then there may be little value in transitioning from EDI to the Web in this particular dyadic exchange. That is, there may be only incremental connectivity savings in choosing one "pipe" over another; that is, in "Webifying" an already EDI-based exchange. If one assumes a broader view of the hospital seeking links with multiple distributors and vendors to develop access to broader portfolios of products, then there is greater value in transitioning to the Web since you no longer need multiple proprietary linkages. Moreover, there may be savings as you shift from the batch-mode processing characteristic of EDI to real-time marketplace transactions using the Internet. In addition, if one adopts an even broader supply chain view, there may be greater savings as you link up multiple hospital customers with manufacturers and the original equipment manufacturers (OEMs). The biggest savings, however, may derive from long-term changes among providers as they redesign business processes to align with Web-based solutions.

Regardless, the Internet has yet to pervade product distribution channels. In a recent survey of distributors cited previously, only 37 percent currently offer an Internet site with e-commerce capabilities, only 42 percent offer an on-line catalogue of the products they distribute, and only 8 percent report experiencing any disintermediation due to e-commerce. Distributors further report they accept customer orders using a variety of forms, with e-commerce being one of the least used:

Phone and fax	90 percent
Salesperson order entry	80 percent
EDI	70 percent
E-mail	59 percent
Internet site	41 percent
Proprietary order-entry technology	33 percent

As for revenues, e-commerce accounts for only 1.7 percent, while EDI accounts for 22 percent.[27]

Perhaps the most palpable threat posed by the Internet and B2B portals is the loss of control over the information regarding where products go. The loss of such control may eliminate some of the fees and rebates earned by distributors. With Web-based purchases and recording of those purchases, manufacturers may have less need to pay distributors tracing fees to find out where their products go. Moreover, with Web-based promotions manufacturers may have less need to pay distributors marketing fees for promoting their products to providers. Consequently, it may be hard to convince distributors to participate in and link to any B2B marketplace that they themselves do not control.

Despite these threats, larger distributors are likely to make (and indeed are making) the needed investments in e-commerce linkages (see Chapter Ten). Given their existing contracts, linkages with manufacturers and customers, and capital, they are likely to maintain their competitive advantage over B2B firms. Across a variety of industries, distributors expect to see a large percentage of their sales revenues derive from Web-based transactions over the next few years. They see a huge opportunity to plug themselves into e-commerce but little threat from B2B firms that lack physical fulfillment (product delivery) and service integration.[28] As a result, they may not abandon EDI for regular, high-volume transactions in their acute care markets. Rather, they may utilize the Internet for the alternate site marketplace, for irregular or low-volume orders, and as a supplement to their telesales force.

A more interesting question is the areas in which distributors will make their e-commerce investments. As noted earlier, the product manufacturer has become the major customer of the distributor. Indeed, distributors exchange data electronically with 80–90 percent of manufacturers, compared to 75 percent of their hospital customers and only 40 percent of GPOs.[29] In the future, distributors may use the Internet to integrate with manufacturers to lessen their costs (for example, sales force automation), provide real-time information on market share, and develop innovative ways to help them bring their products to market on a global basis.[30]

The Web-based firms face some imposing competitive advantages enjoyed by incumbents. Cardinal Health, for example, employs 1,500 information technology (IT) personnel and spends $250 million on its IT operating budget. It also has established on-line relationships with 3,000 suppliers and 55,000 customers, accounting for $18 billion in EDI transactions. Cardinal also expected to complete $100 million in Internet-based sales in the year 2000, and developed a comprehensive Web strategy (Cardinal.com) covering procurement, service extension, and IT management. The latter performs data compilation and information reports for customers (for example, accounts, invoices, contracts, product usage, service levels, supply costs, and so forth). In March 2000, Cardinal outlined its Internet strategy: to create a separate business focused on expanding Cardinal.com, including the planned launch of "entelligence" to help providers make better purchasing decisions. Cardinal also offered Encounter, a Web-based clinical information management system that integrates information from multiple sources into a single analytical platform that allows hospitals to benchmark their outcomes.[31]

Summary: Threat of Distributor Disintermediation by E-Commerce

Overall, there appears to be little short-term threat of disintermediation of distributors, particularly in the "replenishment ordering" of commodity items and high-volume, low-value products. This area represents the bulk of the distributors' sales volume. There is not a great deal of further efficiency gains to be made here. Moreover, Web-based firms lack the service infrastructure (product delivery, handling requirements for narcotics, product installation and service, and product returns) to compete. Finally, established distributors have two strategic assets that are hard to appropriate and imitate: established relationships with both manufacturers and customers, and a long history of supply chain management.

On the other hand, Web-based firms may have an advantage in specialty ordering of capital goods and equipment where ordering, purchasing, and pricing issues are more complex and user specific. There may also be potential for garnering a share of hospital purchases that are made ad hoc and off-contract (for example, to deal with event-specific incidents, or for less commonly ordered items), estimated to be up to 50 percent of hospital purchases. Finally, there may be a huge potential for e-commerce firms in the ASM, due to a lack of practice consolidation and relatively lower levels of distributor concentration.[32]

Thus, in the near future, B2B firms are likely to engage in a variety of distribution strategies. They may *compete* by virtue of carving out one or a small number of the distributor's functions, *partner* in some functional areas by providing virtual sales and service systems, or *substitute* virtual GPOs for the existing purchasing alliances.

Willingness of Integrated Delivery Networks to Supplant Distributors and GPOs

When hospitals come together to form systems or consortia, they pool their logistics costs, which form a larger number, and they ask themselves, What can we do here? Every ten to fifteen years, the answer has been, Let's buy direct, let's build our own warehouse, and let's get away from GPOs and distributors. What is potentially different this time is the presence of 3PLs telling hospitals not to invest in the bricks and mortar of such operations, but to outsource them to the 3PLs. That is, "make it an expense decision rather than a capital decision." In this section, we consider some of the burgeoning efforts of IDNs to act as their own GPO and distributor.

Two Supply Chain Disintermediation Strategies

Disintermediation is the elimination of middlemen firms in supply chains.[33] In health care supply chains, several innovative IDNs have sought to (1) bypass group purchasing organizations and contract directly with manufacturers and (2) oust traditional distributors in favor of regional self-distribution. We interviewed materials managers at four IDNs about their direct contracting and regional self-distribution initiatives:

The Lee Memorial/Sarasota Hospital Purchasing Cooperative, a joint venture by Lee Memorial Health System, a three-hospital system anchored by Lee Memorial Hospital in Fort Myers, and Sarasota Memorial Hospital.

Promina Health System, a network of five local integrated delivery systems (DeKalb Regional Healthcare System, Gwinnett Health System, Piedmont Health System, Southern Regional Health System, and WellStar Health System) that provides geographic coverage across the greater Atlanta area. (In November 1999, WellStar announced its separation from Promina, but will continue to participate in direct contracting).

Sentara Health System, a system of six hospitals and other caregiving sites in southeastern Virginia and northeastern North Carolina.

Continuum Health Partners, a seven-hospital network in New York City. Initially formed as an alliance between St. Luke's

Roosevelt Hospital Center and Beth Israel Medical Center, it has expanded to include Long Island College Hospital and New York Eye & Ear Infirmary.

In addition, we analyzed published case studies of other hospitals engaging in similar initiatives. The next two sections of this chapter describe the motivations, perceived key success factors, and anticipated financial results for each of these strategies. Following this description, we assess the sustainability of these strategies and the generalizability of the four cases.

IDN Strategy #1: Direct Contracting

IDNs have pursued direct contracting for several different reasons. Executives cite several factors associated with the success of these efforts and several financial benefits.

Motivations   E-commerce linkages have enabled these IDNs to pursue direct, long-term, sole-source, high-compliance, GPO-independent contracting with manufacturers. Interviews suggested several leading motivations for direct contracting. One motivation is to increase flexibility in contracting and purchasing by exiting "lockstep, one-size-fits-all" national GPO supply contracts, in which hospitals are required to follow committed purchasing agreements. The hospitals want to combine the GPO's price with the customization desired by an IDN. Continuum Health Partners, for example, launched their own buying organization when their GPO (Premier) balked at using them as a beta site to test a more customized purchasing arrangement. The hospitals also recognize that larger members in national GPOs subsidize the smaller members and thus forgo the pricing they could get themselves.

A second motivation is to leverage manufacturers' willingness to underprice national buying groups in order to secure regional market share through high-compliance, sole-source agreements. Some of these networks were striving to add value for manufacturers in several ways. At Continuum Health Partners, for example, 85 percent of product lines purchased consist of only one SKU. In this manner, the network can deliver high volume on a committed contract to a single supplier. Networks were also seeking to integrate all levels of purchasing (acute inpatient, primary care, long-term care, and hospice) to further drive volume for manufacturers. Networks also consolidate their member hospitals' warehouses, allowing manufacturers to direct ship to one location using bigger trucks. In this manner, there is the possibility that networks can turn distribution into a profit center and/or create for-profit, shared operational systems for nearby hospitals in the areas of central sterile supply, blood banking, laboratory, or food. These may be fruitful areas for IDN collaboration since they do not typically compete on materials management acquisition prices.

A third motivation is to generate new sources of revenue. One innovative strategy is to develop a patient product guide, which is made available to patients upon discharge. Patients requiring home health services, medical, and personal care products can order them over the phone or, more recently, on a computer given them by the network, with twenty-four-hour delivery. This enables the network to integrate the hospital and retail markets by "following the patient," driving product usage and volume to patients postdischarge, and increasing manufacturers' share in the home health and durable medical equipment markets. Because the profit margins are larger on home care versus acute care products, manufacturers may realize significant new revenues without incurring any additional marketing or inventory expenses. Networks seek to participate in these revenue streams or, alternatively, reap bigger discounts on the acute care supplies they purchase. Another revenue source is to capture bulk purchase rebates that otherwise flow to middlemen firms.

A fourth motivation is to further reduce medical supplies costs by eliminating GPO margins and contract administration fees. Some networks do not require the payment of CAFs, but may consider doing so in the future to help recover some of their investment in the buying organization. Several networks mentioned that reduced supply costs was viewed as a means to gain advantage in HMO contracting in the local market.

Key Success Factors   To succeed in direct contracting, respondents mentioned the importance of several key factors. These include guaranteeing and consistently delivering high levels of contract compliance. For example, in order to belong to one of these buying groups, hospitals have to commit to purchasing 85 percent of disposable products through the group. Compliance rests largely on standardization efforts (for example, agreeing to have only one SKU per product line). This requires that physicians be actively involved in vendor selection and product standardization decisions. One means to facilitate this is for the buying group to partner only with leading manufacturers with preferred products. At Continuum Health Partners, for example, these leading vendors included Abbott Labs, Medtronic, and Tyco Kendall. In addition to compliance, networks should also have sufficient bed size to drive sufficient volume to interest manufacturers.

To make the follow-the-patient strategy work, these vendors should also supply the home care market and have the ability to service the retail market. Networks should also use the same warehouse and inventory for both their hospital inpatients and their home care patient catalogue. The networks also look for manufacturers that can assist the network with information technology, consulting, and disease management efforts. For example, the computers given to discharged patients are often funded by grants from either vendors or managed care payers. When patients go to order their home health supplies, they are first required to answer some questions and supply some clinical data useful for developing targeted disease management interventions. Moreover, these data serve to automatically notify physicians and nurses when patients are not complying with their home care regimen.

There are other capabilities needed to make this buying group strategy work. First, the network needs highly motivated materials managers with expertise and abilities in contracting, negotiation, and physician-nurse relations. Second, it needs senior management support and commitment. Third, the group needs to be careful that the costs of standardization and centralization (for example, conversion to a uniform, fully integrated information system across IDN customers) do not outweigh the associated benefits. Thus, for example, the network may not be able to standardize products across all sites of care. As one respondent commented, "Because standardization must not compromise customer need, different products (with different price and quality levels) are sometimes carried for the acute care, nursing home, and physician office environments. Therefore, an IDN may standardize on more than one product within a product category."

Anticipated Financial Results The Lee/Sarasota Cooperative was launched in 1997 with the assistance of Coalesco, a Texas-based purchasing consulting firm. The cooperative reportedly had fifty vendor contracts for $60 million in products. The cooperative's materials managers found that brand-name manufacturers were much more flexible on pricing and terms than they had originally anticipated, and reported a first-year cost savings of 17 percent. One-time signing bonuses helped boost first-year results, but management expected long-term annual savings on medical supplies to average ten to twelve percent.[34,35]

At Continuum Health Partners, the reported savings achieved were small ($1.2 million) relative to the overall costs of purchases ($150 million).[36] These efficiencies represented savings on purchasing. Executives at Health Works, the buying group for Continuum Health Partners, believed the potential might reach as high as $50 million. Published reports indicate that they anticipated a reduction in inpatient medical-surgical costs by 7 percent over GPO prices, another 7 percent on distributors' fees, and $1 million in savings (that is, cut warehouse FTEs) by outsourcing all warehousing functions.[37]

IDN Strategy #2: Regional Self-Distribution

All four IDNs pursuing direct contracting also operated regional self-distribution centers. The two strategies thus seem intertwined.

The Lee/Sarasota Cooperative opened its 52,000-square-foot distribution facility in September 1998. National Healthcare Logistics, a division of National Healthcare Manufacturing Corporation, assisted in designing the "hub and spoke" distribution network and arranged a five-year contract to manage it.[38] The LeeSar Regional Service Center was a hospital-owned ADA for medical-surgical products that offers LUM distribution and just-in-time service at (reportedly) a margin below commercial distributors. A cooperative executive described the Lee/Sarasota distribution concept:

> We've developed a commercial distribution center, LeeSar, that has supplanted Allegiance and Owens & Minor. The commercial distribution center buys and sells to the two health systems. Product goes from the manufacturer directly to LeeSar. The products are then resold and shipped to the two health systems. The distribution company is using an Internet-based system to perform functions such as product utilization tracking and reorder signaling. One result is that the hospitals have much lower levels of owned inventory. At present, there are four acute care delivery sites. Sales and delivery to affiliated nursing homes, physician offices, and clinics is planned. Medical Transport Services (MTS) is under contract to perform and coordinate transportation and delivery for the distribution center. Because we own the supply chain all the way back to the manufacturer's back

door, all the fees and markups due to GPOs and distributors are avoided and retained in the organization. However, developing and implementing a direct contracting and independent distribution center strategy isn't for everyone. The political and organizational pressures (for example, from management, physicians, and the existing GPOs) were intense. In the future, movement toward increased vendor-managed inventory is planned. The longer-term vision is to link inventory and supplies utilization with the entire billing and revenue cycle.

Sentara Health System opened its own distribution facility in February 1997 and staffed it with a full-time operations manager (not a third-party contract). To further reduce its logistics costs, Sentara also centralized mail processing and hospital records at its distribution facility. Promina Health System developed its distribution center to "perform warehousing, breaking product down into low units of measure, and transporting cheaper than Owens & Minor or anyone else can."[39]

At Continuum Health Partners, manufacturers shipped directly to CHP and retained ownership of the inventory. CHP outsourced its warehousing and distribution to two local distributors: one for medical-surgical products and one for pharmaceuticals. At the same time, it consolidated the warehouses of its member hospitals to achieve efficiencies, permit manufacturers to make delivery to one point, and turn the warehouses into a "profit center." To facilitate efficient delivery to both the inpatient and home care market, the local distributor (Caligor Medical, the hospital division of Henry Schein) used LUM. Caligor served as the logistics provider and manager of the warehouse.

Motives for Regional Self-Distribution   Interviews suggested four leading motivations for regional self-distribution. The first was to improve service levels (for example, delivery of LUM directly to hospital departments and physician offices). The second motivation was to reduce medical supply costs by eliminating distributors' price increases, margins, and fees. A third reason, as stated previously, was to capture bulk purchase rebates that otherwise flow to middlemen firms. Fourth, and finally, the networks wished to gain more flexibility than is permitted under traditional distribution contracts.

With regard to the improvement of service levels, one respondent commented, "Levels of quality and service from traditional distribution were not meeting the needs of IDN customers. The distributors tend to treat IDNs and IDN customers the same way. They don't provide individualized service. The reality is, however, when you've seen one IDN, you've seen one."

Key Success Factors   One key success factor in regional self-distribution is a relatively tight geographic clustering of IDN customers. Geographic proximity is needed because distribution costs increase with the number of miles between delivery points. IDNs must have also the capabilities to (1) order and receive large quantities of product at the central location, (2) break down and assemble high-volume shipments from vendors into smaller customer-specific shipments, and (3) deliver orders to IDN customers. A third requirement is electronic communication linkages connecting all IDN customers in the distribution network. Such linkages are particularly critical for developing the follow-the-patient strategy, and may spur the development of hospital Web sites for *two*-way communication (not just hospital promotion).

IDNs are cautioned to conduct their own discounted cash flow analysis comparing self-distribution to traditional distribution before embarking on self-distribution. As with purchasing, they are also cautioned to elicit physician involvement in product standardization efforts; to recruit and retain highly motivated materials managers with logistics and supply chain management expertise; and to curry senior management support and commitment, especially during initial implementation.

Anticipated Financial Results   The Lee/Sarasota Cooperative expected its distribution center to be profitable by fiscal year 2000 and to net long-term annual savings of 5–7 percent.[40,41] Another IDN reported, "The financial benefit to our IDN for direct distribution (compared to traditional distribution) was over $1 million in the first year, and the projected annual benefit in five years is $5 million to $7 million. Continuum Health Partners believed the potential from its joint purchasing and distribution model to be upward of $50 million, or one-third of its total supply costs. This sum includes $4–5 million savings in distribution, $7 million in revenues generated by product distribution, $20 million in revenues from the home health market, and another $14 million savings from the sharing of operational services (for example, laundry, file storage, central sterile supply, blood, and laboratory) across hospitals in the network using the centralized warehouse platform. They also stated that their distributor had a 99 percent fill rate.

Sustainability of Disintermediation Strategies

Since the time of our interviews at these four sites, we have been unable to locate any additional information or updates on several of these initiatives. However, at least one of the four models has entirely collapsed. HealthWorks, the contracting and buying group for Continuum Health Partners, dissolved in the fall of 2000. Earlier that year, senior management at Continuum noticed that HealthWorks was not only incurring high labor expenses (due to twenty-five to thirty FTEs), but had also failed to take out nonsalary costs. HealthWorks had executed purchasing contracts that reportedly achieved lousy pricing and little leverage over vendors, thus yielding higher supply costs for its member hospitals. Officials from Broadlane, the firm that oversees Tenet's GPO BuyPower, were brought in to conduct pricing audits and found a 17 percent difference between what HealthWorks negotiated for products and what Broadlane achieved. These excessive product costs were removed when Continuum outsourced the management of its Enterprise Resource Planning (ERP) system and purchasing department to Broadlane in spring 2001.

Broadlane executives stated that HealthWorks was primarily a "revenue ploy" (focus on CAFs) as opposed to a strategy to reduce costs (focus on product prices). As for the other features of Health-Works' approach, they state that the firm had developed some thought-provoking ideas but were not sure if any of the reported strategies (such as, follow-the-patient) had actually occurred or moved beyond pilot testing.

Conclusion

The materials managers interviewed for this portion of the study made the following predictions. For the next five to ten years

- GPOs will have to "figure out how to compete against or work with IDNs pursuing direct contracting with manufacturers."

- Large, urban IDNs, whose facilities are clustered geographically, will move to self-distribution.

- Traditional middlemen firms will be selling to entities such as smaller systems, rural providers, and stand-alone hospitals.

As proponents, they argue that the philosophical strength of their approach should win adherents. While GPOs rely on an inflexible, centralized system that compels hospitals to commit to purchasing contracts, IDNs rely on a flexible, decentralized system that customizes purchasing arrangements for their hospitals.

The case for acting as one's own GPO seems the stronger of the two. IDNs see many financial incentives to contract by themselves.

First, there is the lure of getting better prices than those obtained by GPOs, especially from smaller or regional vendors not on GPO national contracts. Second, these price discounts may serve as a source of cash flows that are hard to generate elsewhere and can be invested for developing strategic advantage. Moreover, such discounts may not be quickly competed away in other GPO contracting since the IDNs are small and local. Some have suggested that the savings from self-contracting may also provide sufficient "glue" to cement together burgeoning hospital networks and enable them to survive and grow.[42] The number of IDNs with the capability to act as their own GPOs may also be large. According to SMG Marketing Group, by April 2000, 416 multihospital systems qualified as GPOs by virtue of being able to negotiate contracts for joint purchasing, as did 334 IDNs (57 percent of total IDNs), an increase from 216 in 1995.[43] Moreover, 499 out of 599 IDNs in their spring 2001 database indicated they have "integrated purchasing (contracting) among any of their member facilities."[44]

The case for self-distribution is not so clear-cut. Some recent survey data suggest that the self-distribution wave may have crested. In a survey of 361 hospital pharmacists and materials management executives, an astounding 40 percent reported they currently do self-distribution; of the 60 percent that currently use distributors, only 2 percent said they planned to self-distribute in the future. The major barrier reported here were the capital costs involved.[45] Another study of four hospitals compared the cost of procurement in hospitals operating their own warehouse with hospitals relying on medical-surgical distributors. Those pursuing self-distribution incurred 33–40 percent higher procurement costs per bed.[46]

Moreover, there are some shortcomings in the self-distribution movement among IDNs that may yet suggest the need for a distributor partner. Presbyterian Health System in Albuquerque created its own distribution company in the mid-1980s—accumulating 6,000 product lines in a 40,000-square-foot building—to service its own hospital system and nonsystem entities. The system had no problem getting the right product to the right place at the right time—the avowed goal of distribution. However, what it lacked was data on product utilization after products reached the nursing floor. Thus, it could not understand utilization and could not pursue standardization. These proved to be two big areas for cost containment in a market that had become heavily penetrated by managed care. Since Presbyterian lacked the time, skills, and infrastructure needed to tackle these issues, it partnered with McKesson/HBOC Medical Group to gather the data using the latter's bar-code technology, and thereby track medical supply usage and facilitate electronic order replenishment.

One executive posed an interesting question in discussing the issue of self-distribution. He asked, "What difference does it make if a hospital gets one truckload of fifty pallets from a distributor, or if it gets fifty deliveries of one pallet each direct from the manufacturers?" Another executive answered in this manner:

> If you use the distributor, there is one purchase order and one invoice for many, many items. So there is a huge savings there in terms of accounts payable and receivable. You are also rationalizing the number of supplies you have to deal with and everybody agrees that is a good thing. All those direct shipments from manufacturers may allow a little more price flexibility, but then you have got to negotiate pricing with all those manufacturers, and that is not static; it is dynamic, and you don't have anyone helping you with that. So you need to have people doing this stuff for you and that costs money. Also, the distributor's margin of 4 percent is not a lot of money for the value of one truck, one invoice, and one customer service center to follow up on questions like Where's the order?, Why is it back ordered?, etcetera. Finally, if you get all these things direct-ship

from manufacturers, and you don't have a relationship with a few of those guys [FedEx or UPS] with prenegotiated per-pound charge or whatever, there is an upside there that has to be tackled.

Regardless of the arguments, IDNs need to conduct their own make-versus-buy analyses before deciding whether or not to vertically integrate into one or both of these intermediary functions.[47] Indeed, the make-buy decision is often referred to as the classic issue in strategy. What are the relevant considerations here? First and foremost, IDNs need to compare the savings from self-contracting (for example, reduction in vendor prices and elimination of GPO membership fees) with the costs of acting as their own GPO. Such costs are incurred not only today but also into the future as contracts are monitored and come up for renegotiation. Thus, any cost savings gleaned from negotiating better contracts today may get swamped by future expenditures in monitoring and negotiating contracts for thousands of items after contracts expire. Data gathered in some of Novation's studies (see Chapter Four) suggest the number of man-hours involved here. Novation executives also claim that it costs them an average of $25,000 to execute a contract. While Novation can spread this cost across 1,800 members to achieve a low per-hospital cost, the individual hospital member cannot. Novation estimates the cost of executing a comparable contract by the hospital to be as much as $4,000.

There are several other considerations in the make-versus-buy decision. IDNs need to assess whether the level of savings is sufficient to warrant efforts to standardize vendor and product choice, whether physicians are willing to alter their preferences, and whether purchasing and materials management executives are capable of leading this transformation. IDNs need to consider the value added of other GPO services beyond group purchasing (for example, consulting, benchmarking, insurance, and technology assessment) and whether such services can be obtained elsewhere. IDNs should consider whether the products they want to acquire directly are available from second-tier suppliers willing to grant the price discounts sought. IDNs need to assess just how many products for which they can self-contract to achieve the promised cost savings and what volume they can drive over those selected products. GPOs claim that such savings are tiny compared to the savings they can generate with lower price discounts but much greater product volumes. Finally, IDNs need to assess the advantages of self-contracting that extend beyond group purchasing, such as the enhanced ability to contract locally with payers on more favorable terms. Alternatively, IDNs should consider whether their contractual arrangements infringe on member hospital autonomy and local control.[48,49]

For both strategies, a key variable will be the degree to which member hospitals within the IDN are in geographic proximity. Research strongly suggests that geographic concentration of facilities enables hospitals to successfully engage in consolidation strategies ranging from mergers to clinical integration.[50] The other key variable is the ability to pursue SKU consolidation and standardization activities.

Finally, IDNs should consider ways to have the best of both worlds: (1) to use their current GPO or distributor to achieve economies of scale and access their capabilities, and (2) to employ self-contracting and self-distribution that promotes IDN flexibility and advantage. How might this be accomplished? IDNs might seek to utilize their GPO membership and contracts for the commodity items that are over 40 percent of purchases, and then utilize self-contracting strategies for a portion of the remainder (for example, high-cost physician preference items) where the IDN may have an advantage over the GPO in driving standardization. In the same vein, IDNs might commit to using the GPO's contracts on a highly compliant basis in exchange for the GPO agreeing to leverage deals with vendors for noncontract items. Finally, rather than complete self-distribution, IDNs might maintain their own centralized warehouses and yet outsource the management and logistics functions to their distributor partners.

Endnotes

1. Buttrick, Brian. "Big Savings Can Come in Small Packages." *Hospital Materials Management* 25(11) (2000): 15.

2. Cespedes, Frank, and Kasturi Rangan. *Becton Dickinson and Company: VACUTAINER Systems Division.* HBS Case 9-592-037. Boston, Massachusetts: Harvard Business School, 1991.

3. Marino, Anthony P., and David J. Edwards. "Give Logistics Its Own Place in the Price Equation." *Hospital Materials Management* 24(5) (2000): 10–11.

4. Thill, Mark. "Where Have the 3PLs Gone?" *Repertoire* 7(9) (1999): 58.

5. Consedine, Tom. "Melding Supply Chain Links." *Repertoire* 8(8) (2000): 26.

6. McFadden, Christopher D., and Timothy M. Leahy. *U.S. Healthcare Distribution: Positioning the Healthcare Supply Chain for the 21st Century.* New York: Goldman Sachs, 2000.

7. Fein, Adam. *Macro Shock: How Wholesale Distribution Industries Are Being Revolutionized.* New York: Lehman Brothers, 1999.

8. Marhula, Daren C., and Edward G. Shannon. *EHealth B2B Overview.* Minneapolis, Minnesota: U.S. Bancorp Piper Jaffray, 2000.

9. Egger, Ed. "Tenet, Columbia/HCA Invest in Online Procurement Companies." *Health Care Strategic Management* 18(2) (2000): 10–11.

10. Temkin et al. *Distribution Reconsidered.* www.forrester.com, 1999.

11. Narayanan, V. G. *Owens & Minor, Inc. (A) and (B).* Case # 9-100-055. Boston, Massachusetts: Harvard Business School, 2000.

12. Thill, Mark. "Minor Miracle." *Repertoire* 8(10) (2000): 8, 10–11.

13. Fein, Adam J. *Leaning on the Promise: Online Exchanges, Channel Evolution, and Health Care Distribution.* New York: Lehman Brothers, June 1, 2000.

14. Ibid.

15. McFadden, Christopher D., and Timothy Leahy. "U.S. Healthcare Distribution: Overview Comments." Presentation to the Wharton School. December 7, 2000.

16. Repertoire. "Distributors Remain the Low-Cost Solution." *Repertoire* 8(4) (2000): 36–37.

17. Savas, Stephen D., and Jordan S. Kanfer. *Connectivity/EDI.* New York: Goldman Sachs, 2000.

18. See Note Eight.

19. Everard, Lynn J. *Blueprint for an Efficient Health Care Supply Chain.* White Paper. Norcross, Georgia: Medical Distribution Solutions, 2000.

20. See Note Seventeen.

21. Boehm et al. *Sizing Healthcare eCommerce.* www.forrester.com, 1999.

22. Millennium Research Group. *Online Opportunities in the Medical Products Marketplace.* Stream 1, Issue 1. (July 2000). Toronto: Millennium Research Group.

23. WEDI. *The 1993 WEDI Report*. Workgroup for Electronic Data Interchange (October 1993).

24. See Note Twenty-One.

25. McFadden, Christopher D., and Timothy Leahy. *E-Distribution Update and Survey Results*. New York: Goldman Sachs (March 10, 2000).

26. Healthcare Business. "Reinventing the Health Care Supply Chain." *Healthcare Business* Special Supplement (June 2000).

27. See Note Twenty-Five.

28. W. Daniel Garretson et al. *Redefining B2B Channel Roles*. www.forrester.com (2000).

29. See Note Twenty-Five.

30. See Note Fifteen.

31. McFadden, Christopher D., and Timothy M. Leahy. *Cardinal Health Inc.* New York: Goldman Sachs, 2000.

32. See Note Eight.

33. Hughes, Jon, Ralf, Mark, and Bill Michels. *Transform Your Supply Chain: Releasing Value in Business*. Boston: International Thomson Business Press, 1998.

34. Hensley, Scott. "Materials Management: Going It Together: Four Florida Hospitals Find Success with Direct-Purchasing Cooperative." *Modern Healthcare*. June 22, 1998, p. 35.

35. Hospital Materials Management. "Florida Hospitals Form Mini-GPO by Joining Purchasing Operations without Merging." *Hospital Materials Management* 23(12) (December 1998): 8.

36. Foulke, Joanne. "Bypassing the Traditional GPO—An Alternative Approach to Purchasing and Distribution." Presentation to Strategic Sourcing and E-Commerce Solutions for the Med-Surg Supply Chain. Philadelphia, Pennsylvania: October 28, 1999.

37. Healthcare Cost Reengineering Report. "Hospital System Creates Compelling Alternative to GPO." *Healthcare Cost Reengineering Report* 3(12) (1998): 177–181.

38. Reed, Stephen G. "Supply Center to Serve Hospitals: Sarasota Memorial and Lee Memorial Are Opening Distribution Center to Save Money." *Sarasota Herald-Tribune*. September 18, 1998.

39. Hospital Materials Management. "Kentucky Hospitals Share Distribution Center Under New Outsource Agreement." *Hospital Materials Management* 24(5) (1999): 3.

40. Hospital Materials Management. "Shared Distribution Center Lets Hospitals Deal Directly with Vendor, Save on Fees." *Hospital Materials Management* 24(1) (January 1999): 5.

41. See Note Thirty-Eight.
42. Appel, Gary. "Integrated Delivery Systems Purchase More Competitively." *The Business Word* (January 8, 1998). The Health Care News Service.
43. SMG Marketing Group. *Multi-Hospital System (MHS) and Group Purchasing Organizations (GPOs): 2000 Report and Directory*. Chicago: SMG Solutions, 2000.
44. SGM Marketing Group. Personal Communication. From Lisa Garavaglia, 2001.
45. McFadden et al. *Hospital Executive Survey*. New York: Goldman Sachs, 2000.
46. Integrated Cost Management Systems. *Hospital Procurement Processes*. Arlington, Texas: ICMS, 2001.
47. Wall Street analysts suggest the following criteria in making the make-versus-buy decision: the size of the market, salience of product obsolescence, number of alternatives, the number of customers and drop-off points, number of deliveries, customer preferences regarding deliveries, product carrying costs, transportation costs of delivery, and use of nonclinician buyers. If these factors are "high," then the recommendation is to "buy" rather than make. Marsh, Lawrence, Feinstein, Adam, and Joshua Raskin. *HealthCare Information Technology and Outsourcing/Distribution Guidebook*. New York: Lehman Brothers, 2000.
48. Appel, Gary. "The IDN/GPO Relationship." *The Health Strategist* 6(6) (1999): 1–5.
49. Smith, Charlie R. "Determining When Integrated Delivery Systems Should Belong to GPOs." *Healthcare Financial Management* 52(9) (1998): 38.
50. Shortell et al. *Remaking Health Care in America*. San Francisco: Jossey-Bass, 1996.

Part III

· ·

The Manufacturers

7

· ·

Pharmaceutical Manufacturers

Lawton R. Burns and Patricia M. Danzon

Introduction

Pharmaceutical products represent one of the major categories of health care costs. In 1999, retail prescription drugs accounted for $99.6 billion, or 8.2 percent of national health expenditures.[1] These figures do not include drugs sold through institutional settings like hospitals, which are estimated to account for 25 percent of total pharmaceutical sales and 10–15 percent of prescription drug costs.[2,3] As noted in Chapter Three, IDN drug costs consume 15–23 percent of total contracted supply expenditures and total an estimated $13–15 billion annually. Taken together, total pharmaceutical sales for 1999 are estimated to be roughly $122 billion.[4]

Not only are the costs high, they are also rising quickly. As a percentage of total expenditures, retail drug costs have been increasing much faster than other components of health care, rising 16.9 percent between 1998 and 1999, from 7.4 percent to 8.2 percent of total spending.[5] Drug sales in the United States have also been growing faster than gross domestic product.[6] A primary driver of this increase is increased unit sales of drugs, which itself is due to the substitution of drug therapy for other therapies, the aging of the population, the introduction of new products and new product formulations, and the changing mix of available products being used.[7]

Rising drug costs have attracted a lot of attention from the payers and providers of health care, as well as from their purchasing agents: the HMOs acting on behalf of employers and government, and the GPOs acting on behalf of hospital systems. Buyers and their agents have consolidated and become more aggressive purchasers of these products.

These pressures have challenged the pharmaceutical manufacturers at a time of great change within their industry. Since the 1980s, several major features of the industry's structure have changed, engendering greater competition.

Generic drug manufacturers have grown in prominence, and by 1998 accounted for 45 percent of drug units sold (but only 19 percent of revenues).[8] Their ascendance is due to the Waxman-Hatch Act of 1984 (Drug Price Competition and Patent Term Restoration Act) that exempted generic drugs from clinical trials, and virtually eliminated the period between patent expiration and the market entry of generic competitors. Generics have also grown due to Medicaid's and HMOs' refusal to pay for more than the price of a generic, leaving patients to pay the additional cost to get branded drugs.

At the same time, the industry has been consolidating. Between 1990 and 1999, the top four pharmaceutical (pharma) firms grew their combined worldwide market share from 14 to 22 percent, the top eight firms grew their share from 24 to 38 percent, and the top thirty grew their share from 57 to 70 percent.[9] Similar figures hold for the U.S. market, which accounts for the largest portion of the worldwide market.[10] Normally, consolidation might reduce rivalry in an industry. However, in pharma, no one firm has more than a 7 percent market share worldwide. Moreover, as a result of the horizontal combinations, different firms are likely to have product portfolios that overlap with one another.

The expiration of patents of many blockbuster drugs introduced in the 1980s and 1990s has increased marketing competition, and given firms incentive to develop close therapeutic substitutes or generic versions of each other's drugs. The result is pervasive therapeutic and generic drug competition.

Finally, the rise of over-the-counter (OTC) medications offered a lower-priced alternative to branded drugs. OTC medications were subject to less expensive and less time-intensive FDA approval, and fewer FDA restrictions on their advertising. Their appeal to HMOs induced many large pharmaceutical firms to enter the OTC market and produce less potent versions of their branded drugs.[11]

Pharmaceutical firms compete in over twenty different therapeutic categories. The sale of pharmaceutical products varies across these categories. In 1999, the top therapeutic classes (based on sales) in the United States were central nervous system disorders (23.1 percent); neoplasms, endocine system, and metabolic disease (19.7 percent); cardiovascular system (19 percent); digestive and genito-urinary system (13.9 percent); respiratory system (11.1 percent); and infective and parasitic diseases (11 percent).[12] Drugs sold to hospitals tend to address a slightly different mix of therapeutic areas. The top drugs sold in hospitals are used to treat clinical conditions such as anemia, bacterial infections, neutropenia, deep vein thrombosis, and ovarian cancer, as well as support various procedures such as stents and balloon angioplasty.[13]

The foregoing analysis suggests several important points. First, the hospital trade is only one market served by pharma and certainly not the largest. Second, the drugs sold to the hospital trade differ somewhat from drugs sold to other market segments (such as pharmacies or the alternate site market). There can be overlap between hospital inpatient and outpatient markets, and between hospitals and specialty physician clinics (such as oncology). Third, pharmaceutical firms compete within therapeutic areas; firms tend to dominate in one area or another based on their development of a blockbuster drug. Indeed, the market concentration (share of prescriptions sold by the top four firms) in therapeutic areas tends to be quite high. Fourth, the pharmaceutical firm's competitors in one therapeutic area are not likely to be the same across all areas. As a result, any sample of pharmaceutical firms (such as the one used in this study) provides a limited perspective on the pharmaceutical market and supply chain.

This chapter analyzes the role of pharmaceutical firms within that portion of the health care supply chain that manufactures, purchases, and distributes drugs to the hospital market. We begin first with a short description of the organization of the pharmaceutical firm that is oriented to this portion of the market. We then describe how one large pharmaceutical firm contracts with other supply chain participants (for example, GPOs, distributors, and hospitals) for the launch of a new drug. We then analyze in detail several important topics in the sale and distribution of pharmaceutical products to the hospital market. These include (1) the differences between branded versus generic drugs in manufacturer-GPO contracting, and thus the importance of product innovation in this contracting process; (2) the tension in this contracting between cost versus quality and total cost; (3) who is the customer; and (4) the role of the hospital or IDN and its understanding of pharmaceutical products.[14]

Sales and Marketing Organization of Pharmaceutical Firms

Sales and marketing account for a large portion of the pharmaceutical firm's cost structure, estimated as high as 30 percent of sales in the early 1990s.[15] The marketing function is typically concerned with the firm's patented brands and their promotion (for example, advertising), while the sales function is concerned with the firm's sales representatives (drug detailers) who call on major accounts. A pharmaceutical firm will typically have hundreds of organized customers spanning the supply chain: federal and state governments, employers, HMOs, pharmacy benefit managers (PBMs), hospital systems and large medical centers, GPOs, drugstore chains, behavioral health organizations, home health organizations, and wholesalers. The sales staff will also call on individual physicians in hospitals and in their offices. The number of sales representatives has grown dramatically due to the number of new products introduced over the past few years and an increased emphasis on marketing competition.

Within their sales organization, pharmaceutical firms often seek to separate the business functions (such as contracting and negotiations) from the clinical functions (such as relaying information on product safety and efficacy). This is done for three reasons: to maximize the amount of clinical contact time between their detailers and physicians, to develop the economic case for their drugs among customers, and to provide sales representatives with a single point of contact within the firm to resolve business issues. To accomplish this, they often appoint account managers for their large organized customers (for example, a single manager or a national team of account managers for larger GPOs operating in different regions) that seek to represent all of the firm's brands as "one face" to the customer. They seek to market the firms' products at each account by "accessing thought leaders, those people who help make the decisions regarding formulary contracting and the availability of our products." These managers also seek to coordinate their efforts with the managers and teams promoting individual drug brands to "clinical thought leaders," as well as with the district managers for sales representatives serving those accounts.

Sales and marketing thus operate in a matrix structure. Certain sales individuals focus on specific customer accounts, while certain marketing personnel focus on specific brands and clinical products—with a defined corporate entity to integrate them. This

entity is viewed as a solution to the growing complexity and differentiation in the firm's products and customer base. As part of this
matrix, pricing and contracts are developed on a consensual basis
between the account managers and the brand teams.[16]

The sales function works differently for branded items versus
generics. The customer for the branded items is typically the specialty physician in the relevant therapeutic area (for example,
oncologist for a cancer drug or cardiologist for a heart disease drug).
Sales representatives deal directly with these specialists to build
acceptance for the drug and gain physician support for its being
placed on the hospital formulary. For generics (for example, brands
that have gone off patent), on the other hand, the sales organization
deals more with the GPOs and other organized buying agents
in negotiating terms for a portfolio of such products. The two
parts of the sales organization come together at certain times, such
as when the firm's patented brand drug faces competition from new
competitors in its therapeutic area that may be cheaper in price.
Faced with lower-cost alternatives and administrative pressure
to reduce spending, physicians and/or their purchasing managers
may request price discounts or more value from the contracts to
justify paying a higher price for the firm's drug. The account managers try to lend support to the sales representatives by helping to
make a combined clinical and business case for the firm's drug. This
case is often based on the drug's "total cost" (see the following).

Illustration of Manufacturer, GPO, and Distributor Contracting Process

Pharmaceutical firms estimate that 90 percent of their products to
the institutional market go through distributors. The Pharmaceutical Research and Manufacturers of America estimate that only
2 percent of drug sales are made directly to hospitals.[17] One major
exception here are vaccines, which manufacturers ship directly to
physician offices and thus maintain some infrastructure for direct

purchasing. These firms also estimate that 80 percent of their products to the institutional market are negotiated with GPOs; there are a handful of contracts with individual provider organizations that can "perform at the same level as GPOs." To the extent that the pharmaceutical company's portfolio includes a lot of products going to the institutional market, GPOs are an important set of buyers.

In the past, pharmaceutical firms dealt with GPOs using a bidding process and short-term contracts. Today, there are more long-term contracts and reportedly more partnering arrangements based on shared vision and goals and willingness to work together beyond contract price to help the profitability of each other's business. In practice, this can mean GPO efforts to move market share and increase compliance, integrate information across their membership, understand how their providers use the pharmaceutical firm's products, and communicate to their providers. Pharmaceutical executives emphasize the importance of GPOs that inform providers who their GPO is; what firms the GPO has contracted with; and what products they are using, and with what clinical results. They also value GPOs that emphasize care management as much or more than cost management. They would also value GPOs that can transmit vendor and product information to providers in ways that support the efforts of sales representatives.

Nevertheless, due to the overlap in the product portfolios of pharmaceutical firms, GPOs often pit one manufacturer against another at contract negotiating time: "We are all getting large. Our portfolio is broad. Most of us have something that somebody else has that is similar. It is pretty easy for any GPO to say, I don't need you—I can get everything you have even if it's from eight different vendors. Mostly that is what the contract negotiation is to a point—pitting one against the other. That is just the nature of the business."

How do these negotiations proceed? Do GPOs seek preferential pricing from the pharmaceutical firm in exchange for exclusivity in contracting? There is no simple answer to this question. The answer varies by therapeutic area and by contract. Most of the major GPOs contract with most of the large manufacturers in some way. GPOs that succeed in obtaining preferential pricing have to document control; that is, the ability to perform at certain levels, typically in terms of market share and compliance.[18] GPO size can also be an important, but secondary, factor in terms of negotiating discounts and rebates. For the same level of control, larger customers get better pricing; for different levels of control, the customer with the higher level gets better pricing even if it is smaller in size. A GPO can end up contracting with more than one pharmaceutical firm in a given therapeutic area if the vendors differ in their contract requirements for control and the GPO can satisfy both sets. A variety of contracts can develop based on what GPOs can deliver to vendors and what vendors are willing to negotiate on.

Some of the pharmaceutical manufacturers now rely on their matrixed sales or marketing organization to help in these negotiations with GPOs. In the past, when confronted with GPO demands for lower price or greater value, some account managers who were promoted from the ranks of sales representatives tended to "try to keep everybody happy, buy them a cup of coffee, and try to solve the GPO's problem." Instead, the new contracting entity seeks to take a "more honest approach with GPOs—push back more, ask them where we win in this deal, call their bluff, and ask how we can increase shareholder value for both companies."

After the contract is signed, the GPO notifies its institutional members about the contract terms and pricing. At the same time, the manufacturer publicizes the contract to its sales representatives, who then contact providers within these accounts to convey the news about the contract with their GPO and ascertain what they need to do to make the contracted drug available to patients. Some hospitals do not permit the sales representative to discuss a product unless it is on contract and GPO formulary; others do not have such rules. In the latter case, the representative's job is often to build up awareness of the drug among providers and build demand for the GPO to have the drug on formulary and contract for it. In general, according to one executive, "The representative's plan of action (POA) is to get formulary approval, and acceptance and availability for that product to be marketed and dispensed within that institution." To the extent that the GPO has one formulary that all member hospitals adopt (rather than design their own), the manufacturer has less leverage.

As noted earlier (see Chapter Four), GPOs select the distributors that their members will utilize. For their part, pharmaceutical manufacturers contract with all distributors to help increase the penetration of the products into the market. Pharmaceutical manufacturers look to distributors for assistance primarily in the areas of pick, pack, and ship. They are viewed as "efficient order takers," efficient distribution points for bulk shipping that reduce the number of customers to be served, and proficient at multiple deliveries and just-in-time delivery. Especially with new products, manufacturers want to get their products to market quickly and have sufficient quantities to aid product launch and reach as many customer outlets as possible. They therefore contract with virtually all drug wholesalers and eschew exclusive contracts.

In general, wholesalers perform a commodity-type service that is a "nondescript part" of the manufacturer's business. In the market for branded drugs, wholesalers exert little influence on customer demand, and thus the manufacturer's business, since the products are "pulled" by clinicians rather than "pushed" by the distributors. While distributors might wish to act like PBMs and exert influence over what drugs are ordered, they lack a scientific base for rationalizing such decisions and thus would encounter strong physician opposition. As a result, distribution is not an important topic to sales executives in pharmaceutical firms concerned with branded drugs. Moreover, they are not concerned with the topic of "supply chain management," since they frequently equate this with product distribution.

Branded Versus Generic Drugs

The GPO's influence over the pharmaceutical manufacturer varies by type of product. For branded items where the manufacturer has the only drug candidate in that therapeutic area, the GPO and manufacturer negotiate a single-source agreement. While such drugs can be very expensive, the GPO will accede to the manufacturer's price when physicians within their member institutions want it. As one GPO executive explained, "There is nothing you can do as a GPO. If you look at the drugs that we spend the most money on, you can't get contracts for those because they are branded and the price is what the price is, and the suppliers don't care." A pharmaceutical executive put the issue differently: "Basically, what it all comes down to in our contracting is medicine wins first. Regardless of what the situation is, medicine wins first. The best product wins."

In such situations, GPOs may ask to work with the manufacturer on price, but the manufacturer states it makes no sense to them to discount their product. Instead, to manage the product's expense, the manufacturer and GPO will work together to educate providers on how and where the drug should or should not be used. For example, GPOs may develop incentive programs for their members to use the product in the appropriate way and on a committed purchasing basis. They may also develop clinical protocol programs and treatment algorithms, prepare and distribute "white papers" on appropriateness to providers, and work with the manufacturer on pharmaco-economic issues. In this manner, the GPO supports the new product from both a financial as well as clinical standpoint. For pharmaceutical manufacturers with strong brand positions, GPOs are not an important intermediary. Instead, manufacturers view their importance as an information channel to help them influence physician decision making.

Relationships between the manufacturer and GPO become more interesting when additional branded drugs enter the market in that therapeutic area (therapeutic competition or "fast followers"). This is where negotiations become more pronounced and filled with threats of walking away from the table ("We're going to switch to your competitor.") This may be particularly true when the newer brands are much lower in price. The Lilly-Centocor drug *Reopro,* for example, is a monoclonal biologic product that cost $1,300–1,500 per patient; the therapeutic competitor subsequently introduced by a competitor cost only $400 but was "less efficacious" (according to Lilly, it required more follow-up visits and had higher patient mortality). The higher-cost drug, especially if it accounts for a large percentage of the hospital's drug expenditures, becomes a target. The contracting equation now has to balance cost with other product benefits. The manufacturer of the initial, higher-cost product seeks to educate or persuade GPOs that its product justifies the higher cost in terms of its clinical profile and capability to treat the disease better than other drugs (for example, it offers a "death benefit" in terms of lower patient mortality and greater efficacy). Sometimes the GPO will go back and talk to clinicians in their member hospitals to determine if they perceive the same benefits touted by the manufacturer. If clinicians do recognize these benefits and prefer the higher-cost product, the GPO may still contract with that vendor.

Finally, as branded drugs go off patent, they are faced with lots of generic competitors and lower product prices. The latter enter the market at prices 40–70 percent of the market leader, whose price may remain unchanged. However, generics typically capture 50 percent of sales within six months after patent expiration. Generic drugs are typically purchased by GPOs as part of a multi-source arrangement with several vendors. Relationships with GPOs regarding generics tend to be less face-to-face and more based on telephone calls and occasional visits "to see how things are going." Drug manufacturers acknowledge that they may not be as good in dealing with GPOs on the generic side as on the patented side, since they have less experience and leverage here.

Compared to the branded drugs, generics fall off the radar screen of drug manufacturers a bit. "We have no sales representatives running around promoting them. They show up on our sales sheets and we track them, but really at the end of the day it's kind of a below-profile product because the dollars just shrivel." This does not mean that generics are unimportant to manufacturers. As noted previously, the rise of the generic drug market has induced some drug manufacturers to enter. However, most brand manufacturers have given up trying to enter this market in the United States. They continue to sell their branded products (in competition with the generics) to the shrinking "brand loyal" segment, but do not promote them because pharmacists are legally authorized to substitute unless the physician indicates "dispense the brand."

The large GPOs help with product push for generic drugs by simplifying the sales effort to thousands of hospitals: "If you are dealing with commodities, the large GPOs are usually pretty helpful because you have only one place to go for a contract." They also have much greater ability to deliver high compliance on commodity items and to switch market shares for a generic drug since clinicians do not have to be consulted. Finally, as drugs face therapeutic competitors entering the market, or go off patent, the manufacturer has to work with both the sales force and the GPO to transition the contracting relationship from one based heavily on value to one based more on price.

Thus, as their products—both branded and generic—become more multisource (that is, as there are molecules with several manufacturers), manufacturers are forced to work more with the GPOs. Their avowed strategy is to have a continuous stream of innovative and sole-source products that clinicians want, and thus lower the barriers to entry in the hospital market. They explicitly state that GPOs do not drive drug sales but rather can be a barrier or nuisance factor for them. One barrier they pose is counter detailing; that is, disseminating publications that tout the advantages of competitors' products. They thus try to work with the GPOs and "try not to inflame them." The goal here is to keep the negotiations focused on more than just price (for example, marketing attributes of the products).

We should note that these bargaining relationships are also shaped by personalities of the CEOs, organizational learning, and dramatic events at each party. One manufacturer noted it had no dealings with one large GPO due to "bad blood" between their CEOs in the past. Learning also plays a role in negotiations, as parties demonstrate what each can deliver through their contracts. Another mentioned the increasing uncertainty about how to deal with Columbia/HCA after the latter's implication in a Medicare fraud and abuse investigation. "Some Columbia managers (for example, in materials management) may continue to be focused on price, while their clinical staff may argue the best path for them is to emphasize quality and thus the best drugs on the market."

Manufacturer-GPO bargaining situations can resemble a "game of chicken" in which each side threatens to walk away from the relationship. In essence, each side tells the other, You need us more than we need you. The pharmaceutical manufacturer can prevail in such situations to the extent that it is the market leader. One executive said

> Where the relationship always sours is when it is all price. A great example is [GPO X]. They come in with some astronomical "Give me this price or else." Well, we look at them and say you have got to be kidding. Very quickly you know you have an antagonistic relationship. Either side can walk. You might take the position that if [GPO X] wants to walk, it is at their own peril. They would probably say the same thing about us. But, a real interesting piece of working with GPOs is that we know we can still have a relationship with their individual hospitals. So if we cannot go in the front door, we will go in the back door. What you find is that each of their hospitals has their own set of needs, metrics, and responsibilities—regardless of whether they are all in the same GPO or owned. Moreover, the clinicians are not always centered the same way, and they have their own beliefs regarding what is proper medical care.

Thus, manufacturers state they do not need the GPO's permission to access their hospitals. Indeed, oftentimes they will negotiate deals with large IDNs that are better than the deals negotiated by their GPO. These deals may be prompted by financial problems at the provider system, often when HMOs press them for discounts. One executive described the scenario this way:

> The classic case is the hospital having some kind of financial issue. Obviously, the first place they always go and swing the axe is in pharmacy, and the pharmacist gets yelled at by the materials management people or some CFO who says, We need to cut X million dollars out of our pharmacy budget. They find it where they can, and they usually look at the top five drugs used in the hospital. We [the drug manufacturer] then get called on the carpet and into the hospital we go.

The manufacturer is willing to negotiate a more aggressive deal with the IDN member because, "While the GPOs preach a big game of being able to drive share, at the end of the day it is really the individual hospital that drives share." It may also be the case that the member designs and implements the formulary.

Pharmaceutical manufacturers thus believe the competition between rival drugs is played out more at the IDN and hospital level than at the GPO level. Moreover, the larger IDNs are often shareholders in the GPOs and use their GPOs when it is to their convenience, but feel free to cut their own deals with manufacturers ("What are they going to do, kick me out of the group? I own it. They need me more than I need them."). In fact, they tell vendors "We better not find out that you give our GPO a better deal than what we get here at our IDN." At the same time, vendors rely on these IDNs for discretion in not divulging the contracts and terms to either their GPO or other IDNs. "For the most part, the IDN is gentlemanly enough to realize you are trying to work with them, so they are not going to go back to their GPO and tell them the details. They know if they did that, nobody will deal with them anymore." Of course, the manufacturer's willingness to go beyond the GPO contract may depend on the size of the IDN or GPO member that is seeking the additional discount. Pharmaceutical executives state that they don't necessarily want to jeopardize a total GPO contract for just one system.

Product Cost Versus Total Cost

Pharmaceutical executives believe that the current emphasis on cost containment poses an enormous barrier to the sales of their branded drugs. At the hospital level, pharmacy directors, materials managers, and CFOs are pressured to "deliver here and now on the bottom line." One executive said

> They are more concerned with making it through the next budget cut rather than trying to demonstrate value in their department's services.
>
> They pay lip service to the importance of new products, getting product information into the hands of clinicians, driving clinical protocols, studying outcomes, etcetera, and there may be a cursory discussion around these things. But it does not come to fruition because it gets lost in the day-to-day pressures to deliver a number.

Hospital executives are thus incentivized on a different set of metrics than are the pharmaceutical firms. Hospital executives are measured and rewarded for reducing costs (for example, in specific contracts or line items) while pharmaceutical firms are looking to increase their market share and product sales. They do this largely through the development of innovative products that add value to patients and their physicians. They acknowledge that their new products are expensive and add costs to hospital systems. However, they argue that they treat previously unmet needs, treat diseases in new ways that improve the patient's quality of life, or substitute for more expensive services such as hospitalization. Thus, taking these factors into account, the pharmaceutical firms argue that their new products frequently contribute to lower total costs.

Despite pressures for short-term cost reductions, pharmaceutical executives mention several facilitators to disseminating the "total cost" message to GPOs and their hospital members. First, the message is reportedly more effective in some managed care markets (such as full-risk capitation) than in others (such as heavily discounted fee-for-service). Despite this assertion, these firms do not believe that risk contracts with hospitals have been successful. Second, the message is more warmly received by some GPOs and IDNs than by others. Executives state that they strike better partnerships with systems oriented to care management and quality rather than just cost management. Such systems may be those that are able to capture their data and understand both their costs and outcomes. They often point to leading IDNs such as Intermountain to illustrate this clinical orientation to provide the best patient care. They also fare well in IDNs where the director of pharmacy reports to a clinical executive (who has a better understanding of pharmaceuticals) rather than someone in finance. Finance executives tend to "view pharmacy as a bucket of expense within the institution and often fail to compare the value of that bucket of expense with other buckets." Pharmaceutical executives state they also strike better partnerships with providers that are oriented to making process improvements based on utilization and outcomes data, and that are seeking to compete in their local markets based on a quality advantage. Such providers have a corporate philosophy of "being at cutting edge of delivering the best patient care." Third, the total cost message is more warmly received by visionary CEOs, visionary directors of materials management, and systems where these directors of pharmacy and materials management executives have the CEO's ear.

Who Is the Customer?

Pharmaceutical firms recognize four broad classes of customers that they deal with: the payer (insurance company), the buyer (selects the product), the consumer (the patient), and the dispenser (the pharmacy). For branded items, pharmaceutical firms clearly see the physician as their key buyer. Clinicians pull their products through the supply chain, based on their own or their patients' preferences, rather than distributors and GPOs pushing them. For generic items, the GPOs may be the more important set of buyers.

As with medical device firms, pharmaceutical firms maintain direct, continuing contact with physicians through their sales representatives out in the field. They call on physicians in their offices and, for drugs used in procedures such as cardiac catheterizations, follow the physician into the cardiac cath lab. The customer is thus not just the specialty physician in the particular therapeutic area (such as the clinical cardiologist), but also interventional cardiologists in the cath lab, physicians in the emergency room, and other specialists (such as cardiovascular surgeons) who treat cardiac patients. Besides physicians, other customers include nurses and clinical pharmacists. Nonclinicians may also be customers when there are issues regarding price or where there is direct contracting between the pharmaceutical firm and the IDN without a GPO intermediary. In such cases, the customer can be administrators and directors of pharmacy and materials management. Finally, pharmaceutical firms recognize that the Health Care Financing Administration (HCFA) is a customer based on its prominence as a payer.

The Role of IDNs

Pharmaceutical firms view IDNs in slightly different ways than do other players along the health care supply chain. For them, standardization of activity can have both positive and negative aspects. On the one hand, pharmaceutical firms like to see GPOs and their member IDNs have certain standardized features, such as contracting compliance, communication of new product and contract information to hospital members, data collection and reporting, the development of care practices and protocols, and other similar means of "managing their institutions in a consistent way that makes it easier for [pharma] to do business with them."

Moreover, they see opportunities for improved sales and utilization of their products among hospitals that belong to systems. For example, Eli Lilly's drug *ReoPro* had traditionally been used in the central cardiac cath lab of the flagship hospital of a local IDN. However, they noticed that their drug was also being used in conjunction with another drug to treat heart attack victims in the IDN's outlying hospitals. The value of an integrated system to them is when the system as a whole buys and stocks their drug in all of their facilities, and also helps to define the protocols for the drug's proper use. In addition, they value a hospital system with a good communications network (for example, Internet linkages and satellite video conferencing) that can allow them to access the system's hospitals and clinicians quickly and make joint presentations about their products, as opposed to reaching each facility individually. According to one pharmaceutical executive, "all of the decision makers are in one place at one time, you know you have compliance across the board, and all of the issues are worked out right there on the spot."

On the other hand, standardization of activity is sometimes synonymous with commoditization of products and services. Thus, pharmaceutical firms prefer to see purchases driven by clinical preferences expressed in the patient-physician relationship and aggregated up to the hospital and GPO level, rather than imposed by GPO decision making on clinicians down below. They believe that standardizing efforts break down when dealing with their branded items. As one executive said,

> In our commodity products area, if we bid our injectable antibiotic line through buying groups [GPOs], we expect

95 percent compliance, and they deliver that. They are
very good at that stuff because you have a very uniform
goal—you've got a molecule, you've got a couple of
suppliers of that molecule, the molecule's got a defined
place in medicine, and we all agree to use this one
instead of that one. But this breaks down when you start
to get uniqueness in the molecule, and you don't have
a defined place for it. It can be nonstandardized from a
medical standpoint or it can be nonstandardized from
a sales and marketing standpoint.

Manufacturers thus recognize variations in product preferences
both within and between IDN members of a GPO. Some institutions may be more focused on the cost issues of the particular drug,
while others may be more oriented to quality and total cost issues.
As a result, pharmaceutical manufacturers are not entirely sold on
the ability of IDNs, let alone GPOs, to do committed purchasing of
branded drugs. They state that some IDNs want a standardized, discounted price for every entity in their system, but not every entity
possesses the capabilities to deliver in terms of compliance. They
state they would like to contract with IDNs that have homogeneous
members and common goals as to how they position themselves in
the marketplace. They point to the investor-owned systems as
examples of member homogeneity, although some of these systems
are too focused on price for their liking. They also point to some
nonprofit IDNs that try to differentiate themselves (and their hospitals) in the market as clinically superior or convenient to access.
Such hospitals are reportedly easy to do business with.

Overall, however, manufacturers state there are not a lot of
partnerships with GPOs and their member IDNs. In their eyes,
the IDNs are "confused" and "unimpressive." As testimony to this
view, some manufacturers experimented a few years back with
separate managers for all IDNs, but have since eliminated these
positions since the IDNs lacked the required capabilities to drive

compliance. According to one executive, "We are very sensitive to not give somebody a price when they don't have the capabilities that [GPO X] has; we base our pricing on the abilities and capabilities of the parties we contract with." When asked to name names, most executives were hard-pressed to identify more than three or four IDNs that truly behaved as integrated systems; that is, with consistency across their members, influence over their clinicians, and so on. The few exceptions mentioned were IDNs in isolated geographic areas, with large market shares, and longstanding partnerships or ownerships with physician groups and health plans.

Manufacturers also believe the IDNs have needs that are too unique to bundle together into a GPO platform, although it may be possible to develop programs to meet the needs of regional groups within a GPO or IDN. According to one executive,

> You can meet some of their needs at a group level, but they end up saying, You know, that's not quite what I need, so can you tweak the relationship for me? And then you have to tweak it for the next person, and pretty soon you're back at the individual hospital level. You have to take individual needs and cobble them into a group, and sometimes that work is real work. Unfortunately, most of the time the group manages to cover only 80 percent of the members' needs, and then you have to go back and take care of the other 20 percent, in which case you might as well have taken care of 100 percent from the start.

In addition, the manufacturer (through its account group executive team) is trying to relay a message about the combined clinical and economic benefits of its product, and is confronted with a buyer with fragmented decision making where the joint consideration of these two issues is unlikely. As one executive expressed it,

"There are too many hands in the cookie jar." Another put it this way:

> The aligned metrics are a huge deal. We go into a sys-
> tem, for example—the clinical people there go, Ooh,
> aah, this is a great product—but pharmacy is incented
> on cutting dollars. Well, the two don't get together, mak-
> ing it hard to find some aligned metric between all of the
> members there. Coupled with that are all of the com-
> peting egos and agendas within the organization. You
> can have an administrator sitting at the table right
> beside the head of medicine and they hate each other.
> Well, we're in trouble if one likes our drug and the
> other doesn't. We're going to get nowhere on that.

The situation gets even more difficult when the IDN has developed an insurance vehicle or other elements of the continuum of
care (such as physician practices). For example, physicians within
one IDN may compete with each other. One IDN can partner with
multiple cardiology groups to work its cath lab, and those groups can
have totally different preferences for the drugs they utilize. This
makes it hard to standardize within a given market. Similarly,
hospitals that have their own insurance company typically execute
separate contracts with the pharmaceutical manufacturer. This is due
in part to the lack of integrated purchasing between these two entities. It is also due to the fact that the HMOs tend to purchase more
branded products while the hospitals purchase more generic drugs.
Finally, the different contracts reflect the reality that HMOs can
influence prescribing and utilization more directly than can hospitals through their formularies. While both HMOs and hospitals have
formularies, they exert different levels of control. One executive said

> One of the control factors is dispensing. The HMO for-
> mulary tells the pharmacist that we don't reimburse this

product. This is a lot more difficult in the hospital because they don't own the patients. The HMO says we are acting on behalf of the patient; hospitals don't have such a contract with the payer. So they would be accepting a certain level of legal risk by restricting access to the product. Another factor are physician incentives. Hospitals don't have as much control over physician incentives as do HMOs. A third control factor is how big it is on the radar screen. Hospitals focus on big products such as sepsis, which HMOs don't. In contrast, HMOs focus heavily on Prozac, which is not a heavily used product in hospitals.

A final control factor is where the initial prescribing decision is made for a patient. Instances where a patient gets prescribed drug A in the physician's office and then gets switched to drug B in the hospital can involve medical malpractice issues. Moreover, after hospital discharge, the patient may revert to the original medication. As a result, drug manufacturers provide bigger discounts to the HMOs than to the hospitals because they exert a greater impact on the patient's drug use.

Vertical integration and other efforts to develop a continuum of care have also added great complexity to IDNs that make it hard for manufacturers to deal with them. First, IDNs bundle and then unbundle themselves of various components. One day they are integrated, the next day they are disintegrated; one day they are centralized, the next day they are decentralized. In the manufacturer's eyes, "That just creates a whole bunch of chaos in the contracting process." At the same time, executives state that providers can be as complex as they want, but they will only get the same deal as a GPO if they can deliver the market share. Second, GPOs tend to present to manufacturers defined purchasing contracts (buckets) for hospitals, for physicians and alternate care sites, and so on. By contrast, IDNs blur these distinctions and then ask for contracts that span the continuum and require each provider to state the same price. As noted previously, manufacturers find it very hard to accommodate such requests.

One area where pharmaceutical manufacturers express a desire for closer collaboration with IDNs is coordination of clinical research activities.[19] Manufacturers view IDNs and centers of excellence as possible partners in the development and clinical testing of products using their patients. Thus, even if the manufacturer does not have any blockbuster products currently serving the hospital market, its pipeline may contain such drugs. Any partnerships with IDNs are likely to be based on that IDN's scientific expertise or experience with a given disease, and are not going to be across the board.

Looking into the Future

Pharmaceutical firms are not exactly sure how prominent hospitals will be as part of their customer mix in the future. Pharmaceutical executives are not sure what their future pipeline of hospital-based products will ultimately be. They do believe that with hospital consolidations and closings they will be dealing with a smaller number of institutional customers in the future. In contrast, they also report strong growth in their alternate site business, although it is a small portion of their total business. As partial validation of these beliefs, industry data show that between 1997 and 1999, the percentage of prescription drug sales going to the hospital market fell from 13.7 percent to 10.5 percent. At the same time, the percentages rose slightly for alternate care sites such as physician clinics (from 5.9 percent to 6.1 percent) and home health care (from 1.0 percent to 1.1 percent).[20,21]

Endnotes

1. Health Care Financing Administration. www.hcfa.gov.
2. PhRMA. *Pharmaceutical Industry Profile 2000.* www.phrma.org, 2000.

3. These figures also do not include over-the-counter drugs and diagnostics.

4. IMS Health. Referenced in NWDA *Industry Profile and Healthcare Factbook*. Reston, Virginia: National Wholesaler Druggists' Association, 2000.

5. See Note One.

6. Northrup, Jon. Presentation to Wharton School, November 2000.

7. IMS Health, referenced in *Pharmaceutical Industry Profile 2000*. PhRMA, www.phrma.org.

8. Scott-Levin. *Source Prescription Audit (SPA)*. December 1999.

9. See Note Six.

10. Kaiser Family Foundation. *Prescription Drug Trends: A Chartbook*. Menlo Park, California: Henry J. Kaiser Family Foundation, 2000.

11. Anita McGahan et al. *The Pharmaceutical Industry in the 1990s*. HBS Case 9-796-058. Boston: Harvard Business School Publishing, 1995.

12. See Note Two.

13. See Note Four.

14. For this study we interviewed executives at several major pharmaceutical firms. Due to issues revolving around competition (for example, trade secrets) and litigation, some firms did not wish to be identified. Executives were typically also wary of divulging too much information about their company's strategies in dealing with market segments.

15. See Note Eleven.

16. Account managers often are experienced sales representatives from the field, who understand the inner workings of the organized customers. They have been promoted to give them more challenging assignments and reduce the burden of travel.

17. See Note Two.

18. Preferential deals entail front-end discounts off list price and back-end rebates. Discounts can only be paid to customers who actually take ownership of the products; rebates can be paid to anyone after the fact for moving market share.

19. Pharmaceutical executives were very guarded and general in their remarks here. They preferred to not divulge the specifics of any research partnerships with IDNs.

20. IMS Health. Cited in PhRMA, 2000.

21. By contrast, the biggest percentage increase in drug sales was evident among chain drug stores (from 28.6 percent to 37.6 percent).

8

Medical Device Manufacturers
Two Broad Categories of Medical Products

Robert A. DeGraaff and Mark V. Pauly

Medical product manufacturers produce two broad categories of outputs: advanced devices and commodity-type medical and surgical supplies. Manufacturers of advanced devices, the focus of this chapter, produce higher-priced, lower-volume, technologically sophisticated diagnostic and therapeutic products and applications. Issues and opportunities for producers of higher-volume, lower-priced, commodity-type medical and surgical supplies are considered in the next chapter. The Bureau of Economic Analysis estimates that shipments of medical devices, equipment, and supplies in 1999 by medical product manufacturers totaled $56.5 billion.[1] This figure, which accounts for 4.67 percent of national health expenditures and .61 percent of GDP, is the sum of shipments from four 4-digit standard industrial classification codes (see Exhibit 8.1).[2,3]

Major Drivers of Competition Among Medical Device Makers

Medical device firms design, develop, produce, market, and sell equipment, supplies, and services for the detection, diagnosis, treatment, and prevention of disease. Based on interviews with study respondents, corporate documents (such as company 10-K reports), and industry profiles (such as Standard & Poor's semiannual industry survey), we conclude that medical device manufacturers can be

Exhibit 8.1   Medical Product Shipments Data

Medical Product Shipments, 1999, in billions*		
SIC Code	Description	
3841	Surgical and Medical Instruments and Apparatus	21.355
3842	Orthopedic, Prosthetic, and Surgical Appliances and Supplies	19.242
3844	X-Ray Apparatus and Tubes and Related Irradiation Apparatus	4.069
3845	Electromedical and Electrotherapeutic Apparatus	11.871
Total Shipments Across 4 Medical Product SIC Codes		56.537

*SIC 3843 (Dental Equipment/Supplies), with 1999 shipments of $2.941 billion, is excluded

Sources: Bureau of Economic Analysis. www.bea.doc.gov, 2001. Health Care Financing Administration. www.hcfa.gov, 2001.

characterized as competing on the basis of five dimensions: product innovation, product performance, pricing and contracting, cost of goods sold, and customer support services.

The first major driver of competition is *product innovation*. To remain competitive in this fast-paced industry segment, medical device manufacturers must—at competitive prices—continually improve existing products and develop new ones. These firms improve their products and capabilities through both internal research and development and through acquisitions. Innovations that (1) improve clinical outcomes; (2) reduce procedure time and operating room costs; (3) enable less invasive procedures; (4) allow patients to reduce or avoid inpatient hospitalizations; (5) shorten recovery time; (6) facilitate patient care in less expensive settings; or (7) extend life expectancy are drivers of growth. The U.S. Food and Drug Administration (FDA) regulates the clinical testing, manufacture, labeling, distribution, and promotion of medical devices. Before a new device can be marketed, the manufacturer must receive FDA approval. Medical device manufacturers also seek patent protection for their technologies.

Second, device manufacturers compete on the basis of *product performance*. Aspects of performance include clinical outcomes, product reliability, and physicians' overall perception of product quality. Device manufacturers work to build physician preference for their technologies through product design and features, ease of use, patient outcomes, product availability, and product line familiarity. Demand for sophisticated diagnostic and therapeutic products is steadily increasing in ASM sites.

The third dimension is *pricing and contracting*. As payment systems have evolved from cost-based, fee-for-service reimbursement to prospective payment and capitation, IDNs and their GPOs have become more price sensitive and more focused on cost containment. As a result, suppliers are awarded purchasing contracts based on the combination of competitive pricing and other attributes such as product performance, ease of use, and customer service. Exclusion from GPO contracts can be disastrous to the revenue streams of suppliers.

The fourth dimension is controlling or reducing the *total cost of delivered products* through production efficiencies and supply chain management. Manufacturers are under pressure to continually improve their internal production processes and cost structures to meet the pricing and service levels demanded by large-volume customers. In addition, supply chain management is driving logistics costs out of products through improved interorganizational coordination of purchasing, order management, inventory management, and physical distribution. One executive said

> IDNs have been working with us on efforts to reduce transaction costs. The primary reduction of transaction costs has resulted from streamlining the use of purchase orders. Instead of submitting a purchase order for each transaction (at an average cost of $48 *per transaction*), IDNs now submit blanket purchase orders. This, in addition to the proliferation of electronic ordering, has allowed the administrative costs associated with the

processing of transactions to be reduced. Additionally, the increased use of electronic ordering has allowed for vendor managed inventory; automatic replenishment; and the collection, analysis, and application of customer-specific information to better respond to and serve them. We are always interested in exploring ways to reduce inventory costs and add speed to product movement.

Customer support services is a fifth dimension of competition. Examples of support services include (1) providing a twenty-four-hour telephone customer service center that offers a single point of contact for customers with problems and questions; (2) collaborative planning and information sharing with provider organizations aimed at improving cost profiles, productivity, and clinical outcomes; (3) consignment inventory—for example, a hospital has a supply of artificial joints in its operating suite, but the vendor retains ownership of the inventory until the devices are used in surgery; (4) equipment training, maintenance, and service; and (5) expediting the contract renewal and expansion process.

Who Is the Device Manufacturer's Customer?

In their supply chain strategy, device manufacturers must simultaneously serve the needs of five downstream groups: patients, physicians, IDNs, GPOs, and sales representatives and independent distributors. The ultimate end customer is the patient, and the end user is the physician (or other caregiver). Each downstream group plays a role in selecting or influencing the brand name or product line used in the delivery of care. Executives made the following comments:

I see three interrelated customers. First, the patient receiving the implant is a customer. However, nine times out of ten, patients are unaware of the manufacturer and type of implant they're receiving. Therefore, second, the surgeon making the buying decision is a customer. Third, hospitals, integrated systems, and hospital GPOs that have standardized purchasing systems and reduced surgeon choice are a customer.

The end customer is clearly the patient. However, the patient is not the one making economic decisions regarding products, etcetera. Therefore, there are different customers at different points in the supply chain. Ultimately, the customer is the person making economic decisions. Who that person is depends upon where in the supply chain the product is purchased and what channel you're selling it through. It could be a buying group, a distributor, or a physician.

Manufacturer-Physician Interactions and Issues

Manufacturers (producers) must consider several issues in dealing with physicians (providers). These include physician preferences, resistance to standardization, product design, and clinical trials.

Physician Preference

The physicians that use or surgically implant the technology are the traditional, principal decision makers in the choice of manufacturer and product. In areas such as orthopedic implants and cardiac rhythm management, physicians often have specific brand preferences for device product lines, instrumentation, and supplies. Preference levels for scientifically advanced medical device systems tend to be much higher than those for lower-cost, higher-volume, commodity-type medical supplies. These brand preferences develop from the physicians' training experiences, product familiarity, establishment of routines, and product satisfaction. One result of establishing brand preference early in the physician's career is that the manufacturer's revenue increases as the practice grows. To maintain and strengthen brand loyalty, manufacturers seek feedback from physicians for use in developing upgrades and the next generation of products.

Resistance to Product Standardization

As part of their cost management and product standardization efforts, GPOs and IDNs are reducing the number and variety of products they contract for. They have sought to heavily involve physicians in evaluating the performance, reliability, and cost of candidate products and in selecting the medical devices and product lines to be included in contracts.[4] Nevertheless, converting physicians from off-contract to on-contract products remains a significant challenge and an elusive goal. The potential for tension and conflict is high when physician preference clashes with product standardization. Yet, the most significant potential improvement in supply chain management for medical devices is getting physicians to be more attentive to the costs of care they generate. Physicians with strong brand preferences are resistant to change; cite switching costs due to differences in device systems and instrumentation; and must be convinced that product effectiveness, reliability, and clinical outcomes are not compromised in switching to less expensive products. Frequently, physicians with strong preferences for advanced medical devices are carved out of standardization initiatives. Executives mentioned a variety of concerns:

> GPOs have overestimated their ability to convert surgeons to on-contract device vendors. GPOs have been more effective in driving compliance for higher-volume, lower-cost commodity items.

> As products become more standardized, it's important to still provide products that physicians want to use. While physician preference is sometimes overridden by economic concerns, for example, GPOs, it is important to make sure that products still possess the features that

make products easy to use and effective. The primary point of contact still remains the physician. We try to influence physicians and satisfy them so that they will influence buying groups.

GPOs must understand that in the orthopedics industry, surgeons sell surgeons. When a new technique or product is developed, we have champion surgeons inform other surgeons. From the manufacturer's point of view, the usual materials-management-oriented purchasing committee process does not work for physician preference items.

Product Design

Device manufacturers routinely engage physicians on product design teams. Physician selection criteria include innovativeness, reputation among peers, affiliation with a university teaching hospital, membership in professional societies, and prior design team experience. Consulting fees or royalties are negotiated on a physician-by-physician basis and reflect the value the physician is adding to the product design process. Device makers also engage selected physicians to travel to hospital sites to conduct on-site education sessions, demonstrate procedures, and observe surgery. Frequently, new products or innovations carry the name(s) of the designing physician. Naming an innovation after its designing physicians adds prestige to the product and helps generate sales.

Clinical Trials

The FDA must ensure the safety and efficacy of new medical devices (and the associated treatment procedures) before full-scale production and selling can begin. In this premarket application process, manufacturers present results of human clinical trials, animal testing data, and manufacturing information. Whereas the FDA reviews and scrutinizes the premarket application, it is the manufacturer that funds, organizes, and manages the clinical trials. To aid in the FDA approval process, manufacturers seek contracts to perform clinical trials at prestigious research institutions such as the Cleveland Clinic, Mayo Clinic, or other leading university medical centers. The physicians at these prominent institutions bring clinical expertise, experience in conducting clinical trials, and knowledge of the FDA approval process. Premarket clinical trials for novel medical devices often take years and many millions of dollars to complete, although the duration is shorter than that for drug testing.[5]

Manufacturer-Field Staff Issues

Manufacturers must also consider several issues in dealing with their own sales forces on the field. These include direct relations with physicians, product distribution, and restructuring the field sales organization.

Physician Relations

The medical device industry remains highly relationship oriented. The field staff, composed of employed sales representatives and independent distributors, serves as a resource and consultant to physicians.[6] In addition to detailing product information, generating new accounts, strengthening physician preference levels, and driving market share, the sales representatives and independent distributors provide training to physicians and nurses, and are frequently present in the operating room to assist the surgical team during implantation procedures. Commonly, the field staff personally deliver the implants and instrumentation to the operating room on the day of surgery. One executive explained it this way:

> Each regional sales office maintains its own inventory of implants and instruments. About 70 percent to 80 percent of implants are delivered to the hospital by the sales representatives. In many cases the sales representatives bring the inventory JIT and attend the surgery.

Therefore, it is not necessary to ship from a JIT ware-house. Only 20–30 percent of implant orders are shipped directly to hospitals.

Orthopedic Implant Distribution

Orthopedic implant distribution differs from the standard distribution of medical products and pharmaceuticals in two ways. First, rather than partnering with large national distributor firms, device manufacturers ship finished products and instrumentation to their regional sales offices (or directly to the hospitals) via Federal Express or United Parcel Service. Each regional center manages its own inventory of implants, instrumentation, and supplies. Second, implant field staff perform customer services that the large national distribution companies do not. While both distributor types offer inventory management, order preparation and packaging, product transportation, and delivery, the distribution of medical devices also entails an unusually close working relationship with physicians (for example, being present in the operating room during procedures).

Field Organization Restructuring

To gain more direct management control over the inventory and product movement processes, device manufacturers are moving toward employed field staff and territory managers, and away from contracting with independent distributors. Under the new management structures, compensation incentives for field staff are being aligned with corporate objectives such as controlling costs through inventory management. Contract administration capabilities and pricing specialists are being developed at the corporate office, and field staff are working more closely with purchasing managers and other nonphysician economic decision makers in an attempt to influence product selection decisions. In competing for business, field staff are often granted a level of autonomy to offer on-the-spot discounts to individual hospitals or integrated delivery networks. Finally, "Sales growth is a key performance indicator among sales representatives. However, generating new accounts is especially difficult for sales representatives in areas with significant levels of national contract business. To ease this tension somewhat, the sales force is compensated to service the national account business."

Transacting with Hospital Systems and Group Purchasing Organizations

Manufacturers (producers) must also consider several issues in dealing with GPOs (purchasers) and hospital systems (providers). These include the criteria that drive contracting and the growth in GPO contracting.

Contracting Criteria

When negotiating with either IDNs or GPOs, eight considerations drive device manufacturers' willingness to agree to discounted pricing or to invest in customer service initiatives that enhance customer satisfaction and retention. The first two drivers are (1) current and potential *purchase volume*, and (2) actual and expected *contract compliance performance*. Buyers combining high levels of purchase volume and contract compliance have the most favorable profile for generating revenue and market share. Device manufacturers are also generally willing to extend favorable contract terms to smaller but high-compliance buyers to achieve pockets of regional market share.

To offset the unit revenue impact of discounted contract pricing, device makers rely on the use of performance measurement metrics to monitor, control, and improve key operational areas. For example, to prevent a buildup of consignment inventory, one device maker closely watches inventory turns on consigned items. If a hospital's consignment inventory turns are below a contract-specified threshold, then the contract calls for corrective action steps and spells out revisions to (or termination of) the consignment arrangement.

For lower-compliance customers (that is, those not able to achieve, maintain, or enforce contract-specified levels of committed purchase volume or market share), manufacturers' willingness to price discount increases with customer size and revenue potential. In many cases, manufacturers design contracts that rebate all or a portion of the price discounts after a buyer achieves predetermined levels of sales volume or market share. Manufacturers also value buyers' flexibility to update, modify, or extend contracts over time as product lines and the competitive environment change. In addition, "Individual health systems such as the Mayo Clinic or universities with large research, patient care, and education operations are large enough to pull as much weight as an entire buying group."

Third, a device maker's willingness to deal depends also upon the buyer's commitment to *partnering for product development and problem solving*. Collaborative partnership opportunities include (1) physician involvement in designing, developing, evaluating, and improving products; (2) institutional participation in planning and conducting clinical product testing; and (3) discussing and working toward solving issues that emerge in the rapidly evolving health care value chain. "Smaller operations such as Johns Hopkins are so involved in the areas of research and development that they are viewed as important regardless of their small size."

The fourth contracting criterion is willingness to commit to operating within *single-* and *dual-source agreements*. Ideally, device makers would prefer to enter long-term, sole-source agreements with IDNs and GPOs. Manufacturers are in the best position under single-source contracts to offer the lowest prices (in exchange for committed volume), provide the highest levels of tailored customer service, build the strongest customer-supplier relationships, and achieve the highest sales volumes. A major component of customer service in sole-source contracting is maintaining safety stocks or qualified back-up vendors in the event of demand spikes or temporary product unavailability. Device makers pursue single sourcing in their own procurement. One explained

> In transacting with our own suppliers, we single source. We single source based on the philosophy that when we team up with a supplier, it's going to be a long-term relationship. Before sole sourcing with a supplier, we evaluate them in terms of quality control processes, financial stability, and management depth. So when we single source, the risk is minimized. But we do have backups identified if need be. Sole sourcing enables the highest volumes, the best service, and the lowest prices.
>
> The decision to single versus dual source is driven by the component's importance from a material standpoint. Components without a lot of engineering or components that involve sheer volume orders, we can single source and still get in a qualified replacement if there's ever a problem.

Under a dual-source contract, buyers engage two preferred vendors. From the buyers' perspective, the advantages of maintaining relationships with two (or more) medical device makers are (1) added choice and flexibility in product line selection; (2) reduced need to convert a portion of physicians from off- to on-contract products; (3) fast access to an alternate vendor if one is unable to promptly fill an order; and (4) customer service competition among vendors (for example, give preference to the vendor(s) that provide free upgrades, weekend service, consignment inventory, freight concessions, twenty-four-hour customer service, product delivery on the same day items were ordered, and so forth). In contrast, from the sellers' point of view, sales revenue becomes more uncertain, discounted pricing for volume is compromised, and development of a strong customer-supplier relationship is inhibited when buyers have multiple suppliers.

A fifth criterion in contracting is the content, sophistication, and maturity of the GPO's or IDN's supply chain strategy, logistics management capabilities, and information technology infrastructure. Executives said

> These elements are key in determining what kind of deal a GPO or IDN can get. If a purchasing entity has its supply chain strategy intact and is set up with streamlined operations to service all of its provider locations, then this partnership with the manufacturer will be more equal, there will be fewer problems, and a more favorable deal will be extended.

> In terms of information systems and achieving information technology efficiencies, individual hospitals, integrated systems, and buying groups are behind the curve. Most facilities lack detailed information about cost per case and outcomes, and do not have a good way to use clinical and financial information to their advantage in managed care contracting, and so forth. Outcomes have been broadly discussed but never really quantified well.

Sixth, the *number of delivery points* influences contract and pricing negotiations with IDNs and GPOs. Device manufacturers are most willing to extend favorable pricing terms for shipping large, consolidated orders to a single, central location. Materials handling, packing, and transportation costs increase with number of delivery points (for example, the loading docks of each member hospital and ambulatory surgery centers). Vendor willingness to ship to multiple delivery points in discounted pricing contracts increases with the revenue and market share importance of the customer. Many IDNs have developed (or are developing) sophisticated internal storage and delivery systems; however, inefficiencies in internal materials handling remain a significant opportunity for process and cost improvement for many providers. One executive stated

> IDNs with consolidated warehouses where we can ship to one location and the ability to distribute products to every floor of the hospital and throughout the health system helps to cut out costs and reduce our staffing levels. Some IDNs can pick up their products from our distribution centers. As hospitals become more organized and efficient, they are able to streamline costs on both ends of the transaction. Thus both the supplier and the hospital witness lower costs.

Seventh, device makers favor buyers with financial strength and *ability to deliver prompt payment*. Lastly, contracting with *teaching hospitals* is important to manufacturers because physicians develop brand name and product line preferences early in their career. When newly trained physicians graduate and move to new areas, they take these preferences with them.

Growth in Device Manufacturer-GPO Contracting

Compared with lower-priced, higher-volume commodity-type items (such as medical-surgical supplies), a smaller but growing percentage of medical device sales volume is flowing through group purchasing contracts. One leading device maker estimated that as recently as 1998 only 15–20 percent of its sales went through GPO agreements. At that time, device manufacturers did not feel the need to enter GPO contracts because most hospitals ordered their physician preference products directly from the manufacturer by telephone or fax, or orders were handled by the manufacturer's field staff. More recently, brand name device makers have become increasingly willing to participate in price discounted contracts with GPOs to grow market share by selling to a contractually consolidated group of member providers, to be represented as best-in-class vendors in disease management portfolios, or to prevent the erosion of market share that would occur if the manufacturer were excluded from a GPO's list of contracted suppliers.

Recent examples of device manufacturers entering GPO contracts are plentiful. In the orthopedic implant segment, Premier signed five-year agreements in 1999 with Zimmer, Howmedica Osteonics, Smith & Nephew, DeRoyal Industries, and Synthes to create an orthopedic portfolio for hip, knee, and shoulder implants; trauma products; and other orthopedic instrumentation and supplies.[7] Novation also announced in 1999 a similar set of multiyear, multi-source orthopedic agreements with DePuy, Howmedica Osteonics, and Zimmer. Under the Novation contract, providers are eligible to receive quarterly incentive rebates equal to 4 percent of purchase volume if 90 percent of orthopedic implants and instrumentation were purchased from one or a combination of the contracted manufacturers.[8] Multisource agreements with two or more top manufacturers permit compliance within a range of physician preferences.[9]

In addition to orthopedics, GPOs have created product portfolios based on cardiovascular, oncology, neuromuscular, and other major disease categories.[10] In the cardiovascular area, for example, Medtronic has signed multiyear partnership agreements with Premier, Novation, Tenet, and Consorta to be a major supplier of cardiac rhythm management devices (such as pacemakers and defibrillators), coronary stents, and other cardiovascular products.[11,12] One executive mentioned that in addition to securing discounted pricing for member provider organizations,

> GPOs are showing increasing levels of understanding about the total service package. That is, they not only think of the price at which they wish to purchase a product, but also think of how quickly it can be delivered, the cost of transporting the product, if substitutes are available, and what will happen if the product is on back order. Still, GPOs are much more prone to focus on price, while doctors are really much more interactive and understand our product and what it can do.

[As a manufacturer we're actively trying to offer more
than innovative product features and price.] Buying
groups that are looking at the whole picture instead of
just price have the right idea. There are many value-
adding services, such as whether a supplier can offer
twenty-four-hour customer service, access to evidence-
based clinical studies, and whether products can be
delivered on the day they were ordered. Buying groups
which consider all aspects of the partnership between
supplier and buying group are entering into the most
intelligent partnerships. Because of this, they will most
likely outlast those which make decisions based solely
upon on the price of a product. Some don't have the
wherewithal to do cost-based and full analysis of services.

An issue of primary concern to device manufacturers is whether
the incremental revenue benefit (that is, market share growth and
increased contract compliance) exceeds the cost of the contract
administration fees paid to the GPOs. GPO contracting reduces the
manufacturer's transaction costs of negotiating with thousands of
hospitals. However, "GPOs bring with them delays of signals of the
customer's need. Therefore, we're not able to respond to the needs
of the end customer as rapidly as possible."

Frequently, smaller device manufacturers are frustrated by GPOs'
tendency to contract with market share leaders. Smaller producers
find themselves in a disadvantaged situation: they are not invited
to join GPO contracts because they do not command significant
market share, and they cannot grow market share because they are
not included in GPO contracts. Often this situation is resolved
when smaller, innovative device makers are acquired by a market
leader. Still, as executives said

Niche players do manage to compete, and many are
regionally very successful. But if the big players cut the

field to two or three suppliers, then niche players might get restricted from doing business.

There continues to be a lot of product purchased from smaller manufacturers off contract. Smaller manufacturers tend to have higher profit margins and don't have to give away discounts. Given lackluster compliance within groups, I'm not convinced that being a smaller manufacturer outside of the contract is a huge detriment.

Recommendations and Best Practices for Reducing End-to-End Supply Chain Costs

Medical device executives advocate six improvement actions (recommended best practices) to downstream partners for curbing health care supply chain costs. The first is to *increase order lead times*. With a few exceptions, implants surgeries are scheduled at least a week in advance; yet a high percentage of product orders are placed by hospitals one or two days before the procedure. Earlier product ordering for scheduled surgeries would enable a substantial reduction in the cost of overnight delivery of implants, instrumentation, and other supplies to the field staff or hospital. Similarly, cost savings can be achieved through improved hospital-manufacturer communication as to whether (1) an order is for a next-day procedure (in which case it needs to be overnighted) or (2) the order is an inventory replacement item that is not yet scheduled to be implanted (in which case it can be shipped at less than half of the priority overnight rate). One executive said

> Each year for the past several years we have driven at least 10 percent of the cost of goods out of the product. We're driving for productivity improvement throughout the supply chain. We're doing things like reducing product movement expense and cutting inventory. We've got to keep improving return on sales and earnings.

Second, *inventory velocity* (the speed at which inventory moves through the supply chain) can be accelerated in downstream customer storerooms and consignment shelves through improved contract compliance performance. Executives explain:

> Avoidable supply chain costs are incurred when customers accumulate substantial inventories in anticipation of on-contract product consumption, but then return large quantities of excess inventory to the manufacturer because they couldn't move it or because it reached its expiration date. This boils down to ability to follow through on the terms of a contract. Poor contract compliance causes additional expense, and these agreements will be revised or terminated.

> It costs a lot of money to maintain heavy consignment in hospitals, with every salesman making sure that when a physician or nurse wants one, there are three to grab. There may be fourteen weeks of inventory out there.

> Device manufacturers must continually assess where costs can be taken out of supply chains and where services should be added or expanded. Perhaps there are areas where in fact you should add some costs in to best serve important customers. Here's a good example: One hospital reduced the size of its O.R. consignment storage area by half and converted administrative and other storage space to revenue-generating clinical activities. Now we ship to this hospital every day via overnight priority. The shipping costs are high, but the hospital holds only three to four days of inventory. So, it costs us twice as much to ship, but we have only a tenth of the inventory. We're working to find the right balance between replenishment processes, inventory costs, customer service levels, and shipping costs.

A third recommendation is to *decrease end-to-end finished goods inventory*. Although consignment and case-by-case ordering of implants and instrumentation have reduced hospitals' inventory levels, they have substantially increased implant manufacturers' finished goods inventories. One executive said

> Finished goods inventory in the *territory offices* can be reduced if hospitals have product shipped directly from the manufacturer to the facility (rather than having it delivered by the sales representatives). Similarly, decreasing consignment inventories (and moving to direct shipment) can reduce finished goods inventory in the *hospitals*. Purchase and ownership of instrumentation by high-volume users may also reduce overall supply chain costs.

Fourth, to reduce the overall cost of implant surgeries, physicians are called upon to be more thorough and complete in *preoperative templating, sizing, and product ordering*. As one respondent put it, "Because implant sizing and instrumentation requirements are somewhat uncertain until the surgery is performed, a large and expensive inventory typically accompanies the patient to the operating suite. Nevertheless, surgeons spending more time reading the X rays and considering other available information before the surgery can narrow the uncertainty and reduce the quantity of carry-in inventory."

A fifth recommendation is to *adopt a retailers' approach to supply chain management*. "Wal-Mart's approach to supply chain management and information systems is a good model for hospitals. At the end of each sales day, Wal-Mart sends inventory data and replenishment orders to its suppliers. In like manner, increased communication between manufacturers and hospitals regarding surgery schedules and product utilization would be of great value."

Sixth, and finally, device manufacturers—especially those that are providing equity investments and subscription fees—advocate wide membership in and utilization of the *Global Healthcare Exchange*. The Exchange aims to streamline its customers' procurement processes and reduce supply chain costs by (1) providing a secure, reliable, and easy-to-navigate Internet site for researching, sourcing, buying, and selling an extensive portfolio of products and services used in patient care; and (2) offering on-line customer service features such as up-to-date product catalogs, product availability queries, contract- or customer-specific pricing information, ordering from multiple suppliers using a single electronic purchase order, order tracking and status reports, customer-directed distribution options, historical purchasing activity reports, twenty-four-hour receipt of customer problems or complaints, and (in the near future) clinical information to support the practice of evidence-based medicine.[13] Future capabilities envisioned by the Exchange include (1) tracking and continuously updating customer-specific order points, lot sizes, inventory carrying levels, and safety stocks; (2) improving production scheduling based on accurate product consumption and inventory data;[14] (3) cost per case and care process reporting (using activity-based costing and management principles) based on point-of-use capture data; and (4) clinical and economic evaluations of alternative treatment strategies. An evaluation of this Exchange is presented in Chapter Ten.[15]

Endnotes

1. Bureau of Economic Analysis. Shipments of Manufacturing Industries by Four-Digit SIC Industry, Three-Digit SIC Industry Group, and Two-Digit SIC Major Group. Accessed at www.bea.doc.gov/bea/dn2/gpo.htm. Product shipment amounts are based on data collected by the U.S. Census Bureau's Annual Survey of Manufacturers, 2001.

2. Bureau of Economic Analysis. National Income and Product Account Table 1.1: Gross Domestic Product. Accessed at www.bea.doc.gov/bea/dn/nipaweb/PopularTables.asp, 2001.

3. Centers for Medicare and Medicaid Services (formerly Health Care Financing Administration). National Health Expenditures Table 1: National Health Expenditures Aggregate and Per Capita Amounts, Percent Distribution, and Average Annual Percent Growth, by Source of Funds: Selected Calendar Years 1960–99. http://www.hcfa.gov/stats/nhe-oact/tables, 2001.

4. Anon. "Premier Announced Coronary and Peripheral Stent Contracts, Others." *PR Newswire* (November 1, 1999).

5. *Standard and Poor's Industry Survey. Healthcare Products and Supplies, 2000.*

6. The two types of field staff perform the same job. The fundamental distinction is that sales representatives are manufacturer employees and the independent distributors are contracted.

7. Anon. "Premier Signs Up Vendors to Provide Range of Orthopedic Implants and Soft Goods." *Hospital Materials Management* (August 1999): 6.

8. Anon. "Novation Awards Hip and Knee Implant Agreements to DePuy, Howmedica Osteonics, and Zimmer and Pilots Committed Initiative." *PR Newswire* (September 8, 1999).

9. DeJohn, Paula. "Selling the Package: GPOs Bundle Contracts by Disease, Not Vendor." *Health Industry Today* (July 2001): 1.

10. Ibid.

11. Medtronic, Inc. Press Releases. September 14, 1998; May 12, 1999; October 27, 1999; October 28, 1999; and November 7, 2000. http://www.medtronic.com/newsroom/news_release.html.

12. Anon. "Tenet Selects Medtronic to Provide Most Pacemakers Under New Two-Year Deal." *Hospital Materials Management* (December 1999): 4.

13. This paragraph draws upon Global Healthcare Exchange press releases available at www.ghx.com.

14. Lancioni, Richard A., Michael F. Smith, and Terence A. Oliva. "The Role of the Internet in Supply Chain Management." *Industrial Marketing Management* 29 (2000): 45–56.

15. The authors thank Nick Braccino, Gordon Brown, Steve Elliott, Tom Gibson, Jennifer Hetrick, Leslie R. Jebson, and Ron Jost for their valuable insights and thoughtful discussions of issues in health care value chains.

9

Medical-Surgical Manufacturers

Lawton R. Burns

Introduction

The manufacturers of medical-surgical (med-surg) products share many characteristics with pharmaceutical firms (covered in Chapter Seven). They focus heavily on developing innovative products that appeal directly to clinicians. They rely heavily on distributors to ship product to their customers. They produce products in several different therapeutic areas. Finally, they are concerned with integrating these product offerings for the customer and developing "total cost" approaches. Unlike pharmaceutical firms, however, med-surg firms are also interested in rendering services to their institutional customers and in bypassing GPOs in favor of direct, bilateral contracts with hospitals. They have also diversified their product lines via acquisitions to broaden their appeal to large customers that want one-stop shopping.

This chapter analyzes these similarities and differences using information gleaned from on-site interviews with executives from these firms. The aim here is to articulate how the characteristics of med-surg firms shape their view of the health care supply chain—from distributors to GPOs and IDNs. As with pharmaceutical firms, the differences among these firms preclude us from making any claim regarding the generalizability of our observations for the entire industry.

Med-Surg Manufacturers and Product Line Diversification

Med-surg manufacturers operate in several different product lines. The largest of these, Johnson & Johnson ($29.1 billion in sales in 2000), has eighteen different operating companies that manufacture products in three major business segments: medical devices and diagnostics, pharmaceuticals, and consumer. The operating companies within these divisions are well known, including Cordis (stents), Ethicon (wound management), Ethicon Endo-Surgery (surgical instruments), Janssen (pharmaceuticals), Ortho-Clinical Diagnostics (hospital laboratory products), Ortho-McNeil Pharmaceutical (prescription drugs), and McNeil Consumer Healthcare (for example, Tylenol and Motrin). Becton Dickinson ($3.6 billion in revenues, 2000) operates companies in three business areas: BD Medical Systems (injection syringes and needles), BD Clinical Laboratory Solutions (blood and specimen collection kits), and BD Biosciences (clinical laboratory products). Baxter International, with $6.9 billion in sales (2000), operates businesses in three areas: Bioscience (blood therapies), Medication Delivery (intravenous solutions), and Renal (kidney dialysis products); its cardiovascular business (heart valves and valve repair products) was spun off in 1999. Some of these operating units formed internally; others were external acquisitions.

There are several rationales behind these acquisitions. As publicly owned for-profit entities, these firms are driven to grow and grow earnings. They are also motivated to increase their cash flow, which is used to fund internal research and development (R&D), which, in turn, fuels future growth. New businesses are developed or acquired to further the aim of growth. Other firms and their product lines are also acquired to build businesses (for example, in pharmaceuticals, cardiology, and so forth) and market-leading franchises. Some of these firms state that their goal is to have the number one or number two position (for example, market share) in each of the product markets in which they compete. There are variations on this growth rationale. Oftentimes the manufacturer has dominant market share in its initial product area, which then becomes a mature industry with decreasing prospects for domestic growth. The manufacturer then turns to international markets for this product and/or seeks to diversify out of this market into others with greater prospects for growth. Such a scenario describes Becton Dickinson's foray outside of its core needle and syringe market (where it enjoys dominant share) into the biosciences.

In all of these firms, innovation is viewed as the key to growth. Similar to pharmaceutical firms' emphasis on branded drugs over generics, med-surg firms emphasize innovative new products over older, commodity-type products. Innovative products are described as higher in value and lower in volume. They command higher prices and yield higher returns, and are less subject to GPO contracts, CAFs, and price discounting pressures. This is because they are valued by clinicians who will (hopefully) insist on their preferred vendor rather than submit to a standardized product choice. As one executive explained, "When you get more into the technology, purchasing becomes more and more diffuse, the customer preference comes into play, and the GPO compliance wavers." Another executive stated, "The last thing you want is your product to become a commodity, so how can you avoid that as best as possible? Keep it out of the large-purchasing type of relationships." It is not surprising that med-surg manufacturers commonly mention specialty-based physicians as their customer. Moreover, across a med-surg manufacturer's portfolio, innovative products may constitute 25 percent of the volume of goods shipped, but as much as 75 percent of customer orders and a sizable share of firm profits.

Med-surg manufacturers desire innovative products for at least six additional reasons. First, these firms seek to sell a mix of commodity and innovative products. Some prefer to bundle these products together in packages whereby the innovative items can "pull along everything else." Thus, for example, one firm seeks to first develop high-share agreements with customers for its market-leading products, and then use that relationship to develop contracts for extensions of the product line or new products that grow those business segments more quickly. Another manufacturer constructed a matrix that cross-classified its operating companies and the product markets (for example, anti-infectives, sutures, analgesics, and so on) in which it operated. It sought to develop hospital contracts where purchases covered more cells in the matrix; that is, the hospital purchased more products from more different operating companies to cover its clinical area needs. In this manner, the firm attempted to "touch on all the value points" for both the customer and its own internal units.

Second, by tying a mix of products together in bundles, these firms seek to recover the GPO-negotiated price discounts they have to offer on commodity products with the higher margins earned on high-technology items. They are even willing to discount the innovative items slightly to pull the commodity items along. Of course, they offer better pricing to GPOs that negotiate deals involving greater breadth across the firm's products along with compliance and volume.

Third, by tying these different types of products together, manufacturers seek to reduce marketing risk across their different product divisions. For example, at any given point, these divisions will be selling items at varying stages of the product's life cycle and industry maturity. Some products will be on the upswing in their life cycle (increasing demand for the technology), while others will be on downswings due to new product introductions and innovations by competitors. The bundling approach serves to protect products and divisions having marketing problems by virtue of tying their sales to the sales of more successful products.

Fourth, innovative products are less likely to be handled by distributor intermediaries and more likely to be shipped directly by the manufacturer (for example, using FedEx or UPS) or distributed using the manufacturer's own distribution network. In this manner, the manufacturer controls the customer relationship, has direct access to sales information, and eliminates the wholesaler margin for the customer.

Fifth, higher-priced innovative items provide one vehicle for manufacturers to engage their hospital customers in discussions of "total cost" and "value" (that is, quality for a given level of cost). Such discussions are important given that hospitals are under pressures from payers to reduce costs; vendors seek to offer hospitals one basis for justifying the higher cost of their innovative products. The challenge here of course, as with pharma, is countering the customer's short-term fixation on price with the long-term consideration of total costs incurred using the technology. Manufacturers recognize this, but hope to engage "progressive" hospitals that are developing disease management programs, continua of care efforts, and episode of care reimbursement models with payers that see value in product bundles.

Sixth, and finally, these manufacturers have witnessed the consolidation of hospitals into systems and IDNs, and the rise and growing concentration of GPOs. They are now confronted by large organized buyers, which may demand broad product portfolios to facilitate one-stop-shopping convenience for their members. Premier is often cited as being the first GPO to pursue this "80/20 approach" (that is, it sources 80 percent of the products needed by its hospital members from 20 percent of its vendors). By virtue of their acquisitions, med-surg manufacturers seek to broaden their portfolios and thereby offer this convenience. Some assert that GPOs want to lower their transactions costs by contracting with a smaller number of large vendors with broad product portfolios. Moreover, by virtue of their own merger and acquisition activity, the manufacturers seek to bargain with large buyers on a more level playing field.[1]

Product Portfolios and Matrix Management

Medical-surgical manufacturers employ several approaches in managing their diverse portfolios of products. These include disease management, matrix management, customer site representatives, and coordinating divisions.

Disease Management

The bundled product approach is part of broader strategies of disease management and matrix management that have been employed by pharmaceutical firms as well as med-surg manufacturers.[2] With respect to disease management, these firms have developed programs and services based on various bundles of their products. These programs are oriented to serve specific population segments or target certain surgical procedures that require pre and postsurgical therapies (for example, combining a hip implant with pain medication, a rehabilitation program, and an overall care map). The manufacturers seek to sell these programs and their associated product bundles to IDNs. The goal is to get the IDN to buy products across more cells in the matrix of operating companies and product categories, and to enter into as many exclusive contracts in these cells as possible, in exchange for better pricing on all products. In this manner, the coordinating division seeks to increase the volume and share for as many of the operating divisions it represents as possible.

Matrix Management

With respect to matrix management, these firms have multiple product divisions that approach hospitals through their separate field sales forces. Each product division may have multiple sets of sales forces for its different products. The result is that the manufacturer may have dozens of sales forces out in the field calling on hospital accounts, each with the company logo on their business cards. The result is that the hospital customer may no longer be able to differentiate who or what product company they are meeting with. Moreover, the customer may be tired of having so many people call on them the same day. Some executives estimate that hospitals may be visited by over 100,000 different salespeople overall.

It is not surprising that, confronted with so many companies (product divisions and sales forces), customers have mentioned to manufacturers that they would prefer to have one person from the manufacturer, whom they can turn to for information, sales coordination, and problem resolution. In terms of organization theory, the increasing differentiation of sales activity necessitates an increase in integrative activity. Matrix management is one such effort to integrate cross-functional and cross-product activities.[3,4] The manufacturers have responded to the request for integration in several interrelated ways. First, they have sought to bring together all of the firm's divisions that sell products to large IDNs by developing account managers, market managers, and customer-site representatives. Account managers assume responsibility for contracts with specific large IDNs and GPOs, market managers assume responsibility for overseeing contract implementation activity across the largest metropolitan statistical areas (MSAs) in the United States, and customer-site representatives (CSRs) coordinate sales-call activity within a specific IDN account on-site. Some combination of these three approaches (but not necessarily all three) is often found within manufacturers.

Customer-Site Representatives

Manufacturers offer their theory behind the CSR approach. Some firms report that they have over 100 different salespeople calling on a single hospital account at any given time. While their salespeople know a little about one product segment, the firms want someone who knows "a lot about a lot" of product segments, such that they can educate providers about the benefits of the continuum and provide a higher level of customer service than the competition. They have also modeled the results of their sales efforts inside hospitals and determined that the additional personnel cost of one CSR per hospital account would require an increment in sales of $150,000 over their base sales. To achieve these savings, they focus the CSR efforts on high-cost, high-visibility procedures at high-volume hospitals (for example, hospitals that do 15,000 or more procedures annually). Such hospitals represent only a few hundred institutions in the country but, due to their system affiliations, account for a large share of the hospitals and the procedures performed. The CSR would thus represent an effort to increase the penetration of the firm's products into these hospital procedures, as well as to decrease the number and cost of visits by sales representatives to the account (estimated roughly at $1,000 per salesperson per year). Manufacturers claim there have been some modest reductions in the number of sales force representatives housed in the product companies as a result of the CSR effort.

While on site, the CSR would work together with hospital managers on critical best practices in OR procedures, inventory management, order processing, and so forth. This is designed to free up the sales representative to focus on sales rather than helping the hospital with inventory management. It may also help hospitals to reduce their levels of inventory promoted by the agents of the manufacturer, who are compensated based on sales commissions. The CSRs would not be commissioned sales agents but full-time employed professionals (for example, clinical nurse or materials manager).

This raises the question whether such specialty-based professionals can actually span several product divisions in their knowledge. One manufacturer that has worked with this concept reported that, as professionals trained in a given functional specialty, the CSRs tend to spend most of their time with their hospital counterparts in that functional specialty rather than with other clinical and functional areas that utilize the firm's products. Manufacturers recognize the difficulty here, and thus plan to phase in their program to initially focus on specialized areas with the CSR's specialized expertise (for example, an OR-based CSR, cath lab–based CSR). A more broadly based CSR program will require better information systems that can electronically (rather than manually) collect product information across each hospital account's clinical areas.

Coordinating Divisions and the Unified Approach to Customer

These integrative approaches are usually directed or overseen by a new corporate division, designed to coordinate the efforts of the product divisions. By doing so, the product divisions become new customers of the coordinating division. At Johnson & Johnson, the integrative unit is Health Care Systems (JJHCS); at Becton Dickinson, it bears the same name (BD Health Care Systems). The similarity reflects the fact that the Becton Dickinson unit was built by former JJHCS executives.

JJHCS is charged with centralizing contracts and pricing across all of the firm's product divisions, as well as centralizing orders and revenue management. For products that get shipped directly to customers without using outside distributors, JJHCS also performs centralized supply chain management functions using its own regional warehouses. Such centralization is believed to contribute economies of scale and thus greater efficiency in performing these functions. The centralization of functions also enables the firm to offer a "united face" to the customer, both in terms of rendering service as well as in terms of bargaining power. The overlapping of effort and responsibility within these matrices is intentionally designed to foster joint consideration and resolution of conflicting corporate interests (for example, goals of product division versus goals of corporation, or interests of sales representative versus interests of firm).

At Becton Dickinson, the Health Care Systems division centralized the customer service groups originally located at each product business, followed by their transportation and warehousing groups, production planning and scheduling functions, and then some of their sales and marketing staff (national accounts). The goal is to "make all of the customer-facing assets seamless," to offer a unified bundle of products to the customer, and to optimize on the firm's "total costs" covering production, warehousing and inventory, and transportation. Obstacles encountered here have been disrupted reporting relationships and career ladders (for example, in sales and marketing), and issues over "who owns the sales numbers and the expense numbers, whose bonus is tied to hitting or not hitting a certain number."

The "united face" approach can also be applied to distributors as well as hospital accounts. At Becton Dickinson, for example, there are dedicated "detailers" to whom distributors can go with questions or requests for information on product pricing, promotion, and logistics. In this manner, the firm seeks to improve customer service, product quality, and customer efficiency. According to one executive,

> Distributors are a big portion of our supply chain, since a large quantity of our product flows through them to the end consumer. We have to make sure we package and deliver product to them which [sic] allows them to handle it, ship it, and deliver it in a way that it is not damaged at the point of use and maintains its sterile product quality and integrity all the way through. So we have people here who are assigned and meet frequently with specific distributors to ask them about claims handling, damaged products, order cycle times, loading and unloading, etcetera. We are always trying to probe the methods of ordering and shipment so as to improve those processes.

The dedicated representatives also work with distributors on combining orders across the firm's product divisions to minimize the number of orders, shipments, and deliveries of product pallets to hospital customers (for example, a smaller number of larger deliveries that meet minimum order requirements). In this manner, the firm believes it can assume responsibility for the entire supply chain down to the hospital customer and ensure delivery of its products based on its own quality standards.

Internal Challenges to the Unified Approach

Manufacturers face several internal and external challenges in pursuing this strategy of bundling and presenting a "unified face to the customer."[5] One internal challenge is the lack of demonstrated success among some of their peer organizations. Baxter attempted the strategy several years ago, operated it for three to four years, and then discarded the approach and returned to each product division handling its own sales force.

Another internal challenge to this strategy is its perceived low priority. For manufacturers, supply chain costs may represent only a minor percentage of their net sales (for example, less than 10 percent), and thus command much less attention than product innovation and R&D issues. Given the high margins they earn on high-technology products, there is understandably little interest in pursuing supply chain efficiencies that might narrow such margins. Moreover, technological investments are viewed as better strategic bets than "customer facing" efforts. Other, more important, issues concern growth in global sales and overcoming foreign trade barriers that hinder the export of their products.

Another internal problem stems from the "silo mentality" in multiproduct firms. One manufacturer characterized its product divisions as "longstanding, independent nation states." As a result, different product divisions may be unaware of the range and synergies among the products they bring to the marketplace. In addition, it may be hard to convince divisions to subsidize the weaker divisions by discounting their products slightly to pull all products in the bundle along. At Johnson & Johnson, for example,

> Historically, operating companies, particularly those with large market shares or high profitability, have been reluctant to give corporate marketing programs the freedom to negotiate pricing, fearful of the impact on an individual company P&L [profit and loss], and concerned that broad, corporate-wide business bundles would only work to the detriment of well-positioned companies.
>
> Companies like Ethicon, in particular, rebelled on the grounds that the strategy was most often used to position weaker companies by leveraging stronger ones

or that customers would only agree to buy products from smaller companies if they received a price concession from a market leader. Whether driven by customer demand or the needs of smaller sister companies, the stronger J&J companies rarely saw sufficient benefit from a coordinated program. . . .[6]

More recently, JJHCS executives have claimed the system works by increasing overall corporate sales volume, share, and profitability; and by currying the support of product company executives who suffered down-cycles in demand for their products but received a boost from contract packages that bundled their products with those of more successful divisions. At the end of the day, however, for such coordinating divisions to succeed, they must be able to demonstrate that their centralized approach outperformed the former, decentralized efforts of product divisions in terms of maintaining share (in highly penetrated accounts and product markets) and growing share (in less penetrated accounts and markets).

External Challenges to the Unified Approach

Manufacturers report several external challenges to this strategy emanating from the hospital customer. For example, the notion of total cost, as opposed to product price, has not been widely embraced. "The price at the pump today is much more visible and more watched than any story you could weave around total cost. The total cost story explains why you may have to spend three times as much on the front end to save on the back end five times what you would have spent. That is a difficult story to weave for many customers."

One explanation offered by manufacturers is the short-term pressure that hospital CEOs are under to maintain financial viability. Very few people are willing to take the risk to spend more today to realize either greater savings or better outcomes in the future. Another explanation is the short tenure of CEOs that prevents them from seeing the long term and/or the results from long-term efforts. Yet another reason is that hospital managers believe it is easier to "beat up on manufacturers for another 1–2 percent on price" than it is to glean efficiencies in the 85 percent of their spending on nonsupply issues (for example, cutting staffing or improving procedures).

Manufacturers also report that there are too many people in the hospital account who have to be connected and "get on the same page" to make the bundle decision work. Executives made the following comments:

> In most places it hasn't worked. The decision making breaks down all over the place. Departments are unwilling to give up their bit of comfort zone or turf around the selection of what product they want, and don't want to have another department determine for them how they are going to operate."

> There have been hundreds of attempts and very few successes. The best places are where we have tremendous equity with physician decision makers—people who have their name on the product and are very influential clinicians. And yet even these people cannot influence what happens in their own clinical area and get others to accept a bundled package. You can have the most influential surgeon in the world demand a particular product or procedural method, and there are other people who are not going to follow that selection. I'm sure that Medtronic goes through the same thing. They have great equity with their pacing physicians [cardiologists using pacemaker products] but they can't get the cardiopulmonary surgeons to do what you want them to do around cardiopulmonary products.

The network of physician decision makers gets more complex as the bundle crosses multiple specialties. Executives cited several examples where bundling broke down in specific IDN accounts when surgeons, anesthesiologists, and pharmacists could not agree on the included items and/or wanted "consideration" from the manu-facturer [for example, pricing concessions] for going along with the deal. Moreover, if the clinicians don't like it or the manufacturer does not accede to these requests for consideration, the various clinical departments may torpedo the effort by sending off memos to other departments criticizing the bundle. Even the presence of powerful CEOs and CFOs may not be sufficient to successfully promote a bundling approach. As one executive asserted, "Many times they are too intimidated [by these powerful physicians] to drive the change."

Another external challenge to this approach is gaining the trust of IDNs. As noted in Chapter Four, buyers are already skeptical of manufacturers' pricing. Here they may be skeptical of manufacturer programs to sell them more product under the banner of "product bundles" or "disease management." They may (rightfully) perceive these to be bundles of contracting convenience rather than bundles of the best products; moreover, given the differences in manufac-turers' portfolios, it is impossible to evaluate one firm's bundle against another's. Clinicians, in particular, may feel that all product choice is taken away from them. To make the program successful, manu-facturers ideally need to bundle together products that are market leaders in each of their own respective areas. Failing this, they can document how well the bundle serves to deliver high-quality care below a budgeted DRG reimbursement, or at least leverage the brand name behind their market-leading products across other items.

Another major challenge to manufacturer-led efforts in disease management may be that they only tangentially touch the doctor-patient relationship. One executive said

Simplistically, disease management has still got to occur between a doctor and a patient. That is where the relationship gets reinforced and why patients are doing what they are doing. That is what it all goes back to. That relationship is key. HMOs have not done very well implementing disease management programs, but not because their programs weren't good. It is hard to get the doctor to do it at the right time with the patient, and that is the critical step: you have to get those two together to communicate about what and how and when and why they should be following a given protocol. I'm not sure anybody else is going to have a huge impact. Manufacturers may know diseases, and I think we can help, but I'm not sure we can fundamentally change the key relationship and who touches the patient.

At a broad level, these strategies are part of an effort to develop a corporate capability in customer service and customer relationship management. The underlying theory here is that firms can develop strategic competencies in relating with their customers that yield sustained competitive advantage. Unfortunately, strategies of customer service and relationship management have not been widely adopted among provider organizations. Moreover, it is not clear that they possess any critical capabilities in these areas.[7]

New Business Initiatives with Hospital Customers

Medical-surgical manufacturers have developed several new initiatives to serve their hospital customers. These include consulting units, point of use technology, and direct ordering.

Consulting Units

Just as med-surg manufacturers have established corporate divisions to provide customers with a unified face regarding their products, they have also established consulting units (usually through acquisitions) to provide an extensive range of services. Johnson & Johnson, for example, acquired McFaul & Lyons (consulting firm specializing in expense management and reengineering), while Becton Dickinson acquired Concepts in Health Care (specializing in materials management). In the former case, the consulting unit is housed in JJHCS. In the latter case, the acquisition constituted the first step in developing a new corporate division for consulting, BD Consulting and Services.

The firms want to transform these consulting units into service units. Such services are not necessarily intended to promote or accompany the use of the firm's products. Instead, the firms state their goal is to "increase their relevance with the customer," "be a better partner," "provide solutions to customer problems and needs rather than create products for their problems," and "fill a void that goes beyond where our product people go." They also state that product supplies account for only 15 percent of the hospital's budget, whereas services account for a larger share of expenditures (see Chapter Two).

The consulting solutions are quite broad, including

- GPO selection and affiliation

- Assessment and qualification of ERP solutions

- Implementation of ERP applications to materials management, pharmacy, and so forth

- IT systems integration and utilization

- Multisite integration of functions

- Make-versus-buy decisions (group purchasing or direct distribution)

- Supply management optimization

- Clinical department management consulting

- Clinical pathways, and product and procedural standardization

- Operational improvement

- Facilities planning and redesign

- Workflow design

- Benchmarking

It is evident that many of the services offered to hospitals compete with similar offerings from their GPOs. One such service is standardization. As an executive put it,

> We'll go out to the physicians, get them in a room at night, buy them pizza or something, and say, 'Come on guys, let's map your process.' Well, you would never design a process that looks like this. Look at hips. We're all using different hips. Look at pacemakers—how many different pacemakers do you really need? We don't care which product they use or which system they use. We're trying to take the emotion[al] and political aspects out of the decision, and put some business decision process behind it.

It is also evident that some of these services may induce hospitals to leave their GPO or join a rival GPO. For example, hospitals that have been individual customers of the med-surg manufacturer have recently merged or combined into systems. In the past, each hospital had its own (but usually different) GPO affiliation. As a new system seeking some greater economies in its group purchasing, it needs to standardize on one GPO, but may have trouble picking one. The consulting unit is then brought into a "GPO shootout": the consulting unit advises hospitals about the purchasing philosophy and approach taken by different GPOs, their respective strengths and weaknesses, and which GPO better suits the newly merged system. While the system makes the final decision, the consulting unit's analysis may lead it to depart or avoid a GPO where the consulting firm's parent corporation has a large portfolio of contracts as a med-surg manufacturer.

In a similar vein, the consulting unit may advise hospitals to establish their own regional contracting organizations that initially contract for services once performed by GPOs and then later on bring them in-house. In effect, the unit helps hospitals to contract directly with manufacturers and bypass the GPO intermediary. According to one unit interviewed, the direct contracting business is growing slowly as IDNs withdraw from their GPOs and learn how to "stand on their own two feet." The consulting firm's involvement here may seem self-serving. As an executive stated, "We enjoy dealing with IDNs that eschew the GPO, and it's not because we don't have to pay a CAF. It is less bureaucratic, easier to manage, and we have formed a direct relationship with the end user." It is not surprising that it also raises the ire of the GPOs the parent firm contracts with.

A major impetus to consulting services has been hospital CEOs and CFOs asking for dialogue with manufacturers about "issues" rather than "products." This desire has spawned a number of forums (for example, Health Care Executive Forum and Healthcare Research Development Institute) where manufacturers, distributors, GPOs, and hospitals get together to discuss broader issues. These issues encompass how to reduce costs of procedures, how to improve process flows, how to develop centers of excellence, how to improve purchasing compliance, and how to improve change management following mergers and acquisitions. Such forums are favorably viewed because they have more broad representation of supply chain players compared to the Health Industry Manufacturers Association (HIMA) and the Health Industry Distributors Association (HIDA).

Point-of-Use IT

Another major business initiative where manufacturers would like to engage hospitals is point-of-use information technology (IT). Such technology permits a better understanding of the current flow of activity and resources in care delivery, as well as a foundation for mapping improvements to these flows. The technology also provides manufacturers with a view of product consumption that enables them to better plan production schedules. However, they perceive very slow movement toward bar coding and scanning at the hospital level due to the high capital investment and the uncertain payback. For example, hospitals are unsure whether scanners will reduce labor costs in terms of the number of nurses or other FTEs, which is their single biggest cost component. They also do not believe that their presence implies their use. "Unless point-of-use systems such as Pyxis and Omnicell are used properly, most implementations will be money losers. That is because people do not exploit what they are intended to do, which is provide point-of-service monitoring of product consumption and continuous replenishment. Instead, people use them as a shelf and they open the door, take something out, and fail to press the buttons."

Catalysts for change may be the presence of aggressive, early adopters of these innovations, the demonstration of productivity improvements, the falling cost of IT, and succeeding (younger) generations of clinicians that are more comfortable with and demanding of such technological capabilities.

Next-Generation Customer Initiatives: Direct Ordering

Finally, some manufacturers have developed task forces called "next-generation customer initiatives" to explore new ways of dealing with hospitals. Many of these task forces have arisen to study the implication of trends toward vertical and horizontal integration among hospitals. Some have theorized what the hospital of the future will look like; others have tried to project the "winners" in each market and, thus, who should be the manufacturers' closest partners.

Many manufacturers have explored the benefits of direct product ordering by their hospital customers—in effect, cutting out the

GPO middleman. They see many benefits to this approach, such as (1) cutting out CAFs and passing some of them along to hospitals in the form of lower prices, more R&D that benefits providers (for example, by lowering future costs), and added customer services; (2) more direct contact with the customer; and (3) greater control over their products and information regarding their consumption. They also believe that hospitals can get access to the same prices and products as GPOs, and can deliver similar or better levels of contract compliance than GPOs. Finally, manufacturers relish the idea of having more direct contact with clinicians who order their high-technology products with less influence exerted by "economic buyers" (GPOs and hospital CFOs). They cite the benefits of dealing directly with hospital systems that have leading-edge centers of excellence in their flagship institution. Clinical practices within such centers, including the products they order, may be imitated by other hospitals and medical groups in the system and around the state.

On the other hand, they also see many obstacles to direct ordering. First, they lack good data on customer product preferences. At present, they assemble these data from various sources and seek to triangulate what they are told by their sales representatives, distributors, and GPOs. Manufacturers state that sometimes the only reliable information they have comes when hospitals direct order expensive devices over the phone.[8] Hospitals themselves, however, lack the information systems to collect the information manufacturers seek. Second, while most large hospitals are connected to distributors via EDI, and while distributors are connected to manufacturers via EDI, there are few direct EDI connections between manufacturers and hospitals. This is due to the lack of equipment setup or delays in connection as one side tries to develop it. This lack of EDI connectivity raises the cost of product ordering. Third, manufacturers will incur higher contracting costs in dealing with individual hospitals than with GPOs.

Manufacturers are not enthusiastic about direct distribution for all of their products. As noted previously, they maintain some regional warehouses to distribute their high-value items, to carefully handle products that are temperature sensitive or subject to damage, and to handle products (for example, bioscience) with shorter shelf life. Some manufacturers suggest that their capacity, logistical know-how, and financial strength pose an implicit threat that they will enter the distribution business if distributors "get out of line."

Nevertheless, manufacturers offer several reasons why this threat will probably never materialize. First of all, they acknowledge that distributors bring critical mass to hospitals from an EDI and information systems perspective. This is because large distributors handle a large percentage of the hospital's deliveries, offer them EDI connections to place orders to the distributor, and offer them software to automate their materials management processes and integrate their IT systems. Manufacturers can only provide these solutions on a piecemeal basis through their separate product companies. Second, many manufacturers report that their hospital customers want products shipped through a distributor so that they have one source to access their products, have product quickly available from a local warehouse, and don't have to own or hold inventory. Manufacturers, themselves, recognize that distributors enable them to increase the breadth of product offered and delivered to the customer. Third, they acknowledge that they do not fully understand the trade-offs between the cost of holding inventory versus the cost of making multiple product deliveries to hospital customers. Fourth, manufacturers acknowledge that they cannot do distribution as cheaply as distributors can.

> Don't think that we're not asked every day to ship direct. We sit there and say, 'You know, if I could do it for four and a half percent I would be in distribution.' But I can't do it for four and a half percent. And, as a matter of fact, if you were smart you would understand that if the distributor is losing money [on the shipping portion] then that's the best deal you will ever get in your life. As

part of this, manufacturers don't want to duplicate the infrastructure that distributors have developed and tie up capital in warehouses and inventory. Finally, if manufacturers want to exert more control over distributors and their product handling, they acknowledge that they can gain some of this through "distributor rationalization"; that is, partner with a smaller number of distributors, which handle the bulk of product shipments, and promise them greater volume in exchange for not engaging in vendor rationalization or product selection.

Key Success Factors

Perhaps the most important factor in determining the success of these business initiatives between manufacturers and hospitals is the stability of their account people and key hospital staff, and the longevity in these interpersonal customer relationships. Manufacturers note that their most successful partnerships have been where they have sales representatives and account executives dealing with the same hospital or GPO for long periods (for example, up to twenty years). This longevity enables them to develop "customer equity"; that is, trusting and working relationships with clinicians, materials managers, and so on that enable both sides to explore issues of value and total cost in their contracts. The problem here is not so much turnover as upward mobility. Executives had the following perspectives:

> My problem is the representatives are too good and I have to keep promoting them. Right now, if you look at the natural career ladder, this position is considered a stepping stone to higher positions.

> We have to balance making sure that we have a consistent relationship with a customer with making sure the salesperson in the job feels they have a meaningful career and that we can meet the needs of our business here.

Moreover, the travel is such that you just cannot ask somebody to keep that up for ten years. They wouldn't have a family life.

I think we have finally come to the realization that we can get some productivity out of account people if we leave them in assignments for a longer period of time. This could range anywhere from two to ten years.

Moreover, these trusting relationships rest on responsiveness to customer demands for product availability and delivery. Manufacturers place great importance on their sales representatives being forthcoming about back orders and erroneous shipments of product, and honest about when customers might expect their order to be fulfilled.

Opportunities for Efficiencies

There are several areas to target for efficiency improvements in the supply chain. Manufacturers commonly highlight the value of SKU rationalization, reduced duplication, and risk contracting.

SKU/Line Rationalization

Manufacturers commonly point to one area for gleaning further efficiencies in the supply chain: removing SKUs (stockkeeping units). As noted in Chapter Five, distributors have been engaged in a "line rationalization" effort to reduce the number of SKUs they carry, and thus their inventory-holding costs. They prefer to focus on the 20 percent of items that move quickly (high number of "inventory turns") and account for 80 percent of their volume, and let customers source more esoteric items directly from the manufacturer.[9] This threatens manufacturers whose items may not be included among the 20 percent that distributors want to emphasize. Manufacturers dislike distributor efforts to steer customers toward another vendor's products in exchange for a higher margin.

At the same time, manufacturers recognize line rationalization as a good business practice that they should be doing instead. One executive stated

> I think the manufacturers should do it before the distributors do. If you compare the consumer industry with the health care industry, in consumer you find, on average, one SKU moves one unit per week, while in health care it's one unit moves every three to four weeks. So obviously there is something not right in that equation. What manufacturers need to do is challenge themselves to reduce the SKUs before the distributors do it for them. What ends up happening is that the manufacturer still has the SKU, some customer demands it, and the distributor no longer carries it. This means that the cost of carrying that SKU to the end customer grows that much higher. Moreover, as we start to put in our own activity-based costing (ABC) systems and understand that these SKUs with less than a million dollars in sales have logistics costs that are anywhere from five to ten times the logistics cost of a normal SKU, they are going to get weeded out. The same thing happened in the consumer industry.

Manufacturers thus recognize that the distributors' efforts at line rationalization are consistent with their own efforts in SKU or product rationalization: both are oriented to reducing their logistics costs (that is, higher inventory costs for distributors, and higher shipping and inventory costs for manufacturers). In addition, manufacturers face higher production costs from carrying lots of SKUs. This is because they have multiple-machine setups, more machine downtime, and shorter production runs for each of the smaller-volume SKUs they produce.

One avenue manufacturers have pursued to promote SKU rationalization is to develop formularies for medical-surgical products (as exist for drugs). In this model, the manufacturer develops a contract with the hospital that grants average pricing if the hospital wants a full product line, but then offers reduced pricing as the hospital restricts its purchases to the med-surg formulary. As hospitals switch over to the formulary, the manufacturer weeds out SKUs that have low volume. The formulary approach may need to be supplemented by efforts to educate physicians about product standardization (see Chapter Four). Manufacturers acknowledge they have a lot of work to do to get clinicians to accept not having their preferred SKUs on contract.

Barriers to SKU Rationalization

Why have manufacturers been so slow to embrace SKU rationalization? First, they have traditionally been oriented to satisfying the preferences of clinicians who wanted everything customized—that is, sutures of this length or needles of that length, and so on. This orientation is reinforced by the physician's position as the major customer of med-surg manufacturers. This orientation has also been reinforced by a cost-plus reimbursement climate that allowed clinicians to order any product they wanted and have it reimbursed by payers.

Indeed, manufacturers have created the problem of multiple SKUs by actively marketing to physicians and their diverse preferences. For example, when a hospital or its GPO decides on a specific vendor in a given product category, there are other vendors whose products may not have been selected. They do not idly sit by and wait to compete again until the contract with the chosen vendor expires. They actively engage in counter-detailing the current contract by going to the physician or OR nurse.

I'm going to go to the independent contractor and say, 'Look, you're the doctor, what's going on here? Are you going to let some guy down in the basement, who may or may not have a college degree, tell you what the hell to do?' The first thing that guy says is, 'Absolutely not. What the hell, he's practicing medicine for me. I'm not going to let him do that.' And if you think we as device manufacturers are bad, just look at the pharmaceuticals. The drug guys are worse. We are as much the problem as we are the solution.

Indeed, the manufacturers recognize that their counter-detailing efforts are one major reason why hospitals are so disorganized as buyers and weak at clinical standardization. Their efforts also explain why GPO efforts to gain IDN compliance achieve limited success. In fact, the med-surg manufacturers view these disorganized buyers (whom they have helped to create) as a "countervailing force" to the GPO's ability to gain contracting compliance.

Second, manufacturers are wary of eliminating low-volume SKUs that have "strategic linkage" to other, high-volume SKUs. As one executive explained, "I sell only 5 of these a year, but when I sell these 5 it allows me to sell these 50,000 over here." As a result, manufacturers are studying not only the relative volumes of their products but also the volumes of various combinations and interactions of products. Nevertheless, this process may take quite long and yield only limited savings. And one executive urged caution:

We have done some reviews of our product lines where there are 4,000 SKUs. Of these, 2,000 SKUs account for 98 percent of the business, while the other 2,000 account for only 2 percent of the business. A rational person can say even without looking at a number of a specific use that there are too many. And there has got to be a way to take the volume in the bottom 2,000 SKUs and rationalize that some way. But you have got to do it slowly and strategically so that you don't jeopardize any other part of your business or your customer base. If there is no logical alternative to that SKU you may need to have something in your portfolio that says 'I don't make a lot of money on this but it's part of my package and I'm not going to take something out of the hands of a user.'

While an SKU may remain in the manufacturer's portfolio due to lingering physician preferences, it may also remain simply due to inertia: The "lingering practice of just leaving it on the price list and leaving it in the product offering." Only recently have some manufacturers assigned someone the responsibility to cut SKUs. Moreover, they have instructed their forecasting groups to eliminate two SKUs every time a new SKU is added.

Elimination of Duplicated Effort

Another area of possible efficiency gains lies in the reduction of duplicated effort among supply chain participants. It is evident from the previous description of med-surg manufacturers that they are engaged in several GPO-type services: consulting, product promotion and sales, compliance, and sales data collection. For example, as one executive explained

> The GPOs are very demanding in terms of information. With the sales organizations that I've got out there, I wonder why do you need all of this information? It is almost as if they are trying to replace the selling organization, but then they can't because they need the selling organization to convert [providers from one product to another]. If you look at [GPO X's] launch finder for a particular product, you would conclude they have just recreated your entire marketing department, which you worked on for years to create.

Distributors likewise have large sales forces calling on customers, which manufacturers also view as duplicated effort. "It costs a lot of money to have a sales force of 800 people out there calling on all of these places. Hell, I already sold it. Why do I need to go out and sell it again? There are a lot of people out there selling my product or the other guy's product. It costs a lot of money to do that."

Manufacturers cite two major and related barriers to eliminating such duplication. The first is the desire for "channel control"; that is, controlling access to the customer and the data generated by customer sales, and jockeying for position to see who can bring the greatest value to customers. Some supply chain intermediaries try to provide customer value by emulating manufacturers in terms of their sales forces and sales data. As one executive stated, "I can remember sitting down with the chief executives at [Distributor X]. They said, 'You know, we need to walk like J&J, talk like J&J, eat like J&J, drink like J&J. We want to be J&J. Because we know there is value to J&J in that, and we want to bring that same value to our customers.' So they are trying to find ways as a business to operate with more value, so everybody's trying to do the same thing."

The second barrier is fear of sharing information. This fear stems in part from concerns over antitrust and perceived collusion. It also stems from the loss of proprietary knowledge and thus potential revenues and competitive advantage.

Risk Contracting

A third possible source of efficiency might be capitated risk contracts between manufacturers and provider systems. These contracting arrangements rely on providers having capitated contracts with HMOs and passing on a portion of the risk to manufacturers in the form of a per-member-per-month (PMPM) target cost for supplies. Manufacturers that help providers with supply cost and utilization, and thereby stay under the PMPM fee, generate additional savings. Such arrangements have been established in the past. The biggest barrier to their diffusion has been the movement away from capitation and the return to (discounted) fee-for-service reimbursement. Even in markets where capitation is still prevalent, however, the savings from these programs have not been large enough to encourage their spread. A three-year experiment in Seattle between 3M and Group Health Cooperative (closed model HMO with capitation) helped the HMO to reduce its supply costs by one-third. However, because supply expenditures are not a big portion of an HMO's cost structure, the actual dollars were not very large. As a result, the program has not expanded and has been put on the HMO's "back burner."[10]

Endnotes

1. Aguilar, Francis, and Arvind Bhambri. *Johnson & Johnson (A) and (B)*. Boston, Massachusetts: Harvard Business School Publishing, 1996.
2. Cox, Carrie. "Marketing and Sales." Presentation to Aresty Institute of Executive Education. Wharton-Windhover Management Program for Pharmaceutical Executives. Wharton School, April 1999.
3. Lawrence, Paul, and Jay Lorsch. *Organization and Environment*. Cambridge, Massachusetts: Harvard University Press, 1967.
4. Galbraith, Jay. *Organization Design*. Reading, Massachusetts: Addison-Wesley, 1977.
5. There can also be legal challenges to bundling. One form of product bundling that is not covered under the Medicare Safe Harbors is when the manufacturer ties a discount on one item to the purchase of another; that is, I will sell you X at a cheaper price if you buy Y. Manufacturers do not pursue this approach. Instead, they offer GPOs bundles or products from across their divisions: "If you buy from ten divisions we'll give you this, if you buy from eleven we'll give you this plus this, and if you buy from twelve we'll give you this plus this plus this."
6. Cassak, David. "J&J Health Care Systems—Beyond the Supply Chain." *In Vivo* (February 1996): 34.
7. Day, George. "Customer Relationship Management." Unpublished manuscript, 2000.
8. One manufacturer reported that its sales representatives are very protective of their territory and their customers, and want to be the conduit of information regarding customer preferences.
9. According to one manufacturer, the medical-surgical distributor Owens & Minor carries 130,000 items, of which 10,000 (7–8 percent) account for 80 percent of their volume.
10. Haugh, Richard. "Supply Capitation: Proving Ground." *Hospitals and Health Networks* (December 2000): 16.

Part IV

. . . .

E-Commerce

10

• •

E-Commerce in Health Care—Manufacturers, Distributors, and GPOs

Lawton R. Burns and Robert A. DeGraaff

The Promise of E-Commerce in Health Care: The View from Consulting Firms and Investment Banks

The promise of e-commerce in health care can be viewed from many angles. Here, we consider the seven markets of e-health, the relative size of some of these markets, their value proposition, market drivers, and potential savings.

The Seven C's and D's of E-Health

Investment banking analysts and consultants initially classified health care Internet models in terms of the "seven C's and D's" of e-health:[1]

1. *Content* for consumers

2. *Connectivity* with payers, providers, PBMs, and so on

3. *Computer applications*—both Web-integrating desktops and applications

4. *Clinical care*—both technology enablers and disease management programs

5. *Commerce*—business-to-consumer (B2C) and business-to-business (B2B)

6. *Drug discovery*

7. *Drug development*

Hambrecht & Quist estimated that clinical care had the greatest market potential ($700 billion), followed at a great distance by e-commerce ($150 billion), connectivity ($10 billion), and content ($7 billion).[2] We limit our focus here to e-commerce and, in particular, B2B models.

Size of B2B and B2C Markets

The B2B market exceeded the B2C market in size, regardless of the estimates chosen and how inflated they all seemed. Forrester Research claimed that the health care B2B product market would grow from $6 billion in 1999 to $348 billion by 2004 (two-thirds of which are provider claims, one-third of which are supplies, drugs, or equipment).[3] This $348 billion figure represents roughly 17 percent of trade. In contrast, the B2C market would grow during that same period from only $440 million to $22 billion (mostly in prescription drugs). Other analysts estimated the entire B2B market ($43 billion in 1998) was five times the size of the B2C market ($7.8 billion).[4] They estimated that by 2003 the difference would be tenfold ($1 trillion versus $100 billion).

Value Proposition of B2B Models

According to Wall Street analysts, B2B models offered the following benefits:

aggregation of suppliers and their products through electronic catalogues and one-stop shopping capability, which can result in better pricing and lower product costs

connectivity between suppliers and buyers in smaller markets and buyers of lower volumes, which may improve pricing in areas underpenetrated by GPOs

efficiency in pricing for buyers, for example, via access to updated information on pricing and contracts

efficiency in procurement for buyers, for example, by eliminating paper catalogues; paper, phone, and fax ordering; mixing electronic and manual processes; redundant data entry; and incomplete or erroneous information flows from providers to suppliers

exploitation of spot supply market opportunities through auctions

visibility of orders and materials all along the pipeline

improved inventory management on a just-in-time basis across the supply chain, with the potential for higher inventory turns (for vendors) and improved management of used equipment and excess supply capacity (for providers)

reduced cycle times in the fulfillment of transactions

automatic triggers of replenishment through end-use monitoring systems

synchronized databases across supply chain partners

collaborative planning, forecasting, and replenishment with suppliers and customers

dynamic re-planning of schedules and flows to meet customer needs

improved quality of information flows by reducing the number of errors

rationalized reimbursement using electronic payments and automatic reconciliation of rebates at the point of sale

enhanced change management and partnering along the value chain as vendors and providers alike adopt e-commerce technology and share data

infomediaries who understand the customized purchasing patterns and needs of buyers.[5,6]

Some product areas are considered ripe for B2B transactions: specialty supplies, devices, and new and used equipment. These areas are noncommodity products, and thus are not typically included in GPO contracts. Hospitals are estimated to use GPO contract pricing for 80 percent of their pharmaceutical purchases and 50 percent of their medical-surgical purchases—figures which parallel the percentage of purchases in these product categories that flow through distributors—but much less for specialty and device products. Vendors in these areas are less consolidated than they are in pharmaceuticals and medical and surgical supplies, leading to more direct sales to customers. B2B models can help to aggregate buyers in these fragmented markets, lowering their procurement costs.

This is not to discount the importance of B2B transactions for commodity items, however. One problem faced by manufacturers of lower-end supplies is that the sales and distribution functions have been outsourced to wholesalers who call on the end customer. This limits the direct visibility of the product pipeline to the manufacturer, the manufacturer's direct ability to move market share, as well as the manufacturer's ability to directly inform customers regarding new products and innovative changes. The Internet provides a potential remedy to this problem. In addition, it puts the manufacturer into direct contact with motivated buyers, which can reduce sales expenses.

Four Drivers of E-Commerce Potential in Health Care

Investment banks mention four reasons for the power of e-commerce applications in health care. First, the industry has historically underinvested in information technology (IT) compared to other transaction-intensive industries. Health care invests 3.9 percent of its revenues in IT versus 6.7 percent in telecommunications and 10.3 percent in the financial services industry.[7]

This is remarkably low, given that much of health care spending is generated by encounters between patients, providers, and suppliers; and most of these encounters are transactions. Moreover, most of these transactions currently occur over the phone or a fax machine.

Second, decreased hospital reimbursement by the Balanced Budget Act (1997) prompted IDNs to reduce their capital IT budgets by an estimated 40–60 percent between 1998 and 2000. This placed product and pricing pressures on legacy software and hardware vendors, whose IT solutions were expensive, cumbersome to install and use, and offered limited demonstrable return on investment.[8] Such solutions were further hampered by a shortage of qualified IT specialists in the health care industry.

Third, the Health Insurance Portability and Accountability Act (HIPAA) of 1996 contained an administrative simplification section designed to streamline the administration of health insurance. For firms using EDI, this section mandated standards for common financial transactions (for example, pharmacy, physician, and hospital claims; and payments and remittance) and administrative transactions (for example, eligibility verification, precertification, authorization, referral, and enrollment). To meet this mandate, the industry agreed to a common syntax called *X12* to format all data. By virtue of this common standard and access to the Internet, providers could more easily adopt Web-based EDI.

Fourth, the adoption of Extensible Markup Language (XML) as a standardized technological infrastructure has been facilitated by the Organization for the Advancement of Structured Information Standards (OASIS). XML is a data standard that makes data portable and interoperable across systems and firms. It is also a structured language specifically designed for secure Internet-based transactions.[9] This provides formal support for the consolidation of industry information standards, and thus a catalyst for B2B efforts. Users can also push more information through XML compared to EDI.

Projected Savings from E-Commerce

According to Ernst & Young, there exists a potential savings opportunity of 13–27 percent of supply product costs from e-commerce applications to the health care supply chain.[10] These savings derive from

- Decreased external logistics and distribution costs (5–10 percent)

- Improved product utilization and substitution (4–8 percent)

- Increased product standardization (3–6 percent)

- Reduced product shrinkage (1–2 percent)

- Better pricing (0–1 percent)

In this manner, supply costs as a percentage of total operating expenses can be reduced to 12 percent. Thus, for an integrated delivery network (IDN) with annual operating expenses of $1.5 billion, the savings opportunity approaches $18–38 million annually.

What are the strategies Ernst & Young suggests to achieve these savings? Unfortunately, many of them rely on approaches called into question in our previous chapters. These include direct contracting with manufacturers, disintermediation of distributors, the development of "consolidated service centers" to act as the IDN's self-contracted GPO and distributor, manufacturers' use of bar codes on their products, IDN's use of scanning technology for charging and replenishment purposes, just-in-time (JIT) delivery of low unit of measure (LUM) supplies (rather than bulk) to facilitate quick delivery to patient care areas, use of third-party logistics (3PL) firms and the "cross-docking" of supplies (in LUM) at the consolidated service center, and significant IDN investment in information and standardization systems such as Enterprise Resource Planning (ERP).

In contrast to Ernst & Young, Arthur Anderson reported more modest savings available from e-commerce applications in the range of 2–10 percent across *all* supply chain participants, and 1–3 percent of providers' total supply costs (not 13–27 percent). Manufacturers stand to gain the most ($4 billion), while providers might reap $2 billion in savings from using e-commerce solutions for efficient order management and information sharing.[11]

Outsourcing B2B: Application Service Providers (ASPs)

Much of this transition to e-commerce need not entail the same level of capital investment as the legacy systems of the near past. Outsourcing is a real option for IDNs, given the shortage of qualified IT personnel, falling IT budgets, and reimbursement pressures. There are two types of outsourcing: transferring full responsibility for the IT function (including IT staffing) to an external firm, or transferring responsibility for only the software applications.[12] During the last few years, several firms—known as application service providers (ASPs) and business service providers (BSPs)—have emerged to handle these outsourced functions.[13]

ASPs use Internet technology to deliver prepackaged or enterprise software solutions (for example, ERP systems) that are maintained, customized, and monitored by the ASP for businesses across several industries. The ASP either owns or purchases the right to license the specific application software that it hosts in its own data center. It then rents the application to organizations that can access the software from their desktops and process their data using the software at the ASP site. Applications are typically standardized with little customization, and thus are shared with many clients. Full outsourcing, by contrast, entails more of a one-to-one relationship.[14]

ASPs target smaller and mid-sized firms, which have not been already served by the large legacy vendors. Smaller firms find ASPs attractive given their lower cost relative to expensive legacy systems. Such firms never have to deal with the complexities of installing or maintaining software but can still use all of an application's functions by paying a service or subscription fee. Moreover, they may be more willing to forego customized features for the lower cost of ASPs. Such costs are estimated to be anywhere from 33–53 percent less (according to the ASP Consortium) or 50–70 percent less (according to the Gartner Group) than the cost of legacy systems. By contrast, larger firms already have IT departments and need more sophisticated "mission critical" applications, which are not as well served by standardized packages. They also have a variety of legacy systems that must be integrated with one another and customized to meet their specific needs.[15]

ASP Advantages

ASPs offer several advantages over traditional legacy systems:

There are no expensive up-front licensing, purchasing, or implementation expenditures.

They provide a single point of contact to access multiple software applications.

They provide universal access to these applications by virtue of using the Internet.

They provide the firm with access to specialized expertise at the ASP, which focuses on technical issues and best practices.

They allow the client to re-deploy personnel and financial resources to other parts of the firm.

Maintenance costs are low and bundled into the subscription rental fee.

Services are provided on a predictable monthly subscription basis. For the ASP, the presence of recurring sales (rather than one big sale) reduces their revenue risk.

The solutions are modular rather than bundled, thus offering a trial basis for using any application.

Implementation times range from three to six months rather than twelve to eighteen months.

Providers can respond more quickly to HIPAA requirements.

Solutions rely on an "integrating desktop" and "thin-client" technology using Java or a single Web-browser interface to view or exchange information with multiple legacy applications, rather than a large investment in hardware.

They provide upgrades that leverage the latest technology and applications without the need for in-house IT specialists or external consultants.

Providers can maintain their investment in legacy applications; ASPs can take over these licenses.

Switching costs are much lower.

Illustrations of ASP Adoptions

One illustration of the ASP or BSP solution in health care is "OmniBuyer." This application is based on Commerce One's "Buysite" system, an e-procurement technology platform for providers. To implement Buysite, providers must pay $1 million plus transaction royalties. In its place, an ASP firm called OmniCell has co-branded Buysite for health care applications and offered it to providers on a shared-service basis for a subscription fee. By 2000, over 200 hospitals had signed up to use Omnibuyer.[16] Another illustration of ASPs occurred when Talbert Medical Group in California outsourced all of its computer applications to the Trizetto Group. Talbert sought to rebuild its business operations—particularly the tracking of claims for patients referred to specialists and out-of-network—after buying itself back from the failed PPMC MedPartners. The ASP allows Talbert to match claims with preauthorizations to ensure that it pays the correct rate. Group officials state the move reduced their information costs as a percent of net revenues from 6.5 percent to 4.0 percent.

Surveys of hospitals and health systems suggest that provider interest in the ASP market is low but beginning to develop.[17] According to the Eleventh Annual Survey of Information System Trends, only 4 percent of hospitals identified the ASP approach to obtaining software as a priority.[18] The Twelfth Annual Survey conducted the following year found little change in hospital interest levels, with only 13 percent reporting that they currently used ASPs.[19] Similarly, according to PriceWaterhouse Coopers, 14 percent of hospitals or systems have signed or intend to sign contracts with ASPs for clinical data capturing and reporting. Slightly fewer providers have expressed interest in ASP contracts to handle administrative and financial systems (12 percent), departmental systems (10 percent), database and repository services (9 percent), and physician practice management (8 percent). The ASP market for health care is currently estimated at $1.2 billion, and is expected to double by 2002.[20]

ASP Disadvantages

Of course, there are also downsides to ASP solutions that do not receive much attention. First, like B2B, ASPs are hyped as the solution to every problem confronting the industry. Second, there is the question of whether ASP vendors will meet HIPAA standards regarding compliance (for example, security). Third, ASPs may not be designed to handle the heavy volume of transactions that characterize the health care industry. Consequently, providers may encounter sluggish response times sitting at their desktops as they employ these solutions. More critically, the outages experienced in the past by eBay, eToys, and Etrade due to high demand will not be tolerated by health care professionals.[21] Indeed, the key issue facing ASPs may be performance. ASPs may require high bandwidths and/or minimal network delays for high-performance applications. However, broadband pipes are expensive to lease presently and take a long time to install. Some ASPs may be tempted to cut corners and economize by sharing capacity among many customers, leading to congestion and network delays.[22]

Fourth, outsourcing IT functions to an ASP provider is akin to using someone else's software application. A major issue is whether the ASP can be customized to fit the needs of very different IDNs. Some suggest that the costs of customization may far outweigh the fees incurred to license the application. Moreover, providers may lack access to the source code needed to make major modifications. Fifth, the ASP market has become very crowded, with no one firm yet earning profits (as of 2000). Consequently, some industry restructuring is likely. This may pose transition problems for buyers, who may be wary of signing on with ASPs. Sixth, ASPs essentially represent Wall Street's financing of a new pricing strategy. Venture capitalists and investors have financed the ASPs, which have assumed a huge working capital burden in product development. Due to the need of ASPs to develop new products all the time in order to compete, this burden is likely to grow. It is unclear, however, how long Wall Street will finance all of this, especially given providers' low margins. Seventh, hospitals are reportedly reducing their IT budgets by large amounts. They are also reportedly unwilling to capitalize their investments in software when they tap the tax-exempt bond markets. Finally, use of ASPs may threaten the interests and turf of both the IT staff and the chief information officers (CIOs), who feel they are yielding control and worry about whom to contact when problems arise.[23]

Three other questions will need to be resolved before there is any major shift among providers in the use of ASPs. First, who owns the data that is transmitted to the ASP? Can the ASP use it or sell it to others? This hearkens back to one of the first issues raised previously, regarding data security. Second, what is the ASP's domain knowledge in health care? Does it have any applications experience in this industry? And three, how much experience do ASPs have in integrating their software offerings with the legacy systems of providers?

B2B E-Commerce Initiatives in the Health Care Industry

During the late 1990s, a host of e-commerce firms quickly sprung up in the health care supply chain, including Medibuy, Neoforma, MedAssets, OmniCell, and Promedix. Some of these firms have failed; others are still struggling. Their history is profiled next in order to illustrate some of their operating problems and the lessons of e-commerce.

Medibuy

Medibuy.com was launched in August 1998 to be a buyer-centric and vendor-neutral Web site for buying and selling medical and surgical products, commodity items, and capital equipment. The firm initially sought to address two supply chain problems: (1) the exclusion of smaller, nonelite vendors from national contracts and (2) the lack of connectivity between small vendors and large IDN buyers. The firm developed a series of e-commerce products designed to open up the marketplace:

eCatalog, launched in December 1999, to provide product prices and availability via an on-line catalogue.

eRFP, launched in April 1999, to centralize and automate the request-for-proposal process in which buyers submit requests for proposals (RFPs) for desired products, the RFPs are distributed to vendors, and vendors respond with bids.

eAuction, launched in June 1999, to offer an auction site for buying and selling new and used equipment, excess inventory, or refurbished items.

eSpecials, also launched in December 1999, to feature limited-time discounts on selected items.

At the time, Medibuy stated that it did not seek to compete with the national GPOs, since it did not negotiate prices; aggregate buyers to do volume purchasing; or solicit RFPs in product areas covered by the GPOs, such as maintenance and equipment.[24] Moreover, it did not charge transaction fees to contracted suppliers.

The early experience of Medibuy was mixed. The firm reported that it had lined up 1,400 buyers as of January 2000, of which 500–600 were hospitals. Sharp HealthCare was one of the first IDNs to offer its used capital equipment for sale through the eAuction division of Medibuy. There were few options for getting rid of surplus equipment other than storing it in a basement, donating it, or selling it through local brokers who receive huge markups to move the equipment. Sellers in eAuction paid Medibuy a transaction fee of 12 percent of the winning bid. Sharp posted thirty-five surplus items for auction during June 1999, half of which were sold during the month they were posted on-line. Bids received totaled $6,000, an amount four times greater than what Sharp would have received using local equipment dealers. Medibuy officials stated that their auction site had attracted many sellers but few buyers. Two explanations offered were the novelty of the site and the historical absence of a retail market here.[25]

Part of the appeal of Medibuy and its competitor, Neoforma (covered next), lay in the size and fragmented character of the used equipment marketplace. This market is estimated to be $8.5 billion.[26] It is inhabited by "manufacturer refurbishers," and is highly fragmented by geography, product, and capabilities. For example, most refurbishers operate in single-product markets (for example, imaging equipment or rehab equipment) which have only a small volume of sales, no critical mass of buyers and suppliers, and no national players.[27] On an aggregate level, the market sales opportunities may be attractive. Capital equipment purchases in the subacute market (for example, rehabilitation, physical medicine, ambulatory surgery centers, podiatry, and so forth) are estimated at $4.2 billion annually; equipment purchases in the overseas market are estimated at $6 billion annually.[28] There is thus an opportunity to bundle products to develop integrated and customized sourcing solutions for customers. Moreover, there is a further opportunity to combine products with services that support them, such as equipment appraisals, financing, shipping, installation, product support, warranties, and consumable supplies.

Like other B2B firms, Medibuy encountered problems of customer interest and technology development. To solve the first problem, it has revamped its offerings to include

Equipment Services, which documents an IDN's equipment inventory, identifies excess equipment, and uses an extranet to help IDNs relocate excess biomedical and capital medical equipment to other sites within the IDN where they are needed.

Auction, which sells those items not needed by the IDN, using a dynamic on-line trading system linked to qualified buyers and based on a bidding process.

Access, which integrates buyer and supplier systems with the Medibuy Marketplace, and enables end-to-end e-commerce transactions, data capture, and connectivity. Access represents an order processing solution, integrated into the hospital's ERP or materials management information system (using either existing EDI or XML technology), which can channel orders out to suppliers and distributors via EDI.

Freedom, which is a hosted materials management information system (MMIS) that is integrated into the Medibuy Marketplace exchange. It is powered by Lawson Insight software, which allows hospital buyers to outsource their MMIS. Features include on-line desktop requisitioning, purchase order management, inventory management, contract and vendor management, and real-time communication with suppliers.

Reqs, which is a stand-alone procurement solution that can channel orders directly to vendors.

To solve the second problem, Medibuy has allied with several technology partners. The firm partnered with Lawson Software, a leading provider of ERP systems that are now Web enabled for health care, to develop its Freedom materials management solution and provide the e-commece software to power Medibuy's ASP-based marketplace and enable customers to fully outsource their materials management information systems (MMIS). In return, Medibuy will host Lawson's Web-based suite of supply chain management software. Medibuy also signed agreements in early 2001 with Healthcare.com to obtain their integration package SupplyNet. This solution can integrate into hospital MMIS applications and allow Medibuy customers to have a single point of entry for all their purchase orders (POs). Finally, Medibuy partnered with Commerce One to obtain its MarketSite software as the core technology behind its on-line marketplace and its Reqs and Auction services.[29]

In January 2001, Medibuy announced its acquisition of the e-commerce unit of Premier (Premier Health Exchange) as part of a six-year electronic purchasing pact. In February 2001, Medibuy announced its acquisition of HCA's e-procurement company (empactHealth—see the following) and became the exclusive e-commerce provider to HCA's hospitals and alternate care facilities for six years. In addition, Medibuy would become the exclusive e-commerce provider to HCA's group purchasing organization

(Health Trust Purchasing Group) encompassing HCA, LifePoint Hospitals, Triad Hospitals, and Health Management Associates. These deals made Medibuy the sole provider of e-commerce solutions for two large GPOs that purchase on behalf of over 40 percent of U.S. hospitals, and which in turn will promote Medibuy's services to their hospital members. Medibuy will also assist Premier-affiliated hospitals with technical and integration assistance. By virtue of the deal with HCA, Medibuy gained not only HCA's hospital customer base but also its MarketSite e-commerce solution.

Medibuy also developed partnerships with major distributors. In September 2000, Medibuy announced an agreement with Henry Schein to be the exclusive distributor for Medibuy's physician-focused marketplace scheduled to go on-line near the end of that year. This marketplace is supposed to offer physicians the same types of purchasing services already offered to hospitals. In June 2001, it announced a two-year agreement with Allegiance Healthcare Corporation whereby Allegiance will accept orders from hospital members of Premier and Health Trust through Medibuy. Finally, in August 2001, Medibuy announced that Tyco Healthcare would make available its entire product line to HealthTrust and Premier Facilities, using the Medibuy marketplace.

Neoforma

Neoforma.com was founded in 1996, launched its Web site in 1997, and began digitizing supplier catalogues in January 1998. The firm went public and sold more than eight million shares in its IPO on January 24, 2000, netting proceeds of $97 million.

Initially, the company offered four primary services:

Neoforma.com Shop, an on-line site where purchasers (both hospitals and physicians) could locate and buy new medical products, and suppliers could access new customers and markets. Launched by September 1999, this product cleaned up the front-end functions of sourcing, ordering, and inventory management. It did not interfere with traditional functions performed by GPOs and distributors, but instead sought to integrate all market participants and offer a central ordering platform for all of their products. As such, Neoforma attacked the order management inefficiencies noted by EHCR. Revenues here derived from supplier-paid transaction fees of 1–10 percent. The company expected that this service would be the primary source of future revenues.

Neoforma.com Auction, a hospital-based application that offered an auction site for matching buyers and sellers of used, refurbished, and surplus medical equipment. Launched in summer 1999, Neoforma conducted auctions without handling the inventory, and posted digital pictures of equipment on its Web site. Auction had three main features: AdsOnline, which listed the equipment; AuctionLive, which conducted live real-time auctions; and AuctionOnline, which conducted auctions on the Internet. Neoforma acquired General Asset Recovery (GAR), a used equipment specialist, as a wraparound product to help hospitals assess and finance equipment, and assist with equipment and inventory management. Revenues here derived from seller-paid transaction fees (20–40 percent), buyer-paid transaction fees (5–10 percent), and seller-paid asset recovery services. In 1999, the company generated over 60 percent of its total net revenues from this service.

Neoforma.com Plan, another hospital-based application that provided interactive content to health care facility planners to reduce the complexities of planning and outfitting facilities. Launched by July 1998, it served as a one-stop shop for facility construction. Its "room planning guide" helped hospitals design and outfit X-ray departments, operating rooms, and cath labs using floor plans, equipment lists, and specifications.[30] It also allowed vendors to showcase their product setups in prestigious hospital accounts using 360-degree interactive photographs that suggest industry "best practices." Originally marketed as a bundled product approach ("best of breed" solution), Plan became more a software tool that facilitates "room standards" and comprehensive shopping lists; that is, "all the stuff that goes into an OR." Revenues here derived from sponsorship fees (average $5,000 per placement) and subscription and software fees (average $3,000 per user).

Neoforma's Services Delivery Group, which worked with hospitals' existing management systems to integrate them into Marketplace and then connect them with sellers.

Neoforma claimed there was some strategic integration of these services. The first three services together purported to manage the purchasing life cycle from planning to procurement to liquidation.

Between 1996 and 2000, Neoforma's progress as a B2B player was slow. During the first three years of its history, it earned total revenues of only $7,000 from its on-line marketplace for medical supplies. In the first quarter of 2000, thanks to the acquisition of GAR, the firm's auction revenues totaled $725,000. These were live auctions (not Web based), however, in which people stood in a warehouse "looking at CT scanners." Neoforma's CEO estimated that auction revenues constituted roughly 60–70 percent of the firm's total revenues, with 30 percent derived from on-line sales. Other firm executives believed the on-line portion to be even smaller (10–20 percent). Outside observers viewed Auction as a less appealing revenue stream than the other services. Some characterize it as "a one-time deal with no annuity." Others saw it as a market that varied with hospitals' need to raise cash from the disposition of assets; moreover, with BBA relief, there might be less interest in auctions. Nevertheless, the live auctions were considered at the time to be a pathway to obtaining more Web business or, alternatively, a sustaining strategy until Internet business picked up.[31]

Revenues did pick up considerably over the course of 2000. Used and refurbished equipment sales generated $4.6 million, Web-site sponsorship fees from its Plan service generated $2.6 million, and transaction fees generated through its marketplace and equipment sales yielded another $2.3 million. The physician business was also a big contributor to the firm's net earnings. This was expected to change, however, as the firm's revenues increased. Firm officials estimated the potential physician marketplace at $5–8 billion annually, but the hospital market at $30–100 billion. Overall, for 2000, total revenues were $10 million, while losses totaled $209 million!

Neoforma made greater progress in aggregating suppliers and customers. As of December 31, 1999, it handled 120,000 SKUs; by June 30, 2000, it carried 204,000 SKUs from 1,750 manufacturers. Between the fourth quarter of 1999 and the first quarter of 2000, the number of users jumped from 8,000 to 29,000, and the number of transactions jumped from 1,000 to 10,000.

During this period, Neoforma was involved in a spate of technology acquisitions:

In January 2000, Neoforma acquired Pharos Technologies, which developed Internet infrastructure applications and services for the B2B marketplace. Pharos enhanced Neoforma's product search capabilities and catalogue management engine. This allowed vendors to differentiate their products on the Web and avoid commoditization using unique product features.[32] The new technology also allowed vendors to track which customers had visited the Web site and which equipment they inspected. In addition, its Plan feature allowed vendors to showcase products with rich content and thereby serve as a remote sales tool for Internet-based room planning service.

In spring 2000, Neoforma acquired EquipMD, a B2B procurement company dealing with fifty-five suppliers, which provide 85 percent of the purchasing needs of 15,000 physicians

(4,000 practices in forty-seven states) buying off these contracts. The B2B also developed working relationships with several of the major alternate site distributors (Owens & Minor, Physician Sales & Service, and Henry Schein). Subsequently, Neoforma developed two customer divisions— one for hospitals (major portion of revenues) and one for physicians (major portion of profits).[33] Neoforma also announced it was going to leverage Ariba's procurement solution to build its e-procurement solution for hospitals.[34]

In late march 2000, Neoforma agreed to acquire Eclipsys Corporation and Healthvision, a private company that Eclipsys and VHA formed in 1999. This deal followed only weeks after the Medibuy-Premier deal. The new company was designed to offer hospitals a range of services to purchase supplies; manage clinical information; and connect with insurers, physicians, and patients via the Internet. The transaction also included an exclusive ten-year arrangement for the new firm to build, operate, and maintain e-commerce services to Novation (Marketplace@Novation), VHA and UHC's supply company. This was an exclusive one-way commitment from Novation to Neoforma; Neoforma was free to obtain business from other hospitals and markets (for example, long-term care). Novation would pay $200 million in outsourcing fees to the new company, while VHA and UHC would receive 58.6 million and 10.7 million shares of Neoforma.com stock, respectively, and thus control about one-third of the new company. Analysts suggested that the Novation contract was the key to the Eclipsys deal. The theory was that Neoforma could not get access to Novation without agreeing to buy Eclipsys, a firm with which it had little in common.

Following the announcement of the Neoforma-Eclypsis/ Healthvision deal, however, the stock prices of both firms plummeted. The acquisition was subsequently called off. Instead, Neoforma signed a co-marketing and distribution agreement with Healthvision, and purchased a five-year license from Eclypsis to use its eWebIT enterprise application. Neoforma's exclusive ten-year contract with Novation (using Marketplace@Novation) remained intact but, given the fall in Neoforma stock price, was restructured to give VHA and UHC control of 43 percent of Neoforma (57.6 million shares).

By early 2001, given Neoforma's need for capital and VHA and UHC's investment and interest in seeing it succeed, VHA and UHC increased their investment and share of Neoforma stock to a combined 61 percent. In January 2001, the firm received an additional $30.5 million in a second round of funding provided by VHA, UHC, and i2 Technologies.

By early 2001, Neoforma shifted its emphasis from public to private marketplaces. It announced its intention to divest its live auction house, General Asset Recovery, and its content service business due to their failure to generate high revenues. Rather than the full panoply of services it once offered (for example, on-line auctions), the firm focused on (1) its Marketplace initiative, (2) an alternate site product (NeoMD) serving 18,000 physicians and 250 long-term care facilities, and (3) a joint venture with a Canadian GPO representing more than 170 facilities (Canadian Health Marketplace).[35] Such refocusing followed on the heels of Neoforma's deal with Novation and its acquisition of EquipMD. Marketplace software applications include

Access Manager, which controls the services and functions each user can perform within Marketplace

Requisition Manager, which allows users to access product information, create requisitions, and electronically submit POs through the Marketplace

Order Manager, which allows buyers to view the status of orders

Report Manager, which facilitates reports on purchasing expenditures, compliance, utilization, and pricing

Catalog Manager, which allows suppliers to add, edit, or upload their product catalogue directly, along with new product information, product identification, and units of measure

NeoConnect, which provides tools to integrate Marketplace with the legacy systems of both buyers and sellers, and facilitates transactions by supporting both EDI and XML

Like Medibuy, Neoforma developed an array of technology partners. It negotiated a software licensing arrangement with i2 Technologies where customers can access the i2's TradeMatrix collaboration tools to build supply chain management applications. In December 2000, Neoforma and i2 announced a three-year revenue sharing agreement to collaborate on product development, marketing, sales, and service. In February 2001, it announced a strategic alliance with Lawson Software to integrate the latter's Lawson.insight e-procurement service into Marketplace.

The development of Neoforma's Marketplace solution has been gradual but steady. In July 2000, the first set of 19 Novation member hospitals signed commitments to purchase on-line through Neoforma. By October 17, 2000, Neoforma had signed contracts with 159 hospitals to conduct a minimum of 50 percent of their annual purchases through Marketplace. By December, the firm reported success in implementing a fully integrated e-procurement solution to 65 hospitals. Firm executives estimated the implementation process to start transacting through Marketplace to be twenty-two weeks long, at a cost of $30,000–35,000. This cost is currently covered by Neoforma, but is built into the revenue model as far as what suppliers pay Neoforma. The total period required to replace a hospital's traditional ordering system was estimated at eighteen to twenty-four months. Neoforma also reportedly signed up sixty-two manufacturers and distributors, which committed to use Marketplace to list and sell their products. Like Medibuy, Neoforma had not charged transaction fees to contracted suppliers.

In February 2001, Neoforma announced agreements with two large distributors (McKesson and Allegiance), under which both would accept orders from hospital members placed through Marketplace@Novation. By April 2001, Neoforma had signed agreements with over 400 hospitals to participate in its Marketplace. The agreements commit them to transact at least 50 percent of their annual purchasing (estimated at $9–10 billion) on-line. Of these 400-plus hospitals, over 150 are reported to be connected to the Marketplace and transacting purchasing on-line. Neoforma also signed agreements with eighty-three manufacturers and distributors to use Marketplace. Gross volume through the Marketplace in the first quarter was $80 million; the firm's total net loss was $53 million.

MedAssets

MedAssets was launched in April 1999 as an Internet exchange for the refurbishing and resale of used capital equipment. It acquired Comdisco Medical Equipment, a provider of refurbished diagnostic imaging technology, and sought to leverage its base of hospital business (700 refurbishing projects) using its own Internet capabilities. As part of its original service package, MedAssets offered certification and warranty services to hospitals seeking to buy used equipment. These included a Web-based certification program (functionality, maintenance records, and upgradeability) paid for by the seller. MedAssets also assisted the buyer in equipment removal, transport, and reinstallation.[36]

Currently, MedAssets has two divisions. Its "Exchange" division maintains a large fleet of mobile angio, cardiac cath, CT, and MRI systems, and offers used medical imaging equipment at prices advertised as 60 percent below new equipment costs. Its ReMedPar division serves as a multivendor refurbisher and parts distributor for diagnostic imaging equipment.

From this original base of hospitals, MedAssets has sought to become the leader in the alternate site market and aggregate its fragmented buyers and sellers. It now serves the entire continuum of care, including rehabilitation centers, ambulatory surgery centers, physician clinics, and long-term care facilities. As part of this strategy, MedAssets acquired a group purchasing organization, Insource Health Services, which serves both IDNs and freestanding facilities in the acute and alternate site markets. The stated goal was to bring these two markets together for simple purchase and order transactions. Analysts report that 90 percent of Insource's growth is in the alternate site market.[37] The firm intends to aggregate vendors for the hospital market, offer their products to alternate site customers, and use Internet connectivity to facilitate product procurement by providers. One question here is whether the client hospitals of Comdisco will be interested in participating in Insource.

In May 2001, MedAssets pursued this strategy even further by acquiring Health Services Corporation of America (HSCA), a major national GPO serving the hospital market. The combined firm will reportedly wield a combined $4.5 billion in purchasing power on behalf of over 13,000 health care providers. It also supports the firm's goal of providing a full-service procurement business to the health care industry.

OmniCell

OmniCell.com was established in 1992 to automate the cabinet-dispensing business and "the last 100 yards of the health care supply chain." Omnicell's cabinets, first installed in hospitals in 1994, are designed to reduce utilization, stockouts, and inventory, as well as to increase information and staff productivity. According to firm executives, "Medical supplies are wasted all the time. . . . they sit in people's drawers for months, sometimes at the wrong temperature, and then they can't be used at all."[38] The "smart cabinets" require personnel to enter a key code before they can access supplies, which helps to keep track of who takes what items and when. The cabi-

nets then tie into the hospital's local area networks, allowing materials managers to establish automated purchasing rules to facilitate
automatic reordering of supplies.

More recently, the firm has entered the e-commerce arena
in the areas of procurement and distribution. Its two Web-based
platforms, *OmniBuyer* and *OmniSupplier,* are oriented to the
downstream and upstream portions of the supply chain. OmniBuyer
is a Web-based procurement application that uses Commerce One
technology. It offers a customized multisupplier catalogue down to
the hospital department and individual level. The catalogue incor-
porates business rules (for example, spending limits and multiple
types of approval processes—for contract and for noncontract
items) and automates the approval and workflow process. In this
manner, the firm seeks to make process improvements by providing
an end-to-end solution that ties together the purchase order to
back-end systems. For example, there is a controlled enterprise-wide
standardized purchasing program that links to automated supply
cabinets, that connects these cabinets directly to suppliers and automates replenishment and procurement, that automates the requisitioning of noncabinet items, and that generates and integrates
requisitions from multiple departments. All suppliers connect to all
OmniBuyers at a single point.

To date, users of OmniBuyer report savings in personnel time
(for example, ordering or settling inaccurate purchase orders),
improved compliance with GPO contracts, reduced number of purchase orders, reductions in their operating budgets and savings from
returned inventory, and the transition of purchasing from a customer complaint to a customer service department.[39,40] However,
the users report that only a minimal amount of their purchases are
now going through Omnicell. More volume will be generated as
additional vendors come on board. In addition, use of automated
cabinets is higher in some hospital areas (for example, nursing units)
than in others (for example, cath lab, operating room, and pharmacy). Moreover, like the other B2B firms examined here,

OmniBuyer must be synchronized with the hospital's ERP system. Finally, some industry observers are skeptical of the savings, suggesting that OmniCell is "more of a box company than a technology company" and more involved with inventory management. Coupled with the fact that the cabinets are expensive and leased every year, the net gain for hospital customers is uncertain.

With regard to the upstream portion of the supply chain, Omni-Cell's promise is to help manufacturers forecast demand for medical-surgical products using data on product use immediately captured by its hospital systems and transmitted to manufacturers. One problem here is that OmniCell's systems are not pervasive enough among hospital customers to help much. Another issue is whether complete data are even captured. According to one informant, "As with Pyxis machines, people do not exploit these [OmniCell] cabinets for what they are intended to do, which is provide point of service monitoring of product consumption and continuous replenishment. Instead, a lot of people use them as a shell: they open the door, they take something out, and they don't press the buttons. Moreover, they have not signed a GPO partner, which is considered one of the big risks with regard to their on-line solution."

Promedix

Promedix.com was an on-line market focused on middle to high-end specialty medical products (for example, angioplasty catheters and intraocular lenses) procured outside commodity channels.[41] These products account for an estimated 30 percent of hospital supply purchases made via phone and fax orders. There are no national vendors here and no large ("big box") distributors or GPOs handling these products. Compared to commodity products, they are typically made by smaller manufacturers, sold at a higher margin to customers who are less price sensitive in these areas, and distributed to customers using small local wholesalers. The firm sought to bring small and mid-sized specialty manufacturers to hospitals via the Internet, and thus allow them access to large IDN accounts that were not available through the GPOs. In this manner, B2B firms such as Promedix could serve as an "EDI surrogate" for smaller vendors that now don't have to establish EDI linkages with customers (an expense that cannot be recovered with low sales volumes).

The firm also sought to reduce inefficiencies in the hospital ordering process. According to former Promedix executives, the average hospital buys 2,000 nonstock line items on a regular basis. Over time, these line items tend to multiply. Vendors are entered into the hospital systems multiple times with multiple spellings and abbreviations, leading database users to believe they are different firms. The result is that the hospital buys the same product from different vendors at different prices without knowing it. It also means the hospital cannot standardize product selections since it doesn't know the extent to which different departments are duplicating purchases.

There are other inefficiencies as well. Historically, hospitals have purchased surgical devices and specialty products in small lots with direct manufacturer delivery. Sometimes, the lots are so small that the total value of the purchase order (PO) is as little as $40. In contrast, the cost of issuing and processing a PO for the hospital runs anywhere from $15 to $60–70. There are thus savings from consolidating POs.[42] Stanford Hospital and Clinics reportedly issued 43,000 POs for specialty medical products involving 100,000 lines of transactions. Similarly, Mary Hitchcock Memorial Hospital determined that 61 percent of its POs amounted to less than $500 each and accounted for only 4.5 percent of total expenditures.[43]

Promedix pioneered several innovations in on-line markets that differentiated its approach from Neoforma and Medibuy.[44] First, it was not just an intermediary. Promedix partnered with product distributors (for example, UPS) to provide aggregated shipments to hospitals. Second, while it didn't actually hold inventory, it did take title to the inventory and processed all orders and invoicing. This helped to define Promedix's value to vendors. By taking title to the inventory, it took on the accounts receivable (AR) function, reduced the resources vendors expended on managing AR, and gave them more predictable cash flow. Of course, Promedix hoped to improve capital management here as well. Just as with the distributors, Promedix planned to earn revenues from the float period. In the Promedix model, hospitals had thirty-day terms for payment ("the only cost to the customer"); manufacturers gave Promedix net forty-five-, sixty-, and ninety-day terms, as well as paid a transaction fee.

Third, when a hospital purchases a product through the firm's site, it paid Promedix rather than the vendor. In this manner, the hospital executes only one PO for its specialty supplies from multiple vendors, while Promedix disperses the POs. The firm also aggregated diverse, diffuse suppliers of these products (each of whom pays $20,000–25,000 to integrate with the site). Analysts estimate there are 5,000–8,000 manufacturers that do not sell through one of the large distributors, due either to their small volumes or the need for value-added services attached to their products.[45]

During February to June 2000, BD Healthcare Consulting Services conducted a study of the efficiencies created by applying the Promedix buying solution to the procurement of manually ordered surgical specialty items from five suppliers at two hospital members of Intermountain Health Care (IHC).[46] The Promedix solution offered two alternative methods of procurement: Web-based and Integrated procurement.[47]

The study found that the Web-based solution reduced buyer time by 25 percent via order aggregation, elimination of time on the phone, enhanced ability to research product information, and enhanced ability to check order status at any time during the order cycle. When IHC's internal materials management system interfaced with the Promedix solution to offer integrated procurement, buyer time was reduced 75 percent due to reduced phone ordering time, the elimination of double entry of orders (both manual and electronic), consolidation of POs, and electronic transmission of POs. Procurement transaction costs were reduced by 86 percent, and accounts payable costs associated with specialty products were reduced by 83 percent. Some of these savings result from Promedix taking title to all goods ordered through its system, handling multiple invoices from multiple vendors, and handling all payment issues with vendors.

Despite these documented savings, Promedix had difficulty interesting suppliers and providers in its services. Total revenues for the year 2000 were only $1.4 million. In February of that year, Promedix was acquired by Chemdex Corporation, subsequently renamed Ventro. During 2000, Ventro's operating losses from Promedix and Chemdex totaled $524 million. In seeking to explain these disappointing results, Ventro suggested that other players in the market wished to establish their own electronic marketplaces rather than use their's. On January 1, 2001, both firms were shut down by the Ventro parent due to disappointing growth in transaction volumes and revenues. In a veiled statement of their problems, the firm stated that future improvements in transaction volume would flow from "enhancing the speed of transaction processing, reducing [its] substantial human intervention in processing transactions, improved participation by system users and suppliers, enhanced system functionality, successful systems integration with users and suppliers, and successful training of marketplace participants."[48]

Summary of B2B Initiatives

The previous review of B2B start-ups reveals a very rocky history. Several have gone out of business, while others are still struggling to "gain traction" in the industry. Next we review key lessons and several issues confronting these firms.

The first lesson is that "if you make it, they may not come," at least quickly. Despite favorable evidence of their efficiency enhancements to procurement, providers have been slow to sign on (see Chapter Eleven). A second lesson is that the technology is not a slam dunk. Most B2B firms have abandoned their own technology platforms to partner with established technology vendors. A third lesson is that B2B survival and ultimate success may depend on alliance with, acquisition by, or acquisition of GPOs.

There are also a host of issues. One question is whether B2B firms can integrate into hospitals' materials management and ERP systems in such a way as to reduce hospital expenses, minimize disruptions to staff functions, and require as little effort as possible from hospitals. Because hospitals are not likely to adopt a browser-based solution quickly (or at all) in the next few years, any B2B solution must link the ERP systems of suppliers and hospital buyers.

A second issue is whether B2B firms will remain focused solely on the transaction exchange (that is, helping providers to place an order or providing order status information) or will migrate to become more of a fulfillment agency (that is, making sure the product shows up at the door). This issue concerns the degree to which B2B firms might partner with 3PLs and seek to resemble product distributors that excel at fulfillment. Conversely, it is possible that B2B firms will emerge to focus on other discrete functions, such as on-line contracting and negotiations between a hospital and multiple vendors. One new entrant (Intesource) is pursuing the approach of an open, on-line bidding platform.

The issue also concerns whether providers would prefer electronic coordination of multiple orders and deliveries by B2B firms in partnership with 3PLs over aggregated order fulfillment and product delivery now supplied by distributors. For commodity items, providers now get O&M to deliver fifty pallets on a single truck delivery; for specialty items, providers now have UPS or FedEx coordinating fifty different deliveries of one pallet, each using a drop-ship model. The B2B solution requires providers to switch from the former to the latter, although it is unclear which alternative provides greater value to the customer (see Chapter Six).

Response by Supply Chain Incumbents

Regardless of these issues and potential shortcomings, B2B firms have threatened and/or alienated many of the institutionalized players along the supply chain, either due to their price focus or their language of disintermediation. Manufacturers, distributors, and GPOs each have established relationships with hospitals. Each group may consider itself the rightful heir to the B2B technology, and the best-positioned firm to deploy and utilize it. The incumbents have confronted B2B entrants in a variety of ways, ranging from acquisitions (ownership) to strategic partnerships (alliances) to outright competition (market). Large suppliers of medical products, devices, and equipment have banded together to launch their own on-line exchange to reduce administrative costs along the supply chain, as have large distributors of these products. The four largest GPOs (Columbia/HCA, Tenet, Premier, and Novation) now have some involvement in e-commerce. The GPOs may either act as direct competitors with the e-commerce firms, or they may partner with them. Their involvement in B2B is significant, given that they represent acute care hospitals, which purchase up to 55 percent of the total health care supplies marketplace. The following four sections describe the responses to e-commerce and B2B firms by GPOs, suppliers, distributors, and payers.

Competition and Cooperation with GPOs

The e-commerce start-ups face strong competition from incumbent GPOs. At the same time, there is the potential for strategic alliances to form between them.

Columbia/HCA

In December 1999, Columbia/HCA announced it would invest $40 million in a start-up e-commerce firm called empactHealth.com. Commerce One supplied the new start-up with its e-procurement software. Hospitals visiting the empactHealth site would be able to compare prices in on-line catalogues and use electronic invoices and purchase orders. The company would charge access or subscription fees and transaction fees to both suppliers and buyers.[49] The new firm was designed not only to reduce procurement costs for system hospitals, but also to generate new revenues as the procurement model was made available to nonsystem hospitals. In addition, the new firm was designed to protect the GPO's existing business and strong vendor relationships.

Columbia/HCA and its GPO Health Trust agreed to be the first customer of empactHealth. In February 2000, Baxter announced it would join Johnson & Johnson and Medline Industries in selling medical devices and supplies to providers through empactHealth. Contracted suppliers were reportedly charged a .25 percent transaction fee; noncontracted suppliers paid a transaction cost of 1 percent of sales. The following month, empactHealth signed a founding partner agreement with Health Management Associates (HMA), a chain of thirty-two acute care hospitals. HMA became an equity shareholder and agreed to exclusively use "empactBuy" for on-line requisitioning, ordering, and purchasing of all medical and nonmedical supplies and services.

In July 2000, empactHealth signed an agreement to be acquired by Medibuy. The deal created the nation's largest on-line medical supply marketplace by virtue of combining two of the top four on-line procurement companies, the other two being Neoforma and Broadlane (see the following), and by combining customer accounts for Columbia/HCA's group purchasing organization (300 hospitals) and the 1,800 member hospitals of Premier, which agreed to use Medibuy as its e-commerce arm. The two sets of hospitals have a combined $17 billion in annual purchases (2000 data) and account for roughly 30–40 percent of the hospital market. Company executives state the partnership is designed to give hospitals a single solution to e-commerce that is not specific to one GPO or set of contracted suppliers. Like a distributor, the joint operation will manage separate price files for the two GPOs to maintain security. Columbia/HCA will hold a 16 percent ownership in Medibuy after the deal is consummated.

Tenet, Broadlane, and BuyPower

In February 2000, Tenet Healthcare abandoned its own Web site project to partner with Ventro, an on-line supplier that had already amassed three years of experience. The partnership led to the formation of Broadlane, an Internet company designed to sell medical supplies over the Internet to hospitals and physicians. Tenet owned

76 percent of Broadlane, the holding company over Tenet's Buy-Power program (GPO) and Ventro Technology (the e-commerce side). The firm's mission was to position itself as the leading health care supply chain company, by utilizing the efficiencies of the Internet to reduce procurement expenses for both buyers and sellers.[50]

Tenet brought to the partnership the buying power of its GPO (BuyPower), its 111 hospitals, and BuyPower's relationships with 500 other hospitals. Like Columbia/HCA, Tenet brought an estimated $3 billion book of business in medical and related supplies.[51] The acute care hospital market was thus the first market segment to be targeted. Hospital services would include downloaded catalogue prices, RFPs and auctions, capital equipment group buys, e-commerce transactions, and supply chain benchmark data. Ventro brought its purported e-commerce technological capability in procurement, and served as the linkage between Tenet hospitals' MMIS, Broadlane, and product vendors.

Tenet executives believed the key to adding value for hospitals through e-commerce was aggregating vendors. They further believed that vendors would only participate if they could deal with a critical mass of hospitals. Some analysts felt that vendors might fear losing Tenet contracts if they rejected Broadlane.

Another advantage Broadlane hoped to offer its hospital customers was integration of the product procurement function into the provider's existing systems. For physicians who typically lacked legacy systems and thus were considered "underserved," Broadlane offered a browser. For hospital providers, Broadlane could integrate into the hospital's ERP system. Any B2B solution would need to integrate with existing hospital materials management and ERP systems to prevent losses on "maverick buying." Company officials argued that executives of provider systems did not want their personnel buying anything they want from random Web sites.

> Rather, hospitals have a process in place, run by a materials manager and backed by an ERP system, and the hospital CEO 'wants all purchases to go through that

process so that the hospital buys only from certain suppliers and gets all of the pre-negotiated discounts they're
entitled to.' The hospital also wants to make sure that
all transactions are recorded properly . . . so they know
where their money is going and so they can gather the
data needed to later go back and negotiate even better
deals. . . . the value of simply aggregating orders through
a Web site can't compare to the added costs incurred
when the buyer purchases from a noncontract supplier
or doesn't take advantage of the most up-to-date contract pricing available to the institution.[52]

Tenet aimed to harness the e-business procurement solution
offered by Ventro to its own centralized information system spanning its hospitals. In this manner, it could quickly disseminate pricing information and minimize invoice errors, as well as obtain
detailed system reporting on product procurement. It could also use
its information systems to manage hospital supply expenditures,
making sure that the vast majority of products purchased were
under contracts that offered discounted prices. Tenet hospitals purchased 83 percent of products under such contracts, compared to
40–50 percent at other hospitals.[53]

However, in mid-April 2001, Broadlane announced that it was
ending its relationship with Ventro Corporation. According to a
company press release, it became apparent that Ventro had over-
represented the capacity of its exchange and that the Ventro
exchange was incapable of handling the aggregated transaction volume generated by affiliated companies Promedix, Chemdex, and
Broadlane. Broadlane withheld over $4 million in payments to
Ventro, which had effectively stopped providing marketplace services to Broadlane in February 2001. Broadlane structured a deal to
buy back the equity given to Ventro.

Instead of using Ventro, Broadlane turned to its own internal
technology—a private exchange to transact business for Broadlane

customers and suppliers—that was officially launched in April 2001. The Broadlane Exchange allows hospitals to integrate with and order from suppliers in three different ways (EDI, XML, or Web browser) using the Internet, private VANs, or Broadlane's own Web site. It also provides an order routing infrastructure and central repository for purchasing data that links Broadlane's system with the legacy ERP systems of its members.[54]

In May 2001, Broadlane announced that its e-commerce Exchange had successfully processed more than 3,500 hospital POs for 53 Tenet hospitals in its first month and a half of operations. By the end of that month, it expected to have completed the integration of 100 Tenet hospitals with Owens & Minor, its primary distributor for medical and surgical products. Plans then called for integration with other key suppliers. Firm officials anticipated that the integration of its seven largest suppliers with its seven largest customers would generate volume on the exchange of over $1 billion. During the remainder of the year, Broadlane intends to add features such as new transaction sets (invoicing, catalogue updates, and advance ship notification), supply chain visibility (product usage statistics and contract compliance analysis), and enhanced product catalogues (comprehensive product cross-referencing and pricing audit analysis).

Tenet is aware it cannot solely rely on its own member hospitals to sustain its e-commerce business model. Tenet is thus using its e-commerce platform to increase the purchasing volume in its BuyPower GPO by non-GPO members. During 2000, Broadlane formed partnerships with the Cleveland Clinic Foundation (ten facilites), Paracelsus Healthcare (ten facilities), and Universal Health Services (twenty-two facilities), and in December assumed national supply chain contracting for Kaiser Permanente. The firm is reportedly interested in extending selected BuyPower contracts and pricing to non-Tenet hospitals in other GPOs in a few supply categories. Company officials believe hospitals will self-select into these high-compliance purchasing agreements in only a limited manner, and thereby pose little threat to those hospitals' primary GPOs. In this manner, Tenet/Broadlane seeks to consolidate "the other third"—that is, large IDNs that are not contracting with Novation and Premier—under their BuyPower program.

Premier

Premier, the nation's largest nonprofit GPO, announced in 1999 it was investing $50 million in the development of a Web-based electronic catalogue venture. The new company, Premier Health Exchange, would compete with new B2B start-ups in the product areas that most hospitals purchase, and where Premier's GPO had considerable historical experience and leverage. Premier would use an external vendor, Computer Sciences Corporation, to integrate all of the e-commerce software packages. Premier had already begun in spring 1999 to offer this electronic interface with its hospital members through *WebCat*, an electronic catalogue covering 400,000 SKUs providing medical-surgical, pharmaceutical, capital equipment, and food service products. In June 1999, it held its first capital equipment auctions on the Web. The majority of Premier members were using the technology by the end of the year.

Premier's e-commerce strategy relied on integrating aggregated buyers and suppliers. By virtue of being a large GPO, Premier offered the aggregated base (critical mass) of customers and contract pricing—two strategic assets that B2B entrants had difficulty acquiring.[55]

In March 2000, Premier sold its e-commerce unit to Medibuy as part of a six-year electronic purchasing pact. The two entities have only partially integrated. To date, Premier's WebCat has been placed on a section of the Medibuy site. Future plans call for Medibuy to take over the creation of the e-commerce platform started by Premier Health Exchange. The two organizations are still integrating their sites. However, the six-year pact is contingent on the Medibuy IPO, which has been delayed since mid-2000.

Premier received a 44 percent ownership stake in Medibuy (at the time worth $550 million), making it the firm's largest shareholder. Medibuy was to receive $159 million in payments over the six years for infrastructure development and on-line transactions by Premier's hospital members. Medibuy could also earn fees by processing transactions under Premier contracts in excess of predetermined minimum purchasing volumes, and on the sale of all noncontracted products and services sold using Medibuy to Premier members.

Novation

Novation, Premier's chief rival among nonprofit GPOs, engaged in a similar strategy. In March 2000, it announced a ten-year deal with Neoforma, where Novation took a large ownership stake in Neoforma and awarded an exclusive e-commerce pact with Neoforma. Novation announced it would place its entire $14 billion catalogue on Neoforma's site. The subsequent downturn in B2B stock prices after the first quarter of 2000 led to a restructuring of this deal, although Novation officials said their decision to post the catalogue on Neoforma remained unchanged.

The e-commerce solutions for Premier and Novation are similar in that they have both transitioned from public to private (proprietary) marketplaces. The selling proposition for Novation's e-commerce solution differs from Premier, however. When Novation hospitals join the Neoforma Marketplace and begin to transact purchasing through it, they earn equity in Neoforma. With this financial incentive, firm officials hope to entice hospital participation, especially for facilities with poor financial positions. Unfortunately, the Internet crash of 2000 has left the value of stocks like Neoforma at extremely low values, thus calling into question the strength of the incentive.

By June 2001, Novation had linked the internal inventory systems of only 130–170 hospitals to the Neoforma site. Eighty-five suppliers had agreed to post their products on the site for on-line

ordering, but only ten were actually connected. No on-line purchasing had yet occurred, although contract information had been
posted. Some hospital materials managers reportedly griped that to
participate in the site they had to (1) make a large financial commitment for training and systems upgrades and (2) meet a 50 percent compliance target or be financially penalized.[56] Some vendors
also reportedly griped that participation in the MarketPlace was
mandatory if they wished to continue to do business with Novation.
For their part, Novation executives responded that participation is
"like any other contract term or condition—it's kind of a business
parameter we've laid down."[57]

Novation and Neoforma also commissioned a study conducted
by Arthur Andersen to document the savings along the supply
chain generated by e-commerce. The study, released in June 2001,
validated the savings estimated earlier by EHCR in two areas: order
management and information sharing. The combined savings were
roughly $7 billion. The bulk of these savings ($4 billion) accrued
to product manufacturers, primarily in the form of more efficient
use of their sales representatives' time with hospital clients (for
example, less time spent in nonsales activities such as resolving error
resolution), improved data for more accurate production planning
and scheduling, and better integration with distributors (for example, elimination of need to manage separate EDI links with each).
These savings are estimated to reach a minimum of 1.5 percent
of the manufacturer's SG&A costs. The next largest pot of savings
($2.5 billion) accrued to providers, primarily through improved
management of their contract database (for example, elimination
of paper-based contracts and price files, and elimination of manual
entry). The latter savings are estimated to be 1.25–2.45 percent of
the hospital's annual supply cost. Assuming that average hospital
supply expenditures account for 15 percent of total expenses, these
savings amount to .187–.367 percent of total expenses. While small
in absolute terms, the percentage savings may be quite salient to
hospital executives enjoying margins of only 1–2 percent and few
avenues to increase revenues. Drug manufacturers and wholesalers

demonstrated the least savings in this study due to their higher level of automation.[58]

Purchase Connection/MedAssets

Purchase Connection, a California-based GPO renamed Insource Health Services in May 1999, was itself acquired by MedAssets in September 1999. MedAssets now seeks to apply Internet technology to two areas: group purchasing, and capital equipment refurbishing and resale using its MedAssets Exchange. MedAssets purchased the GPO as part of its decision to buy (rather than make from scratch) product contracts with price discounts, and to buy (rather than make) credibility in the eyes of vendors by having customers with proven willingness to utilize those contracts. As a result of the Insource acquisition, MedAssets gained access to $1.5 billion in purchasing volume, 600,000 SKUs, and 400 manufacturing and distribution contracts. In May 2001, MedAssets acquired its second GPO, Health Services Corporation of America (HSCA). By virtue of the acquisition, MedAssets more than doubled its volume of annual purchases to $4.5 billion.

E-Standards Work Group

In June 2000, a consortium of GPOs and affiliated e-commerce and B2B firms formed to develop a common standard for ordering medical-surgical and other nonpharmaceutical products on the Internet. The *E-Standards Work Group* includes Premier/Medibuy, Novation/Neoforma, Consorta, empactHealth, HealthTrust Purchasing Group, InSource Health Services, MedAssets, and (most recently) HealthNexis (covered next). The group's objectives include

- Adopt and promote jointly the use of open data exchange standards.

- Reinforce and promote standards such as Universal Product Number (UPNs) and Health Identification Numbers (HINs).

- Accelerate industry-wide adoption of comprehensive data standards.

- Encourage other industry players to participate.[59]

The driving force behind the E-Standards Work Group is the belief that there can be no e-marketplace without product standards (for example, UPNs or their equivalent). In the computer industry, manufacturers like Dell Computer pushed to formulate standard product codes.[60] In health care, however, distributors have developed proprietary linkages with hospital customers via EDI and have developed ties that are "wrapped up in forty different product coding schemes." The E-Standards Work Group subsequently changed its name to the Coalition for Healthcare Standards (CHeS), and endorsed the product coding efforts of the Electronic Commerce Code Management Association.

Three Phases of GPO E-Commerce Implementation

Some GPOs have conceptualized their Web strategy in terms of "three phases of connectivity."[61] In the first phase, the goal is to get a network of GPO hospitals and their information systems connected to a B2B hub ("marketplace") that can host applications for requisitioning, Web procurement, and contract management, and that can provide order management capabilities (for example, whether the order has been received, billed, and shipped). During this phase the GPO/B2B alliances will link up with distributors. A large portion of the GPO's spending is on products that flow through distributors. While a GPO may have over 400 contracts with 350–400 vendors, five distribution agreements (in areas of pharmaceuticals, medical-surgical supplies, radiology supplies, laboratory supplies, and office supplies) account for roughly 40 percent of the GPO's total spend. These distributors not only have EDI linkages with hospitals but also with major vendors; GPOs, in contrast, have only a handful of direct EDI connections back to suppliers.

The second phase will be marked by data management integration whereby the marketplace will receive data from the buyers, integrate it with the B2B's master datasets, and then map it to suppliers' data sets (for example, products in the vendors' catalogues). During this phase the GPO/B2B alliance will link with the top thirty vendors that ship direct to hospital customers, which accounts for another 20 percent of total GPO spend.

Finally, the third phase is marked by applications implementation, whereby the hosted applications that hospitals use are installed. During this phase, the GPO/B2B will link with the remaining vendors who account for the remaining 40 percent of GPO spend. By virtue of this data integration with distributors, the GPO/B2B alliances hope to be able to send POs directly to suppliers (without going through distributors), which immediately then know what was ordered and by whom. The GPO/B2B firms hope that vendors will prod distributors to cede this function over to them and escape being held captive by distributors over the latter's tracings fees. As one GPO executive surmised, "If the vendor has to pay a fee, they want value for it. They may be more willing to pay it to a GPO/B2B that can transmit product use and user information immediately and accurately (that is, no pricing/invoice errors) rather than wait several months for distributors to sell them old information." Moreover, the data on product usage that vendors receive from GPO/B2B firms may drill down to the provider level rather than just the zip-code level (as in distributor tracings).

Lessons and Issues in GPO–B2B Partnerships

The preceding review suggests several lessons learned about adding B2B functionality to the GPOs. It also suggests the value added by this functionality, the internal challenges, and the external barriers to acceptance by suppliers.

Lessons Learned

Trends in the last few years suggest that there is no selling proposition in stand-alone B2B models in the health care supply chain. That is, the money is not in "Let's go spend $100 million on an e-commerce solution and charge a 1 percent transaction fee." Rather, the margins exist in buying supplies in bulk, a function performed well by GPOs. As one executive explained, "While GPOs do not have a big capital infrastructure—just a couple of hundred employees—they ship out these paper catalogues, people buy off of them, and they get 3 percent of everything. The big GPOs are making boatloads of money and essentially giving it back to their shareholders, all with a paper contract." Given this state of affairs, it seems that the GPOs possess much more power than the B2B start-ups. The B2Bs need critical mass of suppliers and buyers and can only obtain them from the GPOs.

As the GPOs incorporate the B2B solutions, they are not radically transformed by a "disruptive technology" but rather enhanced with a new service option that can potentially add value to their members. The key here is thus not just the technology but also the execution in providing greater customer service. This is an intangible benefit that GPOs will have to work hard on to deliver and document.

At the present, GPOs are challenged to do both. As illustrated previously, most have encountered a bumpy road in developing the technological solution. Some cynics have charged that the GPOs entered the B2B business in hopes of making a lot of money off of B2B IPOs. Since the downturn of Internet stocks, the GPOs are seeking to salvage something from their large investment. "And now it's blown up in their face. E-commerce is hanging around their necks like an albatross."[62]

Value Added of GPO/B2B

When the technology is successfully implemented, the GPO/B2B alliance will be able to perform several additional functions beyond the pure B2B or GPO solution. These value-adding functions include

- Consistent, accurate, dynamic pricing across a system

- Accurate invoices, payments, confirmations

- Automated GPO contract administration

- Improved order tracking

- Reduced time spent on contracting

- Verification of contract adherence by GPO members

- Greater GPO member compliance

- Information on supplies on versus off contract

- Reduction in maverick buying

- Aggregation of member buying needs to facilitate auctions for items not on contract

- Access to more of vendors' product portfolio

- Extend product contracts to non-GPO members

- Potential to place more items on contract buys

- Aggregated information on product usage by members

- Potential information for product standardization

- Reduction in number of one-to-one EDI connections, and reduced number of transactions and POs

The previous review suggests that GPOs will funnel a substantial portion of the supply purchases of their members through the e-commerce platforms they have partnered with using exclusive long-term contracts. The GPOs will thus put a small, select group of B2B start-ups in business by pledging Internet order volume and payments to develop the latter's e-commerce infrastructure over time. The GPOs provide key assets that B2B firms need: a critical mass of order volume from providers, established relationships with suppliers, and discounted prices. The synergy here is obvious: merge the GPO's pricing with the advantages of the B2B's Internet connectivity. Moreover, with the GPO's revenue base, B2B partners will not need to charge as high a transaction fee to vendors. The GPO/B2B alliances should go beyond GPOs and the latter's ability to obtain lower prices by virtue of handling a new set of products not previously contracted by GPOs, by reducing the amount of off-contract and maverick buying by departments, and by improving price transparency and reducing pricing variations within a health system.

Internal Challenges

Of course, these partnerships face several issues and challenges. First, GPOs may be wary of posting their contract terms on the Internet and extending these terms to non-GPO members. Second, they need to demonstrate to themselves and their members that these partnerships actually represent a more efficient model of group purchasing (for example, the dissemination of information actually leads to higher compliance, increased control over purchases, and so forth). Third, enormous time and expense will be involved in integrating e-procurement into hospitals' ERP systems. According to one industry report, hospitals must spend $250,000–300,000 on an interface to use the Internet for purchasing.[63] The solutions must be easily adopted by hospitals with a minimum of cost and effort on their part. For their part, hospitals do not *have* to adopt B2B solutions, and may take a more leisurely approach. Indeed, one survey of hospital materials managers reveals that 71 percent are "very happy" with their experiences with EDI, and many regard the Internet as offering no real improvement in terms of either speed or cost.[64]

Vendor Concerns

Vendors may view the B2B firms as simply another intermediary between themselves and their customers ("channel interference"), and thus the loss of direct customer contact. Moreover, such intermediaries charge another set of transaction fees (as low as 1 percent) for processing orders—fees that vendors cannot control and appear to be unwilling to pay for at present. As one pharmaceutical company executive quipped, "These B2B firms claim to be building a bridge to the manufacturers. But after this bridge is built, they erect a toll booth." This fee comes on top of other fees vendors are already paying (for example, 2–3 percent CAF to GPOs, 1–2 percent discount to distributors for quick payment, and 1–2 percent tracings fee paid to distributors), which total 4–7 percent. Vendors complain they are now required to make a high investment in a critical performance area (sales) for which there is little additional return (that is, they might have gotten the business regardless), with the possible exception of increased sales to the alternate site market. Overall, vendors are not convinced that B2B solutions will deliver greater market share or product sales, which is what they want in return for another transaction fee. Thus, even with B2B technology, can GPOs actually deliver great market share? In addition to sales volume, vendors are not convinced that B2B solutions will allow them to tailor their production schedules to customer ordering and distributors' inventory levels—which constitute "real supply chain management." Vendors may likewise be wary of a renewed emphasis on unit price over total costs and the total product solution they offer.[65] Vendors are concerned over the Internet's promise of price transparency and product comparison, which may lead to price erosion. According to some analysts, vendors dislike open markets and open access.[66] Indeed, the value of the Internet for them lies in closing the marketplace and developing a more favorable market position for themselves and their products. However, with some exceptions, B2B firms may do little to promote product differentiation. Finally, vendors are not convinced by the rationale that they are paying for the implementation of technology to streamline the supply chain. In their view, "Why should we pay hospitals to clean up their act? They are the ones who are inefficient." For these reasons, vendors may boycott the B2B marketplace or seek to circumvent it with their own solution (see the following).

Barriers to Vendor Acceptance

Even if they viewed them favorably, vendors may face barriers in embracing the B2B solutions offered by GPOs. First, they face the challenge of integrating all of their different product lines and divisions into one platform. In some product manufacturers, especially those organized around decentralized product companies that may or may not talk to each other, the cost of integrating multiple information systems may be large. Second, such integration and interface with buyers may entail a short-term increase in FTEs, a visible cost to the manufacturer. The promise of long-term "process cost savings" or even a reduction in sales force FTEs does not convince manufacturers.

> The national account manager at the vendor, who is a sales-type person and who has a relationship with a GPO, really does not understand this e-commerce thing and what is involved with it. Their objective is to increase market share and sales. They do not really care about the operational expenses you are going to reduce back at corporate headquarters [of the vendor]. These operational expenses—for example, the number of FTEs handling orders—have already been accounted for in some fashion. In most cases the vendors do not break that expense out as something that is variable that they can then tie back to sales dollars. "So maybe a B2B solution will save me [the vendor] 25 percent on FTEs, and maybe I can redeploy them to do something else, but unless I can redeploy them to something measurable, I am not going to realize any benefits that can be counted." So the national account manager will not get rewarded for this. So it is a very short conversation with them. So now we [the GPO] are trying to disseminate information on the B2B value proposition back to their corporate headquarters people, such as their VP for

e-commerce, and this is a very long process. And, at the same time, you have to differentiate your story from your B2B competitors.

Several informants mentioned the challenge of educating vendors about the opportunity afforded by e-commerce to reduce the number of sales representatives they have out in the field calling on customers. One issue here is the relative effectiveness of Internet messages versus the sales representative's face-to-face contact, especially for commodity medical-surgical supplies. This challenge is even more acute for branded pharmaceuticals and higher-end medical devices.

> When you talk to your high-dollar suppliers like Johnson & Johnson and the folks who make the clinical preference items and products that are clearly differentiated, they don't follow the typical supply chain model. It is hard to substantiate a transaction fee or the cost of integration with them because they don't really see the value. They go through the GPO in terms of negotiating a price, but the channel is the pacemaker representative or cardiac stent representative who drives around in a Ford Explorer with all this stuff in a bag and talks to the doctor. There is no place on a Web site to look at these data and get it [sic] back to the materials manager. You are talking about completely reengineering that process where department heads and physicians meet with these guys [sales reps], take possession of a product, and then, after the fact, go down and get a purchase order number. The product may be in the patient before a PO has ever gone through the system.

Of course, the real savings here may lie in reducing the manufacturers' cost of dealing with all of their different distributors and their sales forces by virtue of standardization. That is, the manufacturer can develop a standardized Web-based format for services (for example, product knowledge, education, and training) that can be disseminated electronically and customized for each distributor, rather than the old system of giving each distributor its own CD-ROM. Here again, however, the savings may not be apparent to vendors.

E-Commerce Initiatives by Suppliers

Suppliers (producers of products) have responded with their own e-commerce initiatives. While individual firms have developed their own Web strategies, a consortium of suppliers have developed a giant exchange.

The Global Healthcare Exchange (GHX)

Suppliers have had varying reactions to the rise of B2Bs and their alliances with GPOs. Some companies, particularly those that manufacture branded pharmaceuticals and high-end medical devices, have been less concerned about B2Bs given that their products are not prominent in GPO contracts and may not be carried by distributors. Other manufacturers, particularly in medical-surgical supplies, have struck back at B2B entrants using technology provided by Commerce One, Ariba, i2, and their own e-commerce solutions. In some cases, suppliers are partnering with B2B firms just as GPOs are.

In late March 2000, five of the largest suppliers announced their intention to launch an on-line manufacturer exchange (now known as *Global Healthcare Exchange*) to automate product selection, ordering, and tracking; and to electronically process transactions. The five firms include Abbott Laboratories, Baxter International, General Electric's GE Medical Systems unit, Johnson & Johnson, and Medtronic. By October 2000, several more firms had joined, including Becton Dickinson, Guidant Corporation, Boston Scientific,

Sulzer Medica, Tyco Healthcare, Hill-Rom Company, Integra LifeSciences, C. R. Bard, St. Jude Medical, Bayer Diagnostics, Sonora Medical Systems, Utah Medical Products, Varian, and Smith & Nephew. By mid-2001, the number of suppliers participating in the exchange grew to eighty, while the number investing in the exchange grew to seventeen.

The new venture marks an imposing new entry from the supplier side into the B2B market. This is because the initial five partners together claimed to sell enough different products to meet more than 70 percent of the operating needs of any hospital.[67] Their stated goal was to cover 80 percent of the SKUs available to their customers by September 2000. In this manner, suppliers can surmount their limited ability as individual firms to supply only 40 percent of what a hospital needs, and thus to explore distributor disintermediation.

GHX is a public marketplace that allows hospitals to do business with vendors as well as to change vendors. Their cooperative approach is a competitive response to the Internet start-ups profiled earlier and their burgeoning partnerships with GPOs, all of which have migrated to a private marketplace platform (that is, GPO members only) and have relied on commitment to GPO-contracted vendors. The plan is to make the exchange open to all vendors that manufacture hospital products (starting with medical-surgical supplies, and later shifting to devices, laboratory products, and pharmaceuticals), thus providing one Internet site where purchasers can execute and track their orders. The site will educate customers about products and services, provide centralized and direct access to manufacturers' sites, offer the biggest range of products and vendors, provide clinical information on these products, and facilitate global business. The selling proposition for vendors to join is the low transaction fee per member (alternately described as 0.25 percent of the vendor's health care–derived revenues or 1 percent of transactions), which suppliers view as "paying your cost," as "a small cost given the risks and costs of the B2B dot-coms," and as much lower than the 3 percent CAFs demanded by GPOs. GHX is "the easiest way for vendors to pay this cost" and "the lowest cost version of being on the Internet for vendors."

The exchange will not set prices and its site is not an auction, but rather serves as an arena for hospitals and suppliers to come together. Because pricing is not at issue, all pricing and purchase terms must be settled with the manufacturer prior to going on-line. IDNs are thus unable to use the exchange to compare prices, and manufacturers in the exchange will not have access to one another's pricing contracts. The exchange may also reduce sales and distribution overhead costs and streamline purchasing for vendors.

GHX has concentrated on the development of its MasterCatalog, a normalized and standardized product catalogue designed to streamline the buying process. An immediate challenge for GHX is creating the first industry-wide catalogue of products with manufacturers maintaining and updating the information. In 2001, GHX began working with a consulting firm (ECRI) and the Health Industry Business Communications Council (HIBCC) to develop a taxonomy of product names and codes for medical-surgical devices. It also allied itself with a software firm (Aristomed) to clean the master catalogues of hospitals buying from GHX members. GPOs feel that GHX is pushing on this dimension to counter the threat from future GPO efforts to develop a common taxonomy and data classification system that would allow easier comparison of vendors' products. GHX has countered by saying that its taxonomy focuses on non-commodity products that GPOs do not handle, and that it is willing to work with the Coalition for Healthcare Standards (CHeS) and its effort to develop a taxonomy.

In addition to on-line ordering, GHX's services include on-line inquiry regarding order status, order confirmation, access to correct prices and contract terms, and integration into hospital ERP systems. It is not clear how helpful hospitals will find these features.

"Right now, buyers who use the GHX system must request prices from a specific manufacturer, which then pulls the appropriate price based on the status of the buyer—which GPO they belong to and what discounts they are entitled to. To compare costs, a buyer would have to request separate pricing from each supplier. . . . You have competing manufacturers who don't really want people comparing prices . . ."[68]

The selling proposition for IDNs is the convenience of accessing popular products and getting prices comparable to those obtained by GPOs (since there are no CAFs). GHX took out two-page ads in hospital trade journals depicting a fully equipped operating room "furnished by Global Healthcare Exchange," the hospital's "single-source solution for on-line purchasing of medical and nonmedical products and services." Representatives of the initial five firms have stated that they are also seeking to reduce the supply chain costs of their hospital customers by automating orders under already-negotiated contracts, offering catalogue-keeping and product-searching capabilities, and ensuring that customers get accurate contract pricing.

Distributors and GPOs have ascribed other, unstated goals to this exchange. The exchange may serve to

- Increase product sales for the founding members of the exchange.

- Increase sales through the bundling of products and bringing more product through a portal.

- Establish an on-line presence quickly to meet growing provider demand for on-line procurement of medical and surgical supplies (see the following).

- Counteract what the GPOs are doing—"take out an insurance policy" and "make a strategic bet on the future."

- Allow some vendors that have made internal investments in e-commerce to defray some of these costs and/or get some return from their investment.

- Allow other vendors "who lack the capability to do anything on-line (and don't want to admit it) to get up to speed."

Concerns over GHX

There are several concerns about the competitive impact of the Global Health Exchange. Some analysts are skeptical of the manufacturers' motives, stating, "This is the same group that has resisted UPNs, bar-coded products, and a streamlined supply chain."[69] In addition, analysts note that this particular exchange is the only manufacturer exchange focused downstream toward the customer, rather than upstream toward their own suppliers. Manufacturers have apparently decided that e-commerce and exchanges in health care are best driven by manufacturers.[70] The exchange may also (1) be an effort to slow down what is happening in the marketplace, (2) be an exercise in market power to protect their margins, and (3) represent a "war of attrition" to exhaust the dwindling cash resources of the B2B start-ups. With regard to the latter views, some supply chain firms stated, "Exchange members would be happy if the B2Bs disappeared and the exchange did nothing." Others have stated that exchange members may believe that the costs of their participation and investment pale in comparison to the lost margins that would result from pricing transparency arising from a GPO/B2B exchange. GPOs call it the "manufacturer margin protection program."

Others have questioned the feasibility of this alliance. "When have any of these big suppliers ever collaborated on anything that has been successful? They don't necessarily want to work together."

"Guidant, Medtronic, and Boston Scientific have traditionally not been very friendly with each other. They are not going to find a simple solution to working together, integrating, cooperating, and quickly delivering a product." Indeed, the major issue facing the exchange is fortitude in sticking together. The exchange may therefore represent more a delaying tactic that allows manufacturers to "get their arms around the B2B issue."

GHX Partnerships and Hospital Participation

By December 2000, GHX had reportedly signed up fifty hospitals to participate in its procurement solution and had successfully completed live on-line transactions between hospital and supplier pilot member sites. In August of that year, GHX acquired CentriMed, a provider of e-commerce services tailored to medical products, in an effort to catch up with the B2Bs and their ability to integrate into hospital legacy systems. The first production release was scheduled to be launched by spring of 2001. In February 2001, GHX announced an agreement with Omnicell to integrate the latter's OmniBuyer e-procurement platform into GHX. Hospitals that have invested in one system can then leverage that investment to gain access to another. Omnibuyer users will be able to access GHX's panel of manufacturers, while GHX can access Omnicell's extensive hospital membership (for example, hospitals affiliated with the GPO Consortia). That same month, GHX also announced an agreement to connect with Lawson's "insight" e-procurement service, a move that will facilitate integration with Lawson's customers and connectivity with providers that use Lawson. For example, price and product information changes by manufacturers and distributors can be immediately communicated to hospitals' ERP and MMIS systems. All of these initiatives were scheduled for pilot testing and launch in spring 2001.[71]

By early 2001, thirty-eight IDNs (representing 286 hospitals) had registered with GHX to access its catalogue and suppliers. In March 2001, Joint Purchasing Connection (JPC) announced its intention to connect to GHX. JPC assists IDNs in conducting their own GPO services. The firm brings potentially 450 more hospitals to GHX. The Omnicell partnership brings an additional 1,300 hospitals and facilities.[72] Finally, GHX has signed up some independent and regional distributors to help them reconcile changing data on products, contracts, and customers.

The appeal of the exchange is uncertain. One of its selling points (indeed, a selling point of many B2Bs) is the one-stop shopping capability for most medical-surgical supplies an IDN might need. Yet, the historical experience of the pharmaceutical and medical-surgical distributors suggests that bundled packages of supplies are not a paramount need among customers. As further support, a survey of hospital materials managers reveals that 19 percent report that having access to a wider product portfolio is not important, since they are already familiar with most products on the market. These managers further report they do not visit vendors online to have access to more products. What they are interested in is coordinated purchasing, product quality, and purchasing from qualified vendors.[73] To this extent, the manufacturers' exchange may have greater salience for IDN purchasers since it pulls together bundles of top-quality firms and their top-quality products.

Another question regarding customer acceptance concerns trust and value. According to one hospital executive, "They [GHX] are going to manage my supply chain, which makes me uncomfortable. They are also not going to negotiate on price, but only help me with process costs. Why would I work with a company that will not help me with both? They also do not offer equity [as does Novation] and are not portable. What happens if I decide I want to work with a different supplier? It is very hard to substitute, if that new supplier is not a member."

An executive with a major GPO suggested another concern harbored by hospitals: "Will our [hospital] customers flock to GHX? Absolutely not. Both by contract and by culture, hospitals view the members of GHX as suppliers. To have suppliers come in and manage all of this for them is inherently against their culture. This is why GPOs exist. The [hospital] buyers never believed they were getting the best deal. So are they going to ask GHX to come in and take another 3 percent [the amount of the CAF] from our hospitals' already low bottom line? I don't think so."

This is not to say that some hospitals will not be attracted to GHX. However, they may fall into certain categories. First, some likely customers may be those institutions that (1) want to use GHX for off-contract buying, (2) want to do direct purchasing for small commodity items that do not greatly impact their supply expense budget, (3) want to show the CFO how much they saved on a particular contract, and/or (4) currently lack electronic supply chain management solutions (like EDI) and therefore order supplies by sending faxes. GHX may also gain greater traction with hospital members of GPOs that join purchasing groups on a voluntary basis and then circumvent the GPO's contract when (1) it is to their advantage to do so, and (2) their GPO exerts little purchasing discipline over it.

The "Chicken and the Egg" Problem

Finally there is the issue of whether it is more important to aggregate buyers or suppliers—what is referred to as the "chicken and the egg" problem.[74] In the short term, some analysts suggest that buyer aggregation is the more critical activity since it can be used to attract both buyers and sellers and because buyers are needed to implement an e-procurement solution.[75] The formation of GPO-sponsored and GPO-affiliated B2B models might seem to pose some difficulty for any supplier exchange, since the bulk of hospital buyers are now already aligned with a partner. Moreover, for hospitals and IDNs owned by Columbia/HCA and Tenet, there are exclusive arrangements with their corresponding GPOs and B2B solutions (empactHealth/Medibuy and BuyPower/Broadlane, respectively). Finally, any contract between a large GPO and the GHX might seem unlikely since it would obviate the GPO's need for its newly acquired B2B partner.

Nevertheless, in late August 2001, Novation informed its members that their e-commerce site, Marketplace@Novation, would link to the GHX platform as part of a three-year agreement. Both sides agreed to ask their customers to use the other side as the "preferred solution." Some observers speculated the agreement represented a joint answer to the chicken-and-egg problem since each side had experienced difficulty attracting large numbers from the other side. With the agreement, for example, GHX became connected to 280 hospitals already linked electronically to Novation. Neoforma members will be able to access GHX's "Allsource Catalogue" (standardized, electronic product guide), while GHX will license parts of Neoforma's "Neo Connect" application.

Lessons from Manufacturing Industry Exchanges

One might also consider the experience of manufacturer exchanges now occurring in industries beyond health care, such as autos, aerospace, computers, tires, airlines, and agribusiness. These exchanges, collectively known as *NewCos*, have a very short history.[76]

Some problems they are reportedly now confronting include surmounting decades-old rivalries and competing agendas among the consortia members, wariness among their suppliers, Federal Trade Commission concerns over antitrust (for example, coercion of suppliers to use the central site), incompatibility in the software systems used by consortia members (for example, different OEM systems that prevent them from talking to one another), member differences regarding how much to charge future members and how much trading data they are allowed to see, difficulties in agreeing upon a common technology and executable plan, and how much pricing visibility they want their on-line trading partners to see. Another issue is the large member commitment required up front with little information on exchange operating details.[77] Moreover, these exchanges essentially constitute mega joint ventures, which are notoriously difficult to manage. As one B2B executive stated, "The single biggest problem is that joint ventures are hard, joint ventures with many players are twice as hard, and joint ventures with many players who've been competitors for eighty years are nearly impossible."[78]

One of the most visible of these exchanges is in the auto industry. The exchange, called Covisint, includes Ford, General Motors, Daimler/Chrysler, Nissan Motor, and Renault SA, and is powered by Commerce One procurement technologies. The exchange started poorly with each automaker allying with their own technology partner, but developed a standard IT platform due to pressure from supply firms serving all automakers. In September 2000, it cleared FTC and German antitrust scrutiny, and launched its product with more than eighty auctions encompassing $300 million in goods by early 2001. This amount is just a tiny fraction of the $350 billion auto-parts market, however. It remains to be seen what additional revenue sources the exchange will develop, including nonauction services like collaborative planning between suppliers and vendors.[79] Issues remaining to be dealt with include who will be its CEO, which vendor's auction technology software to buy, the size of membership in the buying consortium, the role of distributors versus disintermediation, dynamic inventory control using the Internet, and the possibility of consolidation among exchanges in the future.[80]

E-Commerce Supply Chain Activities of Individual Manufacturers

Individually, supply firms are also entering the B2B space. This is true for both pharmaceutical manufacturers and medical-device makers. Drug manufacturers believe the supply chain is already pretty efficient, although survey data suggest that upstream supply chain strategic alliances with OEMs and raw materials suppliers are underdeveloped.[81] They also have less interest in supply chain management, since there is already a clear distribution channel for branded pharmaceuticals that involve (1) direct advertising to patients and (2) office calls by company sales representatives. In this clear channel, drug distributors do not really influence brand selection or product switching. Industry executives do not believe e-commerce will play much of a role with branded drugs: "New drugs are very expensive and very effective. It is hard, if not impossible, to change formularies away from these drugs to lower-cost, seemingly equivalent therapeutics. All that B2Bs can do here is to make sure that the criteria for drug selection are embedded in the drug ordering process, so that the physician ordering the drug has the information on-line regarding formularies, equivalents, etcetera." Consequently, pharmaceutical firms are also less concerned with pricing visibility and loss of contact with their customers.

The major strategic issues for them are product innovation and R&D (for example, the preclinical drug testing phase and clinical trials) and sales and marketing, rather than manufacturing and purchasing costs. There is thus some interest in e-commerce applications that help speed up drug discovery and recruit patients for clinical trials. As with the B2Bs profiled previously, there is a chicken-and-egg problem here too. To prove that these applications have a positive impact on ROI by shortening the drug development process, big studies are needed that involve big pharmaceutical companies; the latter will not engage in these studies, however, without data from big studies demonstrating their value.

They are also more interested in Web applications for information dissemination and outreach to customers via direct-to-consumer (DTC) drug advertising and direct-to-provider (DTP) information delivery. With the shortage of sales force personnel and the recent full-employment market, pharmaceutical firms have looked to such applications to enhance their marketing efforts by adding another channel. Industry estimates for these two types of spending are $1–2 billion and $30–40 billion.[82] Pharmaceutical firms have also been active in supporting connectivity firms in e–health care (for example, MedicaLogic and Healtheon) through their advertising revenues. Overall, industry experts believe that investments in e-health by pharmaceutical firms will be product specific (rather than across the board) and channel specific (coordinated with other marketing efforts).

Despite these investments, there are some major organizational issues that pharmaceutical firms must confront in incorporating e-commerce. First, it may prove difficult to integrate Web activities into the pharmaceutical firm, given that the latter often lacks a central Internet department. Instead, each division may pursue its own e-commerce activities. Second, as a result, B2B firms may find it difficult to find the right people inside pharmaceutical firms in order to transact business and cut deals. Third, due to the spate of merger and acquisition activity, pharmaceutical firms have become "mass mergerers." In the merger process, projects typically are placed on hold, outsourcing of functions (like e-commerce) get delayed, and merger partners discover they have divergent outsourcing alliances. The incorporation of any e-commerce solution also becomes more difficult in the resulting merged firm, where previous structural issues have doubled or trebled.

On the medical device side, a recent industry analysis suggests that only a small amount of medical device transactions occur over the Internet.[83] Analysts expect materials managers to experiment with e-procurement first with more inexpensive, generic items before they transition to higher-end items. According to one analyst,

> Since high-tech medical devices are generally marketed through direct customer contact on the part of sales representatives, initial purchases of these items on-line will have to wait. Vertical marketplaces will have to increase their product and educational content to ensure that procurement managers are able to adequately familiarize themselves with products despite never having seem them live. Even after e-procurement becomes commonplace in the medical equipment supply chain, it is likely that only those devices that the hospital is familiar with will be purchased on-line. In this market, e-procurement will be used primarily for repurchasing instruments and devices that the hospital has used in the past.[84]

E-Commerce Initiatives by Distributors

Both collectively and individually, distributors have also responded to the B2B challenge.

The New Health Exchange/HealthNexis

In April 2000, five distributors (McKesson/HBOC, Cardinal Health, AmeriSource, Owens & Minor, and Fisher Scientific) announced their intention to launch an on-line marketplace for purchasing drugs, supplies, and laboratory products. The five partners stated they were investing over $100 million in this new marketplace, called *NewHealthExchange.com*, which effectively would serve as a "catalogue of catalogues exchange." The exchange would not compete directly with the exchanges developed by both GPOs and manufacturers. In an April 18, 2000, press release, representatives of the five firms stated that their goal is to

Simplify the product rebate process, which consumes the attention of many of their own employees, and develop contract management tools to assist in contract administration (eligibility and charge-backs).

Establish an industry standard for product information, including the use of common code numbers and electronic systems.

Offer standardized access to thousands of manufacturer product catalogues on the Internet, using a universal product catalogue with up-to-date negotiated pricing.

Simplify order entry and processing procedures for buyers, and improve inventory monitoring by allowing buyers and sellers to obtain information on transaction volume, catalogue activity, and contract activity.

Like the suppliers, the five distributors claimed to act as the middleman for 70 percent of the health care products used by hospitals, physicians, and nursing homes. Collectively, the five distributors process $80 billion of transactions annually, 90 percent of which are handled electronically via EDI or the Internet. Of course, as with manufacturers, there are concerns that distributors are really just engaging in market and channel protection. Faced with already miniscule margins, the distributors may be seeking a means to augment them. And again, as with the manufacturers, the participants are all competitors that are each pursuing their own e-commerce strategy (see the following). However, unlike in manufacturing, distributors in other industries have not collectively set up their own exchange.

Definitive agreements among the distributors were not signed until August 2000, by which point one of the original members (Owens & Minor) withdrew and the remaining four members reduced their financial investment to $50 million. O&M's withdrawal may have reflected differences of opinion over the focus and timing of the exchange's rollout, as well as the firm's desire to maintain an independent stance and flexibility to enter multiple exchanges. From August 2000 to January 2001, the exchange did not pursue contracts with any potential customers (manufacturers, GPOs, or IDNs), although it purportedly wanted to offer a neutral platform where all parties could peacefully come together. The first of their four major services (transaction clearinghouse) was slated for release on March 31, 2001, with subsequent releases planned for the rest of the year.[85]

In March 2001, the exchange renamed itself *HealthNexis*, reflecting its effort to be at the center of supply chain activities. In contrast to other e-commerce platforms, it offers no front-end e-procurement function. It is thus not a marketplace and does not compete with other solutions discussed previously. Its back-end infrastructure platform features four primary service offerings:

Transaction clearinghouse. Launched in April 2001, this is a single point of access for routing and translating POs and invoices using EDI or XML that eliminates VANs companies must pay for to send documents and order.

Product data manager. Launched in May 2001, this is a one-source destination for all product information between trading partners and a management tool for viewing, verifying, updating, and maintaining product information in the Data Repository—a synchronized bank of all product information. It rests on i2 Technologies software.

Contract data manager. Launched in July 2001, this allows trading partners to review and modify contract-related information. It uses I-Many software.

Data reporting services. Expected to be launched by the end of 2001, these are Web-based tools designed to help members examine daily activity reports, error reports, and product updates.[86]

Issues with Distributor Exchange

One issue raised by the distributors' exchange is whether future supply chain transactions take place not only between firms (B2B) but also between exchanges (E2E). The major benefit of E2E is "liquidity"; that is, a large volume of transactions with customer involvement. E2E models multiply the liquidity available through current B2B models, which are struggling with the chicken-and-egg problem. Indeed, along these lines, Health Nexis signed a three-year agreement in late 2001 to merge into GHX in exchange for an equity stake. Nevertheless, at present, the manufacturer exchanges have focused on supply chain costs rather than formulating a new revenue model.

Another issue is whether the Internet will lead to the obsolescence of distributors' proprietary EDI systems through which they have linked to and partnered with hospital systems over the last two decades. Some analysts believe it will, since the Internet will facilitate on-line POs that are not disrupted if a hospital changes its distributor. As suggested earlier, the distributors may not really be interested in product standards that render obsolete their product-coding schemes.

Distributors themselves view the Internet as another choice or product complement (rather than a substitute) alongside their EDI system. In support of this view, recent anecdotal evidence suggests that Internet-based ordering and EDI costs providers roughly the same amount. Moreover, major hospital systems such as Catholic Healthcare West are installing ERP systems purchased from SAP as part of their EDI initiative.

A third issue is whether any industry standards can be established by just a subset of the supply chain participants. The EHCR initiative, which included more representation from the supply chain, failed to produce any such agreement on standards. Moreover, as with manufacturers, some informants questioned whether competitor distributors can really cooperate. "Each distributor in the New Health Exchange has its own formidable supply chain management strategy. Why on earth would they want to collaborate?"

E-Commerce Supply Chain Activities of Individual Distributors

Distributors are involved in a variety of Internet-related activities. According to a recent survey conducted by Goldman Sachs, 42 percent offer an on-line catalogue of the products they distribute. Thirty-seven percent currently have a Web site offering e-commerce capabilities to their customers (hospitals and physicians); of the remainder, 93 percent plan to do so within the year. Moreover, 52 percent of distributors say they have been actively encouraged by their customers to provide or increase their Internet capabilities.[87] E-commerce efforts by specific distributors are summarized next.

Cardinal Health launched its e-commerce initiative, *Cardinal.com*, in March 2000. The firm's Internet strategy encompasses five basic services: ordering and procurement, information services regarding orders and utilization, customization of product catalogues, service extensions, and professional education.[88] The firm is also now seeking to combine Allegiance's order management EDI technology for medical-surgical supplies ("ASAP") with Cardinal Health's own "Choice" program for pharmaceutical product ordering (for example, price catalogue, inventory control, order optimization, and invoicing and credits) into one site with Web-enhanced capabilities. This would provide customers with one-stop-shopping access to a very broad portfolio of products.

Cardinal officials are optimistic that e-commerce may help spur joint purchasing by providers of pharmaceutical and medical-surgical products, something that hasn't happened in the past (see Chapter Five). First, e-commerce may encourage providers to use the Web to tie all procurement to their ERP systems. Even in those IDNs that separate front-end procurement between the pharmacy and materials management departments, they may want to have the back-end functions integrated with all purchase orders routed through their ERP system. Second, there may be an opportunity to automate the estimated 85–95 percent of all hospital purchasing that is "replenishment"; that is, refilling purchase orders on a regular basis. Third, with increasing cost pressures and reported shortages of pharmacists, hospitals may combine pharma and med-surg purchasing in materials management to free up pharmacist time for clinical tasks. Nevertheless, officials do not expect a major integration of pharmacy and materials management purchasing in the near term. This is partly due to the separation of professional domains, and partly due to the greater level of expertise in pharmacy purchasing.[89]

Cardinal is not seeking to replace its large EDI base, which it inherited from the Allegiance acquisition. Allegiance now conducts 86 percent of its orders through EDI, compared to 13 percent through phone and fax and only 1 percent over the Internet. Officials claim that the major difference in cost is between phone and fax, and EDI ($0.65 versus $0.15 per order), not between EDI and the Internet. Rather the Internet provides a complementary set of tools for their customers to *follow up* on orders electronically (for example, source of shipment and date of arrival) instead of using the phone and fax.[90]

As part of Cardinal Health's e-commerce initiative, Allegiance operates an extensive Internet-based order and management system for medical, surgical, and laboratory supplies. In early 2000, Allegiance launched *asap-e.com*, which can be accessed through either Cardinal's or Allegiance's Internet locations. Allegiance customers (hospitals, medical groups, and ambulatory surgery centers) have twenty-four-hour access to the e-catalogue and can order products, check product availability and order status, track shipping, generate reports, and manage contract compliance and usage. This system covers 300,000 medical-surgical supplies, with delivery as fast as two hours, and hopes to link Allegiance's 70,000 customers with its 3,000 contracted product vendors. In March 2000, Allegiance reported that its Internet business amounted to $5 million in revenues.

Owens & Minor (O&M) is pursuing a four-pronged approach in using the Internet to become a provider of supply chain and logistics services and thereby develop business. First, the firm is using O&M Direct, an e-commerce site, to handle customer functions such as order query, order entry, pricing, and product availability. It is working to move customers to this more efficient, cost-effective system of ordering, and has a new product called *Intelli-Order*. Second, O&M has signed on to serve as distributor for various Web-based health sites, such as Neoforma, Medibuy, and MedicalBuyer.com. Third, the company has developed eMed-Express, a small package delivery business targeting nonhospital accounts. This venture essentially represents a 3PL effort in the alternate site market, offering warehousing and distribution for manufacturers that have previously shipped directly to these markets but want to exit the distribution business. Fourth, it made available its internal decision support system (Web Intelligence Supporting Decisions from Owens & Minor, or WISDOM) to both its suppliers and customers to provide them access to its $3.2 billion data warehouse. The warehouse contains current and three-year historical data on customer contracts, sales, pricing details, orders, shipments, and inventory. The "new generation wisdom" here is to allow customers to view O&M purchases, purchases from direct-ship manufacturers, and purchases from specialty distributors—that is, the whole market basket—in order to decide how to convert such items to contract purchases and how to standardize products purchased.[91] O&M expects this service to become a net revenue generator.

E-Commerce Initiatives by Payers

Payers such as health maintenance organizations (HMOs) find themselves confronted by these B2B threats to transaction processing. On the one hand, they have been slow to embrace the Internet due to small IT budgets, low margins in recent years, and physicians' reluctance to partner with them.[92] On the other hand, they have witnessed firms such as Healtheon try to interpose themselves between payers, providers, and patients by offering Web-based claims processing, patient referrals, and prescription management. Indeed, in January 2000, Healtheon acquired Envoy Corporation, the nation's largest electronic medical claims clearinghouse and the electronic middleman used by many HMOs for claims processing. The acquisition was part of Healtheon's strategy of getting physicians to move away from EDI to the Internet and its own stable of Web-based services. Later, in September 2000 the firm acquired Medical Manager to access the physician market using its management software and 180,000 physician customers.

In response, a consortium of seven HMOs—Aetna/US Healthcare, Health Net, Anthem, PacifiCare Health Systems, Wellpoint Health Networks, Oxford Health Plans, and Cigna—formed to launch a Web-based administrative services operation to simplify physician-payer transactions, provide faster reimbursement, and instant approvals. In a public announcement in November 2000, the consortium stated they would provide a real-time transaction system using the Internet to enable providers and insurers to follow a standardized approach for sending and receiving: eligibility and benefits verification, claims submission, claims status, and referrals and authorizations. At this point in time, there are only sketchy details on their collaboration, called *MedUnite*. In January 2001, MedUnite announced a five-year agreement with CSC to serve as its IT support contractor and systems integrator to allow MedUnite to connect in real time with providers. In early June, the consortium purchased the country's second largest medical electronic claims system from NDCHealth. These network services are used by an estimated 10–15 percent of the roughly 100,000 physicians who are customers of NDCHealth's practice management software systems. The transaction closed by the fall of 2001.

While each of the consortium members has reportedly invested $4.2 million to cover start-up costs since its founding, they appear to be hedging their bets by developing claims-processing contracts with other vendors and solutions (for example, Oxford with AthenaHealth.com, or Aetna with WebMD/Envoy). Moreover, the consortium has no agreement with a leading practice management system like Medical Manager, which suggests it will have to develop its own.[93] Finally, NDCHealth's claims system has attracted fewer physician users than WebMD's on-line claims system.[94]

Conclusion

The recent rapid proliferation of e-commerce initiatives in health care supply chains has been an exciting development. The field of new entrants has been crowded, their business models are unproven, provider and customer inertia has been strong, and incumbents have retaliated. Given the fact that freestanding B2B firms lack the ability to generate their own demand, feature capabilities that others are trying to imitate, and impose administrative expenses that may duplicate expenses elsewhere, B2B firms face an uncertain future.

After the first quarter of 2000, the B2B market suffered an enormous contraction. From December 31, 1999 through July 7, 2000, e-health stocks fell 74 percent, compared to 1 percent drop in the NASDAQ composite index and a 1 percent rise in the S&P 500 index.[95] Part of the fall was attributed to Healtheon/WebMD's year-end earnings announcement on March 2, and the market's negative reaction to the news. As the stock slid, it dragged other e-health stocks with it—with firms losing over 60 percent of their market value. Another possible explanation was a negative article published in *Barron's* on March 20, questioning the Internet firms' ability to stay solvent at their current cash "burn rate." Indeed, a stream of analysts lampooned the B2B sector using such headlines as "B2Bluster" and "Healtheon: First Mover Disadvantage."[96,97] Finally, some suggested that the end was inevitable; that is, that B2Bs knew they had a short life span, tried to force changes quickly, and sought to consolidate others, get acquired themselves, and then disappear. Along this path of rapid growth, the B2Bs committed several mistakes made by their dot-com counterparts in industry.[98–101]

As a result, B2B firms will have to focus on what business has always had to focus on—the business model. No rapid change is therefore likely to occur. The success of B2B may come more slowly in several forms. First, only a handful of B2B firms will survive from the once-crowded marketplace. Those that do are likely to be the ones that have partnered with, acquired, or been acquired by incumbents in the supply chain. Incumbents possess the strategic assets that B2B firms lack and cannot quickly develop on their own. Given the fall in B2B stock prices, it is unlikely that B2B laggards and new entrants will be able to use inflated stock valuations as a means to acquire these capabilities.

Second, B2B successes may be observed in those arenas that incumbents do not occupy. These may include the specialty products market, the alternate site market, and the international market. The European market has been characterized as even more inefficient than the United States with greater supply chain management problems. Part of this stems from the numerous small countries (markets) to be served, their different business practices, and the inability to impose a "pan-European solution."

Third, B2B firms may find their greatest opportunity in areas yet to be addressed by automation. Some IDN executives suggest the biggest automation opportunities lie in "the Admins"; that is, completion of clinical forms on patient units and PAR (personnel action report) forms. The latter, which cover payroll, benefits, and other human resource tasks, reportedly entail fifteen to twenty steps, several FTEs, twenty-one-day turnaround, and $20 million in costs at large IDNs.[102]

However, even automation (whether through the Internet, EDI, or other linkage) may not be sufficient. The real need may not be automating steps in provider processes, but rather in eliminating steps in these processes and passing the savings along (downstream to providers and perhaps upstream to manufacturers and distributors). Thus, some real savings may occur in reengineering the procurement process from thirty to forty steps down to ten to twelve steps.[103] Other opportunities for reengineering, some of which have been briefly mentioned previously include managed inventory shelves and cabinets, point-of-use data collection, centralized warehouse management systems, and demand planning.[104]

Overall, to be successful, B2B firms will need to help IDNs and other providers generate new revenues and/or operating savings. The former might include patient recruitment for clinical trials; the latter might encompass reduced labor costs (FTEs), cost of goods sold (COGS), and savings in capitated contracts. What IDNs want most of all, however, is (1) patient volume and filled beds, and (2) closer ties ("sticky relationships") with their physicians. These benchmarks may serve as the ultimate value proposition for B2Bs.

One major challenge for B2Bs, and thus one major trend to monitor, is the devaluation of e-commerce and B2B firms, and the problems encountered with B2B technology among supply chain participants. There may no longer be a perceived "urgency of the times" to propel developments here quickly.

After the dust settles, however, it is not clear how much will have changed in the management of the health care supply chain. Given all of the exchanges being developed by incumbents, there may be the potential for exchanges to efficiently transact with exchanges. Perhaps the real value of the Internet would result from all B2B exchanges consolidating into one large front-end system that would contract with a giant manufacturer exchange (like GHX) as a large back-end system. Such scenarios may represent the real "network effect" of the Internet; that is, reduced need to have multiple parties on-line all at the same time. Such enthusiasm must be tempered by the realization that these start-ups are all competitors whose joint activity is subject to antitrust scrutiny and threatened by self-interest and ego.

On the other hand, the consequence of all these exchanges may be a stalemate between supplier-developed solutions, distributor-developed solutions, and GPO/B2B-developed solutions. That is, at each stage in the value chain, incumbents will have consolidated with one another and/or strategically partnered with B2B firms for their Internet solutions in order to exert power upstream and downstream. The wild card in all of this is the patient (now consumer). The various supply chain players, alliances, and exchanges may ultimately end up competing for the loyalty of Internet-savvy consumers. Thus, in local markets, the competition for the customer's loyalty may be played out among e-health plans and IDNs. More generally, the competition may be between vendors seeking to directly sell their products to providers and consumers (for example, looking for a B2C play using the Internet); and distributor, GPO, and health plan exchanges seeking to mediate or influence those transactions.

Endnotes

1. Goldman Sachs. *Internet Quarterly Review.* New York: Goldman Sachs, 2000.
2. Hambrecht & Quist. *HealthNet Industry Report: Projected Market Size for eHealth.* New York: Hambrecht & Quist, 2000.

3. Boehm et al. *Sizing Healthcare eCommerce.* www.forrester.com (1999).

4. Marhula, Daron C. and Edward G. Shannon. *EHealth B2B Overview.* Minneapolis, Minnesota: U.S. Bancorp Piper Jaffray, 2000.

5. Hochstadt, Bruce, and David Lewis. *Bits of Paper to Bytes of Data: A White Paper on Healthcare Information and Internet.* San Francisco: Thomas Weisel Partners, 1999.

6. Fitzgibbons, Stephen M. *Vital Signs* 1(1): 1–21. Chase Hambrecht & Quist Equity Research, 2000.

7. See Note Five.

8. See Note Five.

9. Savas, Stephen D. and Jordan S. Kanfer. *Connectivity/EDI.* New York: Goldman Sachs, 2000.

10. Ernst & Young. The Health Care Supply Chain Solution (SCS). The Supply Chain Advantage: Driving Vision to Value (Mimeo), 1999.

11. Lacy et al. *The Value of eCommerce in the Healthcare Supply Chain.* Chicago: Arthur Anderson, 2001.

12. LeGrow et al. *ASPs: An Executive Report. Are Application Service Providers Ready for Prime Time?* California Health Care Foundation, Oakland, CA (September 2000).

13. See Note Five.

14. See Note Twelve.

15. See Note Twelve.

16. Barkley, Ronald, and Stephen Bochner. "Hospitals: The Weakest Link in the Supply Chain." *E-Healthcare Connections* 2(Winter 2000): 1–4.

17. Morrisey, John. "Internet Dominates Providers' Line of Sight." *Modern Healthcare* (April 10, 2000): 72–92.

18. Morrisey, John. "Modern Healthcare's 2000 Survey of Hospital Information System Trends." *Modern Healthcare* (February 5, 2001). www.pwchealth.com.

19. Superior Consultant Company and Dell Computer Corporation. 12th Annual HIMSS Leadership Survey, 2001. www.himss.org.

20. Adams, Eric. "Applications for Rent." *Healthcare Business* (January/ February 2000): 55–56.

21. Janah, Monua. "Aspiring to Serve." *Red Herring* (June 2000): 259–266.

22. Heywood, Peter. "ASPs: Hurry Up and Wait." *Red Herring* (September 2000): 368–374.

23. See Note Twenty.

24. Cassak, David. "Hospital Supply's Vapor Chain." *In Vivo* (October 1999): 13–28.

25. Hospital Materials Management. "Hospital Disposes of Its Used Equipment the High-Tech Way, with Online Auction Site." *Hospital Materials Management* (September 1999): 4.

26. Millennium Research Group. *Online Opportunities in the Medical Products Marketplace*. Stream 1, Issue 1. Toronto: Millennium Research Group, 2000.

27. Moreover, there is high variability in refurbishing standards. The Food and Drug Administration (FDA) rescinded its standards in 1997 and have instead made them voluntary.

28. Smith, Loren. "Delivering Intelligent Solutions in Healthcare." Presentation to Medical Equipment and Health Supplies on the Internet Conference. Chicago: May 2000.

29. Millennium Research Group. *Online Healthcare Marketplaces—Player Strategies*. Stream 3, Issue 3. (June 2001). Toronto: Millennium Research Group.

30. See Note Twenty-Four.

31. Gimein, Mark. "Memo from the Promised Land." *Fortune* (May 15, 2000): 189–192.

32. Cassak, David. "E-Health's Second Mover Advantage." *In Vivo* (March 2000): 26–42.

33. Mellenson, Michael. "B–B Commerce: Hot Companies Panel." Presentation to eHealth: B2B Commerce and Connectivity Conference (July 2000), San Francisco.

34. Indeed, Neoforma signed an agreement with HealthWorks (the affiliate of Continuum Health Partners, with $100 million in annual procurement) to develop its first customized e-commerce marketplace and purchasing solution (Marketplace@HealthWorks). This agreement ended when HealthWorks collapsed (see Chapter Six).

35. See Note Twenty-Nine.

36. See Note Thirty-Two.

37. See Note Thirty-Two.

38. Perez, Ken, and John Webb. "Rush Presbyterian and Omnicell.com Collaborate on Automated Supply Procurement." Presentation to Medical Equipment and Health Supplies on the Internet Conference. Chicago: May 2000.

39. Ibid.

40. Hofer, Maureen. "Storage Units Produce $1 Million in Savings." *Hospital Materials Management* 26(4) (2001): 2, 10–11.

41. Industry analysts estimate the high-end device market (for example, implants) at $10 billion, middle-tier products at $7 billion, and lower-tech specialty products at $13 billion in sales.

42. Hospital Materials Management. "E-Commerce Saves by Consolidating Small POs." *Hospital Materials Management* 25(1) (2000): 2, 9.

43. Novation. *Value of Commitment Study*. Dallas, Texas: Novation, 1995.

44. Cassak, David. "Internet Specialty Delivery." *In Vivo* (November 1999): 26–39.

45. Ibid.

46. BD Healthcare Consulting and Services. *E-Commerce Implementation Phase I: Case Study*. Becton Dickinson Healthcare Consulting and Services, 2000.

47. Web-based procurement steps include creating purchase orders (POs) using the IDN's ERP system; printing off copies of the orders; signing on to the Promedix Web site; entering the order; searching for the item by vendor, part number, or description; indicating quantity; and completing the transaction. By contrast, Integrated procurement steps include creating the POs using the IDN's ERP system, creating a file for EDI transaction, transmitting orders via EDI to Promedix in the form of an 850 transaction, and receiving confirmation.

48. Ventro Corporation. Form 10-K. Securities and Exchange Commission. (Fiscal Year Ended December 31, 2000.)

49. Egger, Ed. "Tenet, Columbia/HCA Invest in Online Procurement Companies." *Health Care Strategic Management* 18(2) (2000): 10–11.

50. Pfeil, Steven. "Broadlane, Inc." Presentation to Medical Equipment and Health Supplies on the Internet Conference. Chicago: May 2000.

51. See Note Forty-Nine.

52. Cassak, David. "E-Health's Execution Play." *In Vivo* 18(2) (2000): 14–25.

53. Ibid.

54. See Note Twenty-Nine.

55. Cassak, David. "The New Internet Supply Chain: Issues for Device and Supply Companies." *Start Up* 5(3) (2000): 16–26.

56. Hospital Materials Management. "Novation Marks Three-Year Anniversary with Record Savings, Lagging Dot-Com." *Hospital Materials Management* 26(6) (2001): 6–7.

57. See Note Eleven.

58. See Note Eleven.

59. DeJohn, Paula. "Web Moves Toward Unity as GPOs Push Standards." *Hospital Materials Management* 25(7) (2000): 1, 9.

60. Cf. www.RosettaNet.org.

61. John Burks, personal communication.

62. Cassak, David. "Burden of Proof." *In Vivo* (June 2001): 26–40.

63. Gillett et al. *Hospitals' New Supply Chain.* www.forrester.com (2000).

64. Ibid.

65. Vandermerwe, Sandra, and Marika Taishoff. *Baxter (A): A Changing Customer Environment.* Case #597-039-1. Wellesley, Massachusetts: European Case Clearing House, 1997.

66. See Note Fifty-Five.

67. Winslow, Ron. "J&J, Baxter International, Others Plan Internet Concern for Hospital Purchases." *Wall Street Journal* (2000).

68. Grebb, Michael. "E-Commerce Rising." *Healthcare Business* (April 2001): 24, 72–73. Quoted with permission.

69. Healthcare Business. "Reinventing the Health Care Supply Chain." *Healthcare Business* (June 2000): Special Supplement.

70. Ibid.

71. See Note Twenty-Nine.

72. See Note Twenty-Nine.

73. Millennium Research Group. *Hospital Online Procurement Survey.* Stream 2, Issue 1 (2000). Toronto: Millennium Research Group.

74. See Note Fifty-Five.

75. See Note Twenty-Six.

76. Henig, Peter D. "Revenge of the Bricks." *Red Herring* (August 2000): 121–134.

77. Weinberg, Neil. "Herding Cats." *Forbes* (July 24, 2000): 108, 110.

78. See Note Seventy-Six.

79. Elias, Paul. "Still Trading." *Red Herring* (March 20, 2001): 53–56.

80. Stalkamp, Tom. Presentation to Health Industry Group Purchasing Association (HIGPA) Annual Meeting, 2000.

81. Findley, Richard. *The Pharmaceutical Supply Chain: 1999 Second Pharmaceutical Supply Chain Survey.* New York: AT Kearney, 1999.

82. Bickert, Madeline. "The Impact of E-Commerce on Legacy of Health Care Companies." *Cyber Dialogue* (July 1999).

83. Frost & Sullivan. *The Internet's Role in the U.S. Distribution of Medical Devices.* San Jose, California: Frost & Sullivan, 2000.

84. Millennium Research Group. *Online Opportunities in the Medical Products Marketplace,* p. 15.

85. Becker, Cinda. "No Silver Bullet: Online Purchasing Company Moves Slowly in Hopes of Ensuring Success." *Modern Healthcare* 31(6) (2001): 26.

86. See Note Twenty-Nine.

87. McFadden, Christopher D. *E-Distribution Update and Survey Results.* New York: Goldman Sachs. March 10, 2000.

88. Cassak, David. "Cardinal.com: The New Old Thing." *In Vivo* 18(4) (2000): 11–24.

89. Ibid.

90. Ibid.

91. Thill, Mark. "Minor Miracle." *Repertoire* 8(10) (2000): 8, 10–11.

92. Tschida, Molly. "Getting on Board: Payers Face Barriers as They Move Toward Internet Transactions." *Modern Physician* (May 2000): 60–65.

93. Johnston, Douglas, Michael Barrett and Victoria Sutton. *MedUnite's Debut Doesn't Hold Together.* www.forrester.com (November 15, 2000).

94. Benko, Laura. "Insurers Buy Into Electronic Claims." *Modern Healthcare* (June 11, 2001): 24–25.

95. Frank, Seth. "Wall Street Panel: Comparing Business Models of Today's eHealth Portals." Presentation to eHealth: B2B Commerce and Connectivity Conference (July 2000), San Francisco.

96. Lyons, Daniel. "B2Bluster." *Forbes* (May 1, 2000): 122–126.

97. Setton, Dolly. "Sick Days." *Forbes,* (July 17, 2000): 56, 58.

98. Everard, Lynn J. "Dot-Com Trial and Error." *Repertoire* 8(10) (2000): 18–19.

99. Wise, Richard and David Morrison. "Beyond the Exchange: The Future of B2B." *Harvard Business Review* (November–December 2000): 86–96.

100. Useem, Jerry. "Dot-Coms: What Have We Learned?" *Fortune* (October 30, 2000): 46–64.

101. Kanter, Rosabeth M. "The Ten Deadly Mistakes of Wanna-Dots." *Harvard Business Review* (January 2001): 91–100.

102. Reese, Bert. "Cost Justifying eHealth Solutions for Health Systems: Where's the ROI in the World of 'e'?" Presentation to eHealth: B2B Commerce and Connectivity Conference (July 2000), San Francisco.

103. See Note Sixty-Nine.

104. Pandita, Vinnie. "Centralized Materials Distribution: Is It Right for Your System?" Presentation to Strategic Sourcing and E-Commerce Solutions for the Med-Surg Supply Chain Conference. Philadelphia: October 1999.

. . . .

11

E-Commerce and Integrated Delivery Networks (IDNs)

Lawton R. Burns

Introduction

Previous sections have dealt with manufacturers, distributors, and GPOs. Each of these three parties has demonstrated capabilities and strengths in the health care supply chain. Hospitals and IDNs represent the final customer in the institutional portion of the supply chain. However, as the fourth tire on the automobile, their performance on several dimensions seems to be flat. This chapter begins with a description of the hospital portion of the supply chain and assesses their capabilities to engage their supply chain partners in e-commerce and other improvement activities. Their role is critical. A recent study documented that the logistics practices and internal management policies of automakers as customers of the automobile supply chain strongly influence the ability of their own suppliers to develop lean, efficient systems.[1] That is, the efficiency of the end customer drives the efficiency of the supply chain.

Hospitals and IDNs: The Fourth (Flat) Tire of the Health Care Supply Chain

Hospitals and IDNs exhibit weak capability in several supply chain functions. These include logistics, procurement, utilization, pricing, and support for the materials management role.

Inbound Logistics

To gauge the utility and feasibility of e-commerce for IDNs, it is necessary to understand how the supply chain operates within the walls of the IDN. Several industry reports provide a good overview of this process using both diagrams and analysis.[2,3] On the inbound side, products are typically delivered by distributors to the IDN's central warehouse (if they have one) or to warehouses of each facility in the network. IDNs may have warehouses for both inventory storage as well as just-in-time delivery. Supplies are then transported to the loading docks of each hospital within the IDN. From there, materials management personnel break down the shipments and deliver them to central sterile supply and/or storage areas located on floors throughout the hospital, using exchange carts. Depending on need, carts are exchanged on a daily or weekly basis. From these points, hospital department and ancillary unit personnel may access them. Products are thus handled by a number of different people and inventoried in a number of dispersed sites. When they are used, there are often no bar codes or UPNs that can be scanned to record product utilization and track it by patient or provider. By contrast, ATMs such as Pyxis machines used for drug dispensing on patient units are stocked by the distributor directly without the other intervening steps, and record drug unit utilization when items are removed from the cabinet. Analysts suggest that the hospital distribution process typically contains more steps than the rest of the supply chain put together, and often duplicates activities of other supply chain participants.

Procurement and Transaction Errors

The same thing may be said for the ordering process. Any number of different personnel (for example: physician, nurse, materials manager, pharmacist, and so on) may select the product to be ordered, check for current availability by a manual inspection of inventory, and then manually search for the product using paper catalogues.

Indeed, recent evidence suggests that the number of personnel in the materials management department engaged in procurement-related activities is rivaled by the number of people in other departments (for example, nursing, radiology) performing the same functions.[4] Some GPOs send out catalogues of contracted products on CD-ROMs. From there, the materials manager may check with the authorized distributors regarding product availability, arrange for a purchase order (PO), which may or may not be scrutinized by a separate procurement manager and approval committee, and then order using either a paper requisition, phone order, fax order, or EDI. As noted in earlier chapters, POs are the activities where EDI transaction sets are most heavily utilized. However, other related EDI transaction sets (for example, PO confirmation, catalogue and uniform pricing, and invoicing) are not. These manual entry processes are slower and more error prone than automated entry. The result is that even EDI transactions can experience almost 25 percent error rates.[5] The vast majority of these errors are attributable to inaccurate product information.[6] As a consequence, most of the products are often ordered using out-of-date price information and incomplete information regarding whether they are covered by GPO contracts. When products are ordered, the transactions are entered manually into the hospital's inventory system (front-end integration) but may not be linked to the hospital's accounting or financial system (back-end integration).[7]

Other factors help explain the errors in these transactions. Currently, health care product information resides in multiple catalogue sources and formats, which can be transmitted in either electronic or paper form. There is no centralized, standardized design and management of these catalogues. As a result, it is virtually impossible for manufacturers, distributors, GPOs, or hospitals to maintain an accurate, aggregated "Item Master File" across all vendors. Indeed, some manufacturers have difficulty aggregating product information across their own divisions. Moreover, the master files maintained at each stage in the value chain are likely to vary quite widely, and to increasingly vary as product information and prices change quickly. Every business process and transaction throughout the entire supply chain utilizes information from the different master files. Data disparities between each trading partner's master file causes errors in its transactions.[8]

Variability in Product Ordering and Utilization

Some industry analysts suggest that the entire supply chain process typically breaks down at the front line (that is, point of patient care service). For example, unlike mass merchandisers like Wal-Mart, the point of sale is not well defined in hospital care. Multiple hospital departments may order products using separate processes of procurement (for example, materials management versus radiology). Department heads may engage in maverick buying off contract, physicians are unpredictable in what supplies they will use (for example, in the OR or at the bedside), physicians may take things off supply shelves, three shifts of nurses and staff render care around the clock, and some areas (for example, cath lab or operating room) carry "unofficial inventory," that is beyond the control of materials management. Such activities are exacerbated by the physical distance between the OR and clinical areas, on the one hand, and the hospital pharmacy and materials management departments on the other. That is, there is little daily interaction between clinicians who requisition and use the products and the department managers who order them on behalf of clinicians. These activities make it difficult to centrally record, let alone forecast and manage supply utilization.

This problem has multiple aspects. First, analysts believe that IDNs and their physicians lack information on which physicians order which supplies and with what results. That is, there is little specific information on who the customer actually is, how he or she is using the product, and what outcomes are associated with the product's use. As one observer noted, "The weakest link in the supply chain is the one that does not know its own cost of doing business." Since providers don't know their own costs, they cannot appreciate the process cost savings and capabilities that might exist in new technologies and supplier-initiated efficiency improvements. Manufacturers commonly note that materials managers need to be able to move information as well as products, to invest in IT and scanners that can tell what happens to the product after it is delivered, and to help manufacturers forecast demand. As one executive stated, "You can only kick a box and lick a label so fast." IDNs therefore need to rationalize product demand and utilization. To do so requires that physicians understand the price, quantity, and value of the products they order. IDNs may consider hiring *more* staff for the materials management and pharmacy departments and placing them on the patient units to work with physicians on efficient purchase and utilization. Some analysts suggest that hospitals need to embrace systemwide solutions like activity-based costing, just as some distributors have.[9] Others have called for hospitals to radically reengineer and reduce the number of steps in procurement and distribution. Simply adding an electronic capability to current processes will probably not be sufficient. As one consultant quipped, "This is tantamount to moving garbage at the speed of light."

Part of the problem here is the traditional reliance on "par levels" for maintaining inventories of supplies on hospital units. Some have called par levels the curse of the supply chain, suggesting that hospital staff may order too much product and order it too frequently just to maintain the par levels. Indeed, in a case study of a 300-bed hospital; there were 30,000 EDI transactions; 20,000 phone, fax, and manual transactions; and 150,000 LUM (low unit of measure) transactions just to "fill the bins every day."[10] Half of these LUM transactions are considered unnecessary. Analysts instead recommend the use of "reorder points" that can reduce the number of unnecessary LUM transactions by 50 percent. However, such a system requires buy-in and more disciplined purchasing behavior on the part of nursing staff accustomed to the older system.

Part of this problem may also be a vestige of the old fee-for-service reimbursement model whereby the more expense one generated, the more revenue one earned. Moreover, the problem may reflect impulse buying, which can be exacerbated in academic medical centers by the research needs of scientists ordering products for grants and the prominence of clinical departments. Hospital personnel may practice just-in-case inventory to prevent stock-outs, and "by gosh and by golly" inventory management: "by gosh, I better order it; by golly, I better FedEx it."[11] An executive in a medical-surgical manufacturing firm characterized this behavior as follows:

> I can't tell you how many phone calls I have sat in on where our customer service representatives are taking hospital orders. They start the ordering process with ten cases for UPS for normal ground delivery. By the end of the phone call it has gone to UPS second-day delivery. How could they possibly make a choice in a span of less than sixty seconds to literally increase those shipping costs by 30–40 percent? I have not seen them necessarily have the tools at their disposal to actually make that decision. Maybe they actually did need something, but it would have been better to split the order, with five cases going next-day delivery and five cases going normal delivery.

As just suggested, some hospital staff (for example, nurses) place a big priority on having the product available when needed or when the surgeon requests it. This fosters a "rapid-response mentality" and organization to meet the needs of the moment.[12]

Indeed, the hospital procurement and inventory function bears some resemblance to the "synthetic organization" described more than thirty years ago in the management literature.[13] This model consists of an ad hoc way of dealing with disaster relief that pulls together (1) uncommitted resources—that is, resources that have been stockpiled elsewhere without being targeted for particular situations or patients—accompanied by (2) actors who know how to utilize these resources and (3) information and judgment regarding the need for additional resources. Clinicians are the key actors in the hospital. They form temporary synthetic organizations around each patient that arrives for acute care, and pull down the supplies and other resources needed for that patient from the central supply areas of the hospital. While such organizations "get the job done," they are not necessarily the most efficient mode of organizing.

Variability in Pricing

Other evidence of poor hospital supply chain practices may be found in pricing variances: hospitals within a given IDN pay different prices for the same product, purchased under the same contract, using the same distributor.[14] Some analysts have estimated these variances occur 40 percent of the time, with actual price differences ranging from 2–7 percent.[15] Such variances occur for several reasons, including mismatches between the GPO's negotiated prices and the distributor's and IDN's master price lists, decentralized ordering at the hospital (rather than IDN) level, maverick buying of products by departments without heeding GPO contracts and prices (nonconformances), and pricing errors. The losses sustained in this manner by a fourteen-hospital IDN, because it failed to get the lowest price for each hospital, amounted to $600,000 per year. Moreover, it is estimated that 25–30 percent of the purchasing department buyer's staff time is spent on resolving errors and non-conformances (that is, redundant functions and process delays). Of course, there are no clear incentives elsewhere in the supply chain to correct this problem. Manufacturers reportedly love pricing variances, although they may result in delayed payment (for example, if pricing errors are involved). Part of the overpayment for products may also go to distributors and the GPO the IDN belongs to.[16]

Role of Materials Management Director

Part of the problem may also be attributable to the role of the hospital's director of materials management. This individual must preside over several complex flows of money, products, and information (outlined earlier, in Chapter Three). He or she must also juggle multiple responsibilities that may conflict with one another, such as dealing with pharmaceutical and medical-surgical product sales representatives, complying with and monitoring GPO contracts, processing new requisitions and handling purchase orders for internal constituents and routing them to ADAs, handling off-contract purchases, managing incurred expenses and staying within budget, and so on.[17] Some suggest the materials manager is "run around by surgeons and salesmen." Given the complexity in the ordering and internal product distribution processes of an IDN, as well as the divergent interests of supply chain players, the materials manager faces enormous difficulties in making "value-related purchase decisions."

The materials manager may not be fully equipped to handle this beleaguered role. Some managers lack formal business training, and instead come to their positions by way of "sales rep" experience or having worked in the stockroom. Even if they have formal training, few business schools offer required courses in supply chain management and none specific to the complexity of the health care industry. Product manufacturers are quite blunt in their assessment of some of these individuals:

> There are some good VPs for materials management out there, especially at the bigger hospitals. But you have to think about how they grew up. They grew up from the guy on the loading dock to the manager of the storeroom to the VP. Or she was originally a scrub nurse who then became a head nurse and now is the supervisor of the OR. Where did these people learn materials management? No one taught them that. These people are in

trouble and/or over their head. They're always busy counting boxes or beating up somebody over price. But we [manufacturers] are talking about business systems, about process improvements, about having strategic plans. It is awfully hard to talk to these guys about five years down the road. You wouldn't go into a budget meeting with the executives of my company without guaranteeing 7 percent process improvement in your plants, even during good years.

The role of the materials manager may also be invisible and undervalued. In many hospitals the materials management office is located near the loading dock. The materials manager is trying to be a "presence" in the organization, but may lack the information systems, credentials, and logistics training to succeed. This may change as executives gain a greater appreciation for supply chain management. The experience of human resource managers is both instructive and encouraging. This function is now often located near the executive suite, reflecting the importance accorded to developing human capital resources. Less than two decades ago, the function was called *Personnel* and was often located in the hospital basement.

At the same time, materials managers are under pressure by senior IDN executives to contain costs and keep the IDN fiscally sound, particularly as the cost of new therapies and technologies rises. This alone may command their attention and divert it away from more long-term, strategic actions such as e-commerce and other process improvements. They may not be rewarded for saving unknown process costs in the future. They may not even believe that process costs are the relevant issue, and instead focus on short-term savings on a particular supply item in this year's contract, where results are more immediate and demonstrable. Indeed, any changes they propose in their IDN's supply chain process (for example, switching products or vendors) may involve lots of paperwork and be greeted by clinician resistance. The current situation is not helped by the fact that materials managers can still find vendors that will cut their prices to gain the hospital's contract and incrementally increase their local market share penetration. This reinforces the materials managers' belief that vendors still charge high prices and that focus on unit price is appropriate.[18]

General and Industry Barriers to Internet Adoption by IDNs

Despite the involvement of the powerful actors and forces mentioned in the preceding chapter, the diffusion of B2B solutions may be slow. A recent roundtable of health care executives highlighted the well-known characteristics of their industry that will hamper B2B deployment.[19] These include

- Multiple, complex (and sometimes contractual) relationships: patient-physician, physician-HMO, physician-physician, vendor-provider, and so on

- Lack of alignment among these various parties, retarding the rapid and complete flow of information

- A complex, process-intensive manufacturing model that allows each physician ("line worker") to alter the work process based on their personal experience

- Lack of an integrated and automated customer record, and presence of 7,000 discrete pieces of information contained on a variety of media

- Conflicts between traditional legacy information systems and labor practices versus proprietary processes and innovations

- Decentralized hospital fiefdoms that adopt different solutions without a common underlying platform or infrastructure, and that make it difficult to get all of the moving parts to work together

• Exploding health care knowledge domain and information-intensive work processes

As a result of all of these impediments to change, the revolutionary force of e-commerce may be adopted by providers in an evolutionary fashion. B2B solutions will, by necessity, be implemented as incremental improvements that extend existing legacy systems and accommodate existing stakeholder interests.[20]

In the remainder of this chapter, we analyze some of the specific barriers to Internet adoption among provider organizations. These barriers deal with information technology issues, the limited use of e-commerce for procurement, the decentralized character of IDNs, the lack of integration between IDNs and their physicians, the reliance on top-down strategies to penetrate local markets, and the general breakdown of the supply chain at the provider level.

E-Commerce Initiatives by Integrated Delivery Networks: To B2B or Not to B2B?

IDNs have shown some interest in e-commerce solutions. We first consider their general use of e-commerce and then analyze the application of e-commerce to procurement.

IDN Involvement in E-Commerce

IDNs and hospital systems are beginning to use B2B solutions to automate their transactions with payers (for example, claims submissions). A survey of the "100 most wired" health systems found that they perform 33 percent of eligibility verification tasks on-line, followed by precertification (22 percent of tasks on-line), referral authorization (19 percent), claims submission (16 percent), case management (11 percent), contract performance data (11 percent), and electronic funds transfers (7 percent).[21] Of the remaining "less wired" hospitals, these percentages range only from 0–11 percent.

Nevertheless, IDN involvement with the Internet appears for the moment to be limited primarily to developing patient-oriented Web pages for marketing purposes. These Internet sites typically list directories of the IDN's hospitals and physicians (with directions on how to get there), the IDN's mission and values, health promotion information and classes offered, information on current health topics, and employment opportunities.[22] This may reflect the interest of both patients and health professionals in "content" over "commerce."

Other surveys support this picture. A telephone survey of 350 hospital marketing executives showed that the major Internet applications used are (in order of prevalence) Web site design (91 percent), e-mail (87 percent), employee recruitment (79 percent), health education (70 percent), physician directory (57 percent), Intranet (49 percent), physician referrals (48 percent), communication with physicians (43 percent), information on disease management (42 percent), communication with patients (41 percent), on-line newsletter (34 percent), and discussion groups (10 percent).[23] In surveys of hundreds of health care executives attending the eleventh and twelfth annual meetings of the Health Information and Management Systems Society (HIMSS), over 90 percent said their Web sites are currently focused on external communications, for example, marketing and advertising, employee recruitment, and consumer health information. Their top IT priorities concern HIPAA compliance (over 50 percent of respondents), rather than e-commerce and vendor integration (less than 30 percent).[24,25] Finally, a survey of 320 hospital and health system Web sites revealed that 57 percent were purely informational ("brochureware"), 36 percent offered some interactive features like patient community chat rooms, 6 percent offered some transactional features such as links to payers, and only 1 percent offered some service delivery features such as on-line consultation.[26]

Use of E-Commerce in Procurement

Use of e-commerce for procurement of supplies and equipment, which is central to Web-centered solutions for supply chain management, is much less developed. Recent trend data on Internet use for procurement have been collected by Millennium Research Group using a hospital panel (see Exhibit 11.1).[27] They conducted quarterly interviews with procurement executives (materials managers, purchasing managers, and supervisors) in 100 hospitals during the year 2000. Their data capture the sobered enthusiasm for B2B, with a peak in June 2000, followed by a valley in September and more tempered interest by December 2000.

The data reveal that most purchasing managers (95 percent) use the Internet for professional purposes, but the vast majority (63 percent) use it for five hours or less per week. A growing majority (66 percent) use the Internet to purchase medical supplies and equipment as of December 2000. However, only 5.7 percent of hospital procurement is now transacted on-line, slightly up from 2.6 percent in June. In the June survey, this percentage was

Exhibit 11.1   Survey of 100 Hospital Purchasing Managers

Use of Internet for Professional Purposes			
	June 2000 (Percent)	Sept 2000 (Percent)	Dec 2000 (Percent)
Use Web in weekly work	89	88	95
Use Web for <5 hours per week	67	60	63
Use Web for >10 hours per week	2	7	8
Engage in on-line purchasing	45	54	66
Percent total procurement on-line	2.6	3.5	5.7
Percent expected on-line by 2003	64	47	50
Percent registered with B2B firm	32	29	37
Percent registered with 2 + B2Bs	20	9	7

Source: Millennium Research Group. *Hospital Online Procurement Survey.* Stream 2, Issue 1 (June 2000), Stream 2, Issue 2 (September 2000), Stream 2, Issue 3 (December 2000). Toronto: Millennium Research Group.

expected to rise to 64 percent by 2003, but executives reduced their estimates to 50 percent by the time of the December survey. Finally, roughly one-third of hospitals are registered with one of the on-line B2B firms like Medibuy or Neoforma. This percentage has been fairly stable, although an increasing percentage of hospitals are now registered with just one of these competitors.

While the Millennium data indicate some increase in on-line procurement (from 2.6 percent to 5.7 percent) in just six months time, further analysis reveals that this percentage covers all items purchased. Hospitals are much more likely to procure office and maintenance supplies and IT products on-line than they are to procure medical-surgical supplies. On-line procurement of medical supplies (defined as both lower-end disposables and higher-end devices) is estimated at only 0.8 percent of total purchases in this product area; within this area, 1.1 percent of disposable items are procured on-line, compared to only 0.3 percent of the medical devices.[28] These latter figures represent slight increases from 0.2 percent for both categories of products in 1999.

There are at least three reasons why office and maintenance supplies may experience higher on-line procurement. First, hospitals may lack buying software from their distributors in these product areas, and may thus be amenable to shifting to on-line purchasing. Second, such items do not command any physician interest or require any clinical approval prior to shifting to on-line procurement. Third, they may more easily transition to Web procurement due to product standardization, frequent replenishment, little required service or technical support, and their low share of overall spending. Materials managers may in fact be experimenting with these types of products before shifting to medical products. In contrast, on-line purchasing has failed to penetrate the device market due to the fact that devices are typically less covered by GPO contracts compared to other supplies, are usually ordered in smaller quantities over the phone or by fax, and are delivered directly by the supplier's sales representatives (rather than by distributors).

Moreover, Millennium estimates that only 5–10 percent of this on-line procurement constitutes new orders; the remainder consists of already established business switching to on-line transactions. Thus, there is not a great deal of new business being generated by the B2B exchanges.

Size of the On-Line Market in Procurement

Millennium provides a range of estimates for the actual dollar value of the on-line medical supply marketplace, broken out by hospitals versus ASM. On the one hand, they estimate the total hospital market to be $51.7 billion and the alternate site market to be $16 billion. Given that roughly 0.8 percent of this is on-line, then the total on-line market is estimated at $519 million. Of this, (1) $443 million is spent on disposables and $80 million is spent on devices; and (2) $310 million is from the hospital market (0.6 percent of all hospital spending on supplies) and $210 million is from the alternate site market (1.4 percent of their total supply spend).[29,30] On the other hand, their survey data suggest that total hospital spending on medical supplies and equipment (excluding pharmaceuticals) averages $30 million a year per institution. Applying the percentages just noted suggests that the dollar value of the online purchasing market is $30 million × 5.7% = $1.7 million per hospital, and the value of the on-line medical-surgical supply market is $30 million × 0.8% = $240,000. Across all 6,000 hospitals, the total market value is $1.44 billion. This may provide an upper-bound estimate for on-line hospital purchasing of medical supplies. Even if it is this high, it is not quite the $4 billion that Forrester Research estimated for on-line purchasing for supplies, equipment, and drugs by 2000; and is a far cry from the $124 billion anticipated by 2004.[31]

Sources of Variability in On-Line Procurement

There are several sources of variation in hospital supply spending over the Internet. Millennium classifies hospital e-procurement activity by supply area. Among hospitals engaged in e-procurement,

63 percent use the Web to purchase office and maintenance supplies, 52 percent use the Web for medical-surgical supplies, 24 percent use it for both pharmaceuticals and capital equipment, 20 percent use it for specialty medical supplies, and 17 percent use it for laboratory supplies. As a percentage of total procurement in these areas, Web-based purchasing accounts for 17 percent of office, maintenance, and IT spend; 15 percent of pharma spend; 9 percent of medical-surgical consumables spend; 3 percent of laboratory spend; and only 1 percent of both specialty medical supply and capital equipment spend. The top medical-surgical consumable products bought on-line are custom med-surg pre-packs, gloves, and IV products.[32]

There is also variation in Web-based purchasing by hospital size. It is interesting that smaller hospitals (that is, those with fewer than 150 beds) are less likely to use the Web for purchasing, but conduct more of their procurement on-line.[33] Current on-line purchasing as a percentage of total procurement is 5.9 percent in smaller hospitals versus 3.2 percent in hospitals with 150–299 beds, 2.7 percent in hospitals with 300–499 beds, and only 1.4 percent in hospitals with 500 or more beds.[34] These higher figures for smaller hospitals perhaps reflect their lack of investment in legacy and EDI systems, the higher percentage of lower-end disposable items (and the lower percentage of specialty items and capital equipment) they purchase, more compact and less complex procurement operations, lower percentage spending on capital equipment and specialty supplies, and possibly their greater price sensitivity.[35,36] In contrast, larger hospitals purchase more unique devices and capital equipment that may be harder to source using the Web and for which materials managers may prefer direct dealings with sales representatives. Larger hospitals may also be less willing to risk disruptions to current EDI linkages that work well. Overall, 80 percent of hospitals use EDI for purchasing; the percentage is much higher among larger hospitals.[37]

The Millennium data provide few other clues about hospital variability in Internet-based purchasing. One Wall Street survey of

hospital procurement executives suggests that favorable consideration and evaluation of e-procurement solutions is associated with
IDN membership, region, and certain GPO affiliations, but not
with hospital ownership (for example, for-profit versus nonprofit).[38]

Slow Penetration by E-Commerce in IDNs

There appear to be several reasons for the slow penetration of Web-
based procurement among IDNs, according to the MRG survey:

Many of the survey respondents belong to large GPOs and
report they are waiting for their GPOs to partner with a B2B
before they transition to on-line purchasing. These hospitals
do not want to sacrifice GPO pricing just to purchase on the
Web. They may also be waiting for the GPOs to demonstrate
functionality in their new B2B partners.

Materials managers are waiting for B2B firms that can integrate
with their internal procurement and financial systems. They
want to obtain their GPO prices from the B2B sites, view the
contracts on-line, and credit purchases directly to their GPO.

Materials managers may wait for "automated teller machines" for
medical supplies, like the Pyxis machines they use for drug distribution. These managers may also wait for manufacturers and
distributors to bring this technology to them, just as the distributors brought them EDI and purchasing software in the past.

Many materials managers report they want "high-touch" vendor
relationships to accompany the "high-tech" Internet procurement solutions, especially for the higher-cost items like capital
equipment. That is, B2B firms need to supplement their Web
offerings with extensive customer support and frequent individual salesperson interaction that supports the purchasing
decision. This interaction also serves to build credibility and
trust in the B2B's offering.

Of the 45 percent of respondents engaged in on-line purchasing in the June 2000 Millennium survey, 40 percent report no savings advantage as yet, primarily due to lack of software integration with hospital internal business processes. This lack of interface reportedly necessitates double entry of orders on both the materials management and Web systems. Other respondents believe the savings will come indirectly in the form of quicker product delivery or better use of personnel.

Of those hospitals currently registered with a B2B exchange, barely half (52 percent) report they are "totally satisfied" with the service they have received.[39] Seventeen percent stated they were not satisfied. Causes of dissatisfaction include lack of savings, lack of connectivity with hospital systems, too few qualified vendors, and "illiquid auctions" (that is, not enough buyers and sellers). Hospitals may also want broader product offerings, access to more vendors, and access to capital equipment manufacturers.

Many B2B exchanges lack brand recognition in the eyes of hospital materials managers. For those managers who had not yet registered with an on-line exchange, roughly two-thirds recognized the names *Medibuy* and *Neoforma,* but only one-third recognized *Promedix* and *MedicalBuyer.* Brand recognition is much higher among materials managers whose hospitals have registered with an exchange: 70–80 percent of managers recognize Medibuy and Neoforma, while only 30–50 percent recognize Broadlane and GHX.

On-line purchasing for certain groups of hospitals (for example, municipals) may be inhibited by state contracting laws (for example, open bidding process).

Hospital procurement managers may instead rely on their distributors and their Web sites for e-procurement. In December

2000, 64 percent of procurement managers reported they were buying through the Web sites of manufacturers and distributors, up from 26 percent three months earlier. The most frequently used distributors were Owens & Minor and Cardinal Health/Allegiance.[40]

These somewhat disappointing findings about the cost-containment potential of e-procurement are critical, especially when surveys of hospital purchasing executives suggest that cost savings and efficiencies are the most important perceived benefit of on-line purchasing.[41,42] PricewaterhouseCoopers has presented estimates of these savings as a percentage of supply costs in the range of 6.0–13.5 percent.[43,44] The bulk of these savings lie in order management (consolidated e-procurement) and demand management (oversight of product ordering and stocking), with smaller savings in supplier management (use fewer vendors), logistics management (improved supply distribution), and inventory management (more efficient management of supplies on hand). Their estimates square with Millennium's survey data on the most highly ranked benefits of improved supply chain management on-line (that is, order management and contract management).[45]

E-Commerce: (Too) Radical and Disruptive Innovation in IDNs

IDNs may thus view B2B as too embryonic to make any short-term investments. B2B firms may need to first document the savings from using their platform and demonstrate their long-term staying power before providers invest. For example, can B2B firms help IDNs to reduce the number of FTEs needed or help them move FTEs from order management tasks to more "value work" such as customer management, contracting, and analysis? Can B2B firms reduce manual processing, reduce inventory, improve inventory turnover, improve product tracking, obtain better pricing, provide demand forecasts, and improve overall asset utilization and allocation?

Moreover, IDN migration from EDI to Internet purchasing may be slow. For one reason, hospitals have invested heavily in legacy procurement systems and may be unable to afford their de-installation and replacement. They will also be reluctant to abandon them and face high switching costs unless the transition is smooth and economical. Legacy systems are already paid for; Web-based solutions are not. The EDI component of purchasing is stable and dependable; B2B firms are not. Moreover, materials managers report being happy with EDI and have used it for over a decade.[46] In hospital systems that have adopted ERP solutions, "Everyone knows how to use it, it is still very functional, and, if it is connected to the Internet via our integration, why change it?" As another informant mentioned, "Why do I need an Internet platform? I order 90 percent of my pharmaceuticals via EDI throughout a day. I order 60–70 percent of my medical-surgical supplies through EDI today. I order about that or more on lab supplies through EDI. Why do I need an Internet platform to become electronic and efficient in ordering?"

Another informant stated, "The value of the innovation must exceed the pain of adoption." There are already some reports of the level of pain here. Hospitals switching from mainframes and DOS-based MMIS (for example, Enterprise Systems or ESI's "Nova" system) to Windows-based software on PC-based client-server systems have encountered several problems in searching for products and obtaining reports.[47]

Moreover, according to industry analysts, "It takes several thousand hours to install an interface program so that a hospital's EDI system can receive data from on-line transactions."[48] Estimates for B2B integration at the hospital level range as low as $25,000 (according to one GPO/B2B alliance) to $250,000–300,000 (according to consultants), to as high as $1 million (according to one supplier).[49] Officials at Neoforma state that there is a twenty-four-week implementation period for its Marketplace product. There is also an eighteen- to twenty-four-month period (which includes the twenty-four weeks) needed to replace the existing hospital ordering system with a system that is compatible with Neoforma.

Customization and Decentralization Issues

A related issue is how to deploy B2B solutions to IDNs? Each IDN is different, and each hospital within an IDN is different. Thus, every B2B solution may need to be customized—and customized beyond hospital-specific recognition, the hospital's GPO pricing tier, and preapproved purchasing lists (tools which some on-line vendors employ). According to OmniCell officials, there are at least 800 different health care information systems on the market. Thus, in an IDN with multiple hospitals, any B2B solution requires different interfaces from one facility to the next. Each of these interfaces must also be customized to the IDN customer. Such interfaces are necessary to ensure communication between applications and systems, as well as to ensure proper accounting and control.[50]

B2B firms may mistakenly believe that IDNs typically have centralized materials management and procurement capabilities. Even if the centralized office exists, the IDN facilities may transmit EDI orders electronically from disparate computer systems throughout the system to the central office. Such data are not easily aggregated to yield a picture of consolidated purchasing for the IDN. Moreover, even if centralized procurement exists, the necessary skill sets and buy-in from constituent hospitals within the IDN may be missing. Instead of a central buyer, IDNs may have multiple buyers at each of their hospital members. This may be by default or by design. For example, at Inova, a four-hospital system in Virginia, the purchasing function is pushed down to the hospital level ("the customer/end user") because product purchasing comes out of each hospital's budget.

This messy situation is exacerbated by the recent trend toward hospital systems and networks, which yield an IDN with an odd

configuration of multiple DOS-based and legacy procurement systems that have been cobbled together. Moreover, after the merger,
there are often turf battles over which specific IT systems to use. As
one industry observer explained, "Computer systems represent a
culture." Within a given IDN, hospitals with different computer systems thus have different cyber cultures and allegiances to them.
Efforts to merge these computer cultures encounter much of the
same resistance as corporate-level mergers. The situation is further
complicated by IDNs that include physician offices, which typically
are small in size and dispersed geographically. Such offices may lack
computer linkage with the system, making it difficult to pursue
systemwide change.

The Internet is yet another culture that is foreign to each
hospital's own information system (IS) culture. Novation executives report that some of their hospital members prefer to use the
CD-ROM mailed to them rather than the Novation catalogue
available on-line with regular updates: "That CD-ROM that
Novation mails out is sixty days old by the time the member gets
it and uses it. We want to shoot the CD-ROM, but the members
would throw a fit."

Problems in Partnering with IDNs

B2B firms face several problems in trying to ally with IDNs. These
problems stem from the IDNs' cash shortage, diverted attention,
waiting stance, and physician integration problems.

Cash Squeeze

One problem is the current cash squeeze facing hospitals due to
BBA cutbacks and lower reimbursements from other payers. Hospitals are reportedly cutting their capital budgets by 40–60 percent.
One Boston academic medical center has reportedly decreased its
spending on IT from $34 million to $7 million.[51] All of this follows
massive hospital investments in legacy systems to support "clinical
integration." Analysts estimate this investment at $100 billion,

based on 5,000 community hospitals investing an average of $15–20 million on IT annually over the period.[52] Some of these investments ranged as high as $50–100 million in some systems. Hospitals may thus not be in a position to make the necessary IT capability investments to accommodate e-procurement. Recent surveys suggest little improvement in hospital IT investment plans. *Modern Healthcare's* 2000 survey of information system trends suggests decreased spending on IT (as little as 2.5 percent of hospitals' total operating budget).[53]

Customer Attention

Second, compliance with HIPAA may compete with e-commerce for the IDN's attention and scarce resources. Fitch IBCA estimates that HIPAA compliance could cost three to four times more than Y2K, or up to $25 billion, as hospitals modify their technology, purchase new IT systems, hire and retrain staff in this area, and change existing processes associated with patient privacy. HIPAA will also slow down EDI, as it requires providers to adopt Web standards for several core applications (for example, claims, eligibility, and authorization) if they elect to use electronic communications. Industry observers suspect HIPAA will consume hospitals' dwindling IT budgets for the next two years.[54] Moreover, IDNs are unsure exactly what information they can pool and share for purposes of benchmarking supply chain management that does not violate HIPAA privacy requirements. Nevertheless, once the HIPAA compliance process is underway, providers will set about standardizing EDI transaction formats, code sets, and identifiers that may further spur EDI efforts in procurement.

In the eyes and ears of hospital personnel, B2B, Y2K, and HIPAA may also compete in terms of hype and drama. For them, the urgency of Y2K was followed by the urgency of HIPAA and now by the urgency of B2B. Following the lead of employees in industry who have confronted waves of new consulting interventions, health care personnel may adopt the mantra of avoidance ("wait and see") or the mantra of BOHICA ("bend over; here it comes again").

The e-procurement solutions offered by the GPO/B2B alliances must also compete for the customer's "mind share" with the B2B solutions offered by GHX, HealthNexis, and each vendor and distributor in the supply chain. This has become a crowded marketplace, even if one does not consider all of the B2B start-ups. This situation must contribute to the customer's confusion and lack of understanding about e-commerce. B2B also competes with other electronic solutions at both the firm level (ERP systems) and the patient level (electronic medical records and point-of-use devices like Palm Pilots).

Wait for Shakeout

A third issue facing IDNs is the large number of B2B entrants in the market with little to differentiate them. At the same time, there are no common standards or platforms to allow all B2B firms to partner with all providers. Hence, providers may wait for the inevitable industry shakeout and the emergence of an industry standard before they partner with B2B firms. Recently announced agreements between GHX, HealthNexis, and Neoforma may signal this emerging standard in the future (see Chapter Ten). Moreover, providers comment that the B2B frenzy reminds them all too well of the physician practice management company (PPMC) frenzy of the early 1990s, which induced hospitals to purchase primary care physicians (PCPs). Providers don't want another debacle on their hands. While Wall Street departed the PPMC industry for more profitable lines of investment, hospitals were stuck owning unprofitable PCP practices.[55]

Physician Integration

A fourth issue facing IDNs is their lack of integration with physicians. Many of the promising developments in health care (for example, physician-hospital alliances and clinical integration) have faltered badly due to the lack of alignment between IDNs and their physicians.[56,57] Certain e-commerce initiatives may likewise rest on IDN-physician or B2B-physician collaboration. Recent evidence suggests that these parties may be far apart in their "Net expectations." For example, in one survey, two-thirds of nonphysicians asserted that physician on-line participation was important or very important to execute their own Net plans.[58] In contrast, only a minority of physicians who were active users viewed the Internet as useful or extremely useful for a variety of activities such as providing patient education (25 percent), purchasing products and services (10 percent), obtaining or transferring medical records (10 percent), and processing health insurance claims (10 percent).

Efforts to customize B2B solutions for particular IDNs must take into account variations in physician-institution relationships throughout the IDN, as well as physician receptivity to the Internet, IT, and new technology. With regard to physician-institution relationships, several supply chain participants commented that vendors have an easier time reaching their physician customers in an IDN that has excellent working relationships with these practitioners.[59] When excellent physician-hospital relationships exist, the organization has an easier time of identifying key physicians and opinion leaders, developing disease management programs, and care path development efforts. The presence of such features facilitates the sale of branded products such as drugs and devices. Trust and good working relationships may also be essential for any clinical standardization initiatives.[60] Unfortunately for hospitals, such excellent working relationships are not widespread, according to several national surveys of IDNs and their physicians.[61,62]

Materials managers can play a key role here. These managers need to develop strong interpersonal skills to deal with clinicians. Some analysts suggest they need to actually "partner" with physicians, whom they view as inflexible and difficult, since physicians control the selection of medical devices. Physicians reportedly have closer relationships with the sales representatives from device manufacturers than they do with their own materials managers. The latter may thus need to spend much more of their time with physicians, nurses, and sales representatives in an effort to exert some influence over the process of device ordering. They can provide clear, accurate, and up-to-date information on the supplies that end users are ordering; and access to product codes and prices when orders are placed to help (1) order the desired product, (2) permit cross-referencing and product comparisons, and (3) reduce pricing variations and off-contract buying.

Physician Receptivity to the Internet

Another issue concerns physician receptivity to and participation in Web-based activities. The barriers here are quite familiar:

No compensation structure that rewards them for on-line participation.

Lack of a "cost driver" such as managed care pressures or formularies in the area of medical supplies.

Lack of requirement by either HCFA or HMOs to adopt Web-enabled administrative processes.

Fears of increased liability issues and concerns over security and confidentiality.

Physicians' belief that going on-line will not improve their productivity.

Physicians' belief that on-line applications address the business rather than the clinical domain (for example, ease and accuracy of clinical results obtained).

Possibility that Internet-based clinical solutions will drive administrative solutions (not vice versa).

No evidence that B2B solutions save time, improve physician cash flow, or improve quality of care.

Current inability of B2B solutions to address major areas of opportunity for physicians, such as reduce medical errors and improve patient compliance.

Physicians' primary use of the Internet for e-mail and on-line research, as well as search for non–health care information.[63,64]

The failure of B2Bs to recognize that physicians move on clinical time, not on Internet time or venture capital time— reflected in the fact that most Internet applications ignore the time and financial constraints on physicians in small practices.

The estimated $100,000–500,000 cost to a physician clinic to adopt a full Internet solution (for example, EMR, data sharing with payers and labs, and patient e-mail).[65,66]

The lack of retained earnings and thus disposable income, financial managers, and IT systems in most physicians' offices.

Physicians with computers in their offices use them primarily for billing and scheduling.[67]

The complexity and multiplicity of physician transactions requires multiple interfaces involving potentially incompatible technologies.

Lack of resources to transfer information from legacy systems and/or paper files to Web-based system.

Lack of system IT compatibility across provider settings.

Lack of data and communication standards.[68]

High costs of training office staff in computer use.

Physicians' resistance to having payers, hospitals, or other firms thrust new systems at them, and their preference to decide on new technologies for themselves.

Physicians' mantra of "evidence-based medicine" may create yet another chicken-and-egg problem: physicians want to see a lot of their peers use the technology first before they themselves will adopt it.[69]

Lack of ways for physicians to assess Web products, resulting in physician wariness.

General risk aversion of physicians.

It is not even clear that physicians want an Internet solution to their supply procurement function. One recent survey of 1,200 physicians regarding their use of the Internet found that less than one-quarter purchase medical supplies on-line.[70] Similarly, a recent survey of 221 physician practitioners and leaders of large medical groups found that less than one-third have Web-enabled services for medical product procurement, and that the majority of these use the Web for less than one-quarter of their purchasing activities. Only 17 percent of respondents felt that Web-based purchasing offered their group an "essential advantage."[71] Physicians instead typically hand this function off to their office staff and are not concerned about whether it is electronic or paper based; moreover, their staff are not incentivized to cut costs. Thus, any B2B solution entails short-term costs without any short-term benefits in cost, quality, or physician convenience. The potential long-term benefits in back-office administrative and transactional improvements do not capture the attention or imagination of physicians.[72]

B2B Efforts to Target the Physician Market

Some new B2B startups—such as 1StopMD.com, Medsite, Esurg.com, PhyBuy.com, and Everything4MDs—are targeting the physician office supply marketplace.[73,74] They not only provide supplies on-line but also seek to offer on-line detailing to manufacturers for their products. The B2Bs seek to communicate the manufacturer's product message to MDs, as well as survey physicians regarding their response to these products. Physicians receive free or discounted products (or redeemable certificates) in exchange for their survey participation. The problem they face is the now familiar chicken-and-egg problem: B2Bs need lots of physician interest and commitment to attract manufacturers to support and finance their e-detailing efforts, but manufacturers want to see substantial physician interest before they support these efforts.[75]

Physician surveys suggest they want to be able to (1) access information in clinical journals, (2) access test results and medical records, (3) obtain their continuing medical education (CME), and (4) link to payers.[76] Indeed, some have suggested that the sentinel or watershed event in physician receptivity to the Internet will occur when physicians and payers can easily transmit bills and payments to one another.

The lack of physician participation has been cited as a major reason for Healtheon/WebMD's problems. Healtheon had given away to physicians free subscriptions to its medical portal WebMD in an effort to get them to migrate all of their administrative functions to the site. Nevertheless, only 15 percent of the 100,000 physicians who signed up actually used WebMD for transactions.[77] Moreover, the firm suffered a big drop in sponsored subscriptions from physicians and a reported strategic loss of momentum at physician offices.

The Medical Group Management Association (MGMA) suggests that supply costs are less than 5 percent of a group's total expenses.[78] Group physicians may therefore not be concerned about this element in their cost structure, although concern levels may be higher in ambulatory surgery centers or clinics making greater use of pharmaceuticals (for example, oncology clinics). Physician groups also have no retained earnings and no capital budgets. These considerations have prompted some health care IT firms to give their software and devices (for example, Palm Pilots) away to physicians. This has led analysts to ask the question, "Is free cheap enough?" The question may actually be inappropriate. Given that the adoption of any IT solution requires additional training and supervision of office staff, the supposedly free products may not really be cost free.[79] On the other hand, handheld devices may be one key strategy for capturing supply utilization data at the point of service. The key question here is whether physicians will feel encumbered by taking the time necessary to enter such data.

Indirect Avenues to Target Physicians

Some analysts suspect that B2B firms may never succeed at accessing the physician market directly. Instead, they may need to approach physicians indirectly through the physician's office staff. There are an estimated two million office workers in the health care system. Physicians, especially those in larger practices, have delegated to office nurses and managers the tasks of "communicating"; that is, medical and administrative transactions. B2B firms may need to target their products to these personnel, who may or may not be Web users. As part of their marketing, B2B firms may need to conduct "change management" education and offer product training to demonstrate the value of their products and their cost savings.

> The alternate care market is not known for being computer savvy, as it is estimated that only 40 percent of facilities in this market have computers and only 35 percent have Internet access. Because the purchasers for these facilities are generally inexperienced Internet users, the primary features that alternate care facilities are looking for in an e-procurement solution is simplicity of interface and ease of use. Also, because they typically have to negotiate all of their prices in the off-line world, alternate care facilities are looking for one-stop shopping that provides low prices and the ability to do comparison pricing. To exploit this opportunity, e-procurement sites must step up their educational and training initiatives in the alternate care market.[80]

Since these staff may be heavily engaged in routine and mundane tasks, a significant opportunity may exist for B2B firms to enrich their jobs and thereby partner with them. One B2B start-up has developed a "work flow reengineering" program for office staff.[81,82]

Alternatively, B2B firms may need to access physicians through local market players that have physician networks, deep pockets, and dominant positions in their markets (for example, IDNs, payers, and employers). Given that health care markets exhibit tremendous local diversity, it may be sensible for B2B firms to observe the dictum that "all health care is local" and tailor their strategies to local markets.[83–85] As one illustration, B2B firms may access physicians who are already aggregated into independent practitioner associations (IPAs); such a strategy was followed by Healtheon in selling its solution to Hill Physicians Medical Group in the San Francisco Bay area. Unfortunately, most physicians are not organized into either groups or IPAs.[86]

As another illustration, the PointShare Corporation has successfully penetrated the Yakima (WA) market of physicians (170 physicians now on-line) by virtue of their ability to convince hospitals and payers to jointly plan and participate in an Internet-based community health information network. This network will link together hospitals, payers, physicians, and laboratories that interact daily.[87] The experiment, now under way for two years, has piloted the verification of insurance eligibility (30,000 transactions per month) but has not yet been extended to referrals or lab results. Yakima participants suggest that the experiment has been "a slow process that has been gathering momentum," and that "e-health must learn to walk before it can run."[88]

Why is the PointShare experiment taking so long? There is a three-way sales effort focused on hospitals, physicians, and payers. PointShare targets "bowling pin" players and accounts in each market that can accelerate the diffusion of its solution. Once they reach a penetration level of 25–30 percent of the local physicians, they reportedly reach the threshold needed to attract other practitioners to join. The effort also entails an incremental process of selling software and services to physicians, and then connecting the providers electronically with other parties—a process that must resolve incompatibilities in software and paper-based systems one practice at a time. Part of the firm's activities focus on reengineering the work flow of the physicians' office staff to become not only Web users but also Web savvy. Consultants refer to these activities as part of the "high, last-mile costs" for B2B firms to reach inside provider sites.

Overall, PointShare is working in twenty-nine markets in four states, with a reported average penetration of 23 percent of the local physician market. Some analysts have dismissed PointShare, arguing that their solution is "not scalable" to the rest of the country. However, the failure of national, top-down imposed strategies such as Healtheon suggests that only a grassroots model might eventually succeed. While the Internet and B2B provide the opportunity to have global reach (downstream for vendors, upstream for customers), the provision and consumption of health care remain locally based. B2B solutions may not succeed only on the basis of being neutral intermediaries that tie other parties together. They may also need to be trusted partners that provide business accountability and enjoy provider leadership and sponsorship that emerge from within the markets they serve.

IDNs and the Lessons of B2B

The data presented here suggest a very slow diffusion of e-commerce activity in the health care supply chain at the IDN level. There is little understanding of or appreciation for supply chain management and its potential within the IDN, either at the executive level or at the department level (materials management). It does not help that there is little documentation of either (1) the inefficiencies and costs of the traditional procurement process, other than the dated information from EHCR, or (2) the savings associated with Web-based procurement and managing the value chain. As Lynn Everard has noted, it is hard to sell a product to a customer who does not recognize the need for it.[89]

This slow diffusion has several important ramifications for e-commerce. First, hospital customers may be unable to afford the e-commerce investment, and suppliers feel they should not have to pay the costs of integrating with their hospital customers. Thus, neither party that B2B firms are trying to connect wish to be connected using the B2Bs' technology. Consequently, B2B firms will not quickly gain any traction in the market and may fail to earn any significant transaction fees. To succeed, B2B firms will need deeper pockets than the monies already supplied by venture capitalists and Wall Street, which have soured on their prospects. It remains to be seen just how far the GPOs, manufacturers, and distributors want to go with their own B2B investments, partners, or solutions.

Ultimately, the hospital buyers may have to "step up to the plate" and finance some of this investment, since it directly benefits them. B2B firms and GPOs that give this technology to hospitals for free may reduce the latter's sense of urgency about e-commerce and foster a very low level of commitment to the technology.[90] This may help to explain the low utilization of B2B exchanges for product procurement found by Millennium Research Group. Hospital buyers may also have to make several other, related commitments: external commitment to a specific B2B technological solution, internal commitment to use it, and commitment to integrate purchasing systems across multiple hospital sites.

In a similar vein, consulting firms like Cap Gemini Ernst & Young are now calling for IDNs to take more responsibility for supply chain improvements in four areas: assumption of accountability, management of their information, reduction in product and vendor variability, and end-to-end integration of their supply chain activities.[91] Their specific recommendations in these four areas restate much of what we have learned from our interviews:

Assumption of Accountability

Increase accountability for supply chain performance at executive levels of the system.

Increase central control over product supply usage in key areas (for example, OR or cardiac catheterization lab).

Centralize responsibilities and functions (for example, for materials management and procurement) within the IDN.

Increase level of product standardization across IDN.

Increase compliance with processes and product specifications that influence how the IDN sources the products it buys.

Reduce the number of suppliers used and strengthen relationships with the remaining few.

Utilize a supply chain performance scorecard to improve sourcing (for example, use only one GPO or self-contract and get a higher percent of spending under GPO contracts), to improve logistics (for example, use activity-based distribution, LUM, and point-of-service delivery), and to improve technology (higher percent of electronic spending and Web-based IDN-specific product catalogue).

Management of Information

Create a single IDN-wide MMIS or a system that overlays internal legacy systems to provide aggregate reports.

Create a global e-catalogue that integrates product, price, and supplier data into a single, searchable structure that normalizes varying product descriptions and classifies medical-surgical products (which lack UPNs).

Integrate clinical data (for example, on outcomes, procedural guidelines, and clinical usage patterns) and decision-making support into the materials management process.

Reduced Variability in Products and Suppliers

Identify appropriate product differentiation to justify multiple SKUs for a given item.

Utilize clinical product teams to standardize on a given vendor for a given product, reduce the total number of vendors and distributors, and reduce pricing variations across vendors.

Develop supply chain performance metrics in market-based purchasing (for example, contract and noncontract spending, and adherence to contract terms), national contracting (for example, product category spending by vendor, and physician satisfaction), accounts payable and purchasing consolidation (POs per FTE, payables per FTE, and invoice accuracy), and point-of-use implementation (for example, stock-outs).

Integration of Supply Chain from End to End

Redesign internal processes.

Contract for core technology solution from single vendor with broad set of multiple, tightly integrated solution components.

Form hospital-vendor teams to understand one another's objectives and requirements, and to set mutual performance goals for improvement.

Pursue some "quick cash solutions"—in the areas of contract management, pricing, and inventory management—that provide revenue to support long-term improvements.

The slow diffusion of e-commerce also means that the Internet will not be a revolutionary force in the health care supply chain during the short term. This actually affords IDNs and their trading partners the time to do several important things. First, they need to document the inefficiencies in the current procurement and supply chain management process using more recent data than EHCR figures from the mid-1990s. Second, they need to demonstrate the economic efficiencies offered by B2B solutions, for example, as documented in the 2001 Arthur Anderson study. Both sets of data will be important in persuading top IDN executives about the importance of supply chain management and e-commerce capability. Third, they need to demonstrate the tie-in between product utilization data and cost at the point of service with clinical outcomes. Such information will be critical for obtaining some modicum of physician buy-in. It will also provide the information that suppliers want and may be willing to pay for (for example, in terms of reduced product prices or enhanced customer service). Information on product usage will also help vendors to improve their efforts in demand planning and inventory management— areas that impact their production process directly and lower their costs of business.[92]

Fourth, there must be improved visibility of information, as well as willingness and ability to share this information with supply chain partners upstream. Improved visibility requires IDNs to develop processes and implement technological solutions to capture such information, share it and transmit it internally, and then aggregate it for both internal and external supply chain management players. Information sharing is not automatic, given the level of distrust among supply chain players. Prior experience of community health information networks (CHINs) and the slow diffusion of PointShare's product illustrates the difficulty of electronic linkage among health care organizations.

Of course, other supply chain players will be less interested in the visibility of *their own* data (for example, visibility of manufacturers' prices and contract terms). This will pose a difficulty as long as hospitals see the value of the Internet primarily in terms of shopping for the best price offered by competing manufacturers and then having broad choice among product vendors. To overcome this, hospitals will need to refocus their priorities to include partnership (not just price), long-term focus (not just short-term gains), and more comprehensive ways to reduce spending (not just lowering line-item prices). These ways might include product standardization and/or concentrated business with one vendor; the use of formularies for medical-surgical products; the reduction of costs in high-cost hospital areas (for example, pharmacy, or OR); partnerships between physicians, OR supervisors, and clinical pharmacists; and reduced product use ("the cheapest product is the one not ordered and used").

Product manufacturers should actively engage hospitals in these efforts. Manufacturer-provider partnerships may serve to generate additional revenues for IDNs, help providers reduce utilization, and allow vendors to tailor their products to fit within integrated programs of care that do not necessarily rest on product bundling of one manufacturer's products. Instead, the partnership can seek to develop modularized packages of care for defined treatments, episodes of care, or disease management profiles that include anything from single items to complex product packages.

Finally, rather than wait for some set of future B2B solutions, hospitals may wish to consider the pioneering example of Lourdes Hospital (Paducah, Kentucky) and St. Alexius Medical Center (Bismarck, North Dakota). These facilities have pursued bar coding, handheld scanners, EDI, and par-level management strategies to reduce inventory investments and improve service levels. Instead of making heavy investments in B2B or new software or electronic cabinets, these facilities have sought to improve their processes using available technology.[93]

Endnotes

1. Liker, Jeffrey, and Yen-Chun Wu. "Japanese Automakers, U.S. Suppliers and Supply-Chain Superiority." *Sloan Management Review* (Fall 2000): 81–93.
2. EHCR. *Efficient Healthcare Consumer Response*. Chicago: American Hospital Association, 1996.

3. Marhula, Daren C., and Edward G. Shannon. *EHealth B2B Overview*. Minneapolis, Minnesota: U.S. Bancorp Piper Jaffray, 2000.

4. Integrated Cost Management Systems. *Hospital Procurement Processes*. Arlington, Texas: ICMS, 2001.

5. Cassak, David. "Burden of Proof." *In Vivo* (June 2001): 26–40.

6. Hagemeier, Garren. *The E-Marketplace Case for Industry-wide Electronic Product Data Synchronization*. White Paper. Healthcare EDI Coalition, 2001.

7. DeJohn, Paula. "Main E-Commerce Issue in 2001 Will Be Interface." *Hospital Materials Management* 25(11) (2000): 1, 9–10.

8. See Note Six.

9. EHCR. *Activity-Based Management: A Healthcare Industry Primer*. Chicago: American Hospital Association/Association for Healthcare Resource and Materials Management, 1998.

10. Hughes, Tom. "Integrating Existing Supply Management Process to E-Commerce." Presentation to Medical Equipment and Health Supplies on the Internet Conference. Chicago: May 2000.

11. Ibid.

12. Everard, Lynn J. *Blueprint for an Efficient Health Care Supply Chain*. White Paper. Norcross, Georgia: Medical Distribution Solutions, 2000.

13. Cf. Thompson, James D. *Organizations in Action*. New York: McGraw-Hill, 1967.

14. Similarly, price variances for identical items purchased from different vendors average around 75 percent, that is, an item purchased for $10 might cost only $2.50 from another vendor. (Cf. Grebb, Michael. "E-Commerce Rising." *Healthcare Business* (April 2001): 24, 26, 72.) This provides one avenue for GPOs to demonstrate their value. Novation executives claim these savings vary 6–12 percent, depending on whether the hospital joins its committed compliance program. BuyPower executives state the savings can run as high as 18 percent.

15. Lacy et al. *The Value of eCommerce in the Healthcare Supply Chain*. Chicago: Arthur Andersen, 2001.

16. See Note Ten.

17. Marhula and Shannon. EHealth B2B Overview, Exhibit 16.

18. See Note Twelve. Everard argues that while the focus on lowering unit prices may lower the hospital's acquisition costs, the hospital ultimately fails to capture the savings. This is because falling product prices are matched by falling reimbursement by payers. The result is that any savings get passed on to payers. This may threaten the margin of manufacturers in the long-term and thus threaten the incentives for R&D

investment, new product development, and efforts to educate providers about them.

19. Healthcare Business. "Healthcare E-Volution." *Healthcare Business Roundtable* Section: RT1-19 (1999).
20. See Note Nineteen.
21. Hospitals and Health Networks. "100 Most Wired." *Hospitals and Health Networks* (April 2000): Insert.
22. Flory, Joyce. *Healthcare Organizations on the Net*. Santa Barbara, California: COR Health, 1999.
23. Katzman, Christine. "Cyberspace Use in Infancy." *Modern Healthcare* (January 3, 2000): 44.
24. Tschida, Molly. "Prio-IT-ies." *Modern Physician* (May 2000): 18.
25. Superior Consultant Company and Dell Computer Corporation. *12th Annual HIMSS Leadership Survey, Final Report*, March 2001. www.himss.org.
26. Tieman, Jeff. "Survey: Hospitals Dabble in Internet." *Modern Healthcare* (May 1, 2000): 52, 54.
27. Analysts at Goldman Sachs have also conducted annual surveys of hospital procurement personnel. Their data, based on a sample of 302 respondents (but less than 10 percent of those surveyed), suggest a decrease in the proportion of hospitals considering e-procurement between 2000 (32 percent) and 2001 (27 percent). Christopher McFadden et al. Healthcare: Technology and Distribution—*Annual Survey of Hospital Executives*. New York: Goldman Sachs. September 25, 2001.
28. Millennium Research Group. *Online Opportunities in the Medical Products Marketplace*. Stream 1, Issue 3. (April 2001). Toronto: Millennium Research Group.
29. This is the first of many instances where the Millennium data do not quite add up.
30. Millennium researchers define "alternate site market" to include ambulatory surgery centers, long-term care facilities, and physician groups.
31. Boehm et al. *Sizing Healthcare eCommerce*. www.forrester.com (1999).
32. Millennium Research Group. *Hospital Online Procurement Survey*. Stream 2, Issue 2. (September 2000). Toronto: Millennium Research Group.
33. McFadden et al. *Hospital Executive Survey*. New York: Goldman Sachs, 2000.
34. See Note Thirty-Two.
35. Millennium Research Group. *Hospital Online Procurement Survey*. Stream 2, Issue 1. (June 2000). Toronto: Millennium Research Group.
36. See Note Thirty-Two.
37. See Note Thirty-Two.

38. See Note Thirty-Three.

39. See Note Thirty-Two.

40. Millennium Research Group. *Hospital Online Procurement Survey*. Stream 2, Issue 3. (December 2000).

41. See Note Thirty-Two.

42. See Note Thirty-Three.

43. Internet Health Care Magazine. "Report: Hospitals Will Buy Online, But Cautiously." *Internet Health Care Magazine* (October 2000): 10, 14.

44. The Price Waterhouse estimates lie between those of Ernst & Young and Arthur Anderson, reported in Chapter Eleven.

45. See Note Thirty-Two.

46. Gillett et al. *Hospitals' New Supply Chain*. Forrester Research. www.forrester.com (2000).

47. DeJohn, Paula. "Growing Pains: Glitches Mark New MMI Systems." *Hospital Materials Management* 27(1) (2001): 1, 9–11.

48. DeJohn, Paula. "E-Commerce Poses More Questions Than Answers." *Hospital Materials Management* 25(6) (2000): 1, 9–12.

49. See Note Forty-Six.

50. Thill, Laura. "Right Company, Right Time." *Repertoire* 8(10)(2000): 54.

51. Hochstadt, Bruce. Presentation to eHealth: B2B Commerce and Connectivity Conference (July 2000), San Francisco.

52. Hochstadt, Bruce, and David Lewis. *Bits of Paper to Bytes of Data: A White Paper on Healthcare Information and Internet*. San Francisco: Thomas Weisel Partners, 1999.

53. Morrissey, John. "Modern Healthcare's 2000 Survey of Hospital Information System Trends." *Modern Healthcare* (February 5, 2001). www.pwchealth.com.

54. See Note Twelve.

55. Burns, Lawton R., and Douglas R. Wholey. "Responding to a Consolidating Healthcare System: Options for Physician Organizations." In John Blair, Myron Fottler, and Grant Savage (Eds.), *Advances in Health Care Management*. Volume 1. New York: Elsevier, 2000. pp. 273–335.

56. Burns et al. "Physician Commitment to Organized Delivery Systems." *Medical Care* 39(7) (2001): I9–29. Supplement I.

57. Burns et al. "Make, Buy, or Ally: Impact of Governance Mode on Trading Partner Alignment." Paper presented at Annual Meeting of Academy of Management Association. Toronto: August 2000.

58. Michael J. Barrett et al. *Why Doctors Hate the Net*. www.forrester.com (2000).

59. Mark Leavitt, M. D., and Cindy Derouin. Personal communication.

60. Cassak, David. "Tenet Shakes Things Up." *In Vivo* (July/August 1998): 41–53.

61. See Note Fifty-Six.

62. IDNs may be moving to develop more Web-based relationships with their physicians. Computerized physician order entry (CPOE) systems that facilitate test ordering and results may serve as the new electronic platform for physician-hospital integration in the future. There are already reports of academic medical centers (for example, Vanderbilt University) partnering with large drug distributors (for example, McKesson HBOC) to implement systems that encompass not only CPOE but also interactive evidence-based guidelines, treatment advisors, and relevant content prior to placing orders.

63. Chi-Lum, Bonnie, and Robert Durkin. "Physicians Accessing the Internet: The PAI Project." *Journal of American Medical Association* 282(7) (1999): 633–634.

64. Morrissey, John. "Internet Dominates Providers' Line of Sight." *Modern Healthcare* (April 10, 2000): 72–92.

65. Gilbert, Susan. "Privacy Costs and Wariness Slow One Medical Group's Web Use." *New York Times* (October 25, 2000).

66. Southwick, Karen. "Physician, Wire Thyself." *Forbes ASAP* (November 27, 2000): 249–255.

67. In a survey of 800 practices by PricewaterhouseCoopers and *Modern Physician* magazine, 90 percent used their office computers for billing and 80 percent used them for scheduling. Less than 40 percent used computers for patient reminders and managed care applications; less than 30 percent used them for patient records and referrals; and less than 20 percent used computers for telemedicine, prescriptions, and treatment alerts. (PricewaterhouseCoopers. *E-Connectivity Producing Measurable Results.* November 2000).

68. PriceWaterhouseCoopers. *Survey on Internet Use by Medical Groups.* www.pwchealth.com (2001).

69. See Note Sixty-Six.

70. Hoppszallern, Suzanna. "Physicians and the Internet." *Hospitals and Health Networks* 75(2) (2001): Insert.

71. See Note Sixty-Eight.

72. Dvorin, Jeffrey. "Medsite: Fighting for Physicians' Eyeballs." *Start Up* 5(8) (2000): 21–31.

73. Repertoire. "Dot-Compilation." *Repertoire* 9(3) (2001): 44–49.

74. Conn, Joseph. "EBuy: Practices Save Money Ordering Medical Supplies Online." *Modern Physician* (June 2001): 28–29.

75. See Note Seventy-Two.

76. See Note Sixty-Seven.

77. Setton, Dolly. "Sick Days." *Forbes* 166(2) (2000): 56, 58.

78. The bulk of expenses are physician compensation and the salaries and benefits of the office staff. Considering only office-based costs, analysts have estimated that 10–30 percent may be spent on supplies. Cf. Note Seventy-Two.

79. Roniger, L. Rochelle. "Learning to Love the Web." *Healthcare Business* (July 2000): 34–37.

80. Millennium Research Group. *Online Opportunities in the Medical Products Marketplace.* Stream 1, Issue 1. (July 2000). Page 25.

81. Kilgallon, Timothy J. "B–B Commerce: Hot Companies Panel." Presentation to eHealth: B2B Commerce and Connectivity Conference (July 2000), San Francisco.

82. Of course, education and training assistance from B2B firms may also help them to more deeply penetrate the IDN market. In a June 2000 survey, more hospitals were registered with Medibuy (21 percent) than any other B2B exchange. Hospital materials managers reported they had been approached by Medibuy representatives, who educated them on the Web site and helped them register with the company. Medibuy appeared to have succeeded in overcoming one barrier to Internet use—familiarity and ease of using the product. Several managers stated this was the major reason they registered with Medibuy over its competitors. Millennium Research Group. *Hospital Online Procurement Survey.* Stream 2, Issue 1. (June 2000). Toronto: Millennium Research Group.

83. Ginsburg, Paul B., and N. J. Fasciano. *The Community Snapshots Project: Capturing Health System Change.* Princeton, New Jersey: The Robert Wood Johnson Foundation, 1996.

84. Grossman, Joy. "Health Plan Competition in Local Markets." *Health Services Research* 35(1) (2000): 17–35.

85. Kohn, Linda. "Organizing and Managing Care in a Changing Health System." *Health Services Research* 35(1) (2000): 37–52.

86. See Note Fifty-Five.

87. See Note Eighty-One.

88. Rauber, Chris. "e-Health: The View from Main Street." *Healthcare Business* (May 2000): 60–66.

89. Everard, Lynn J. "Dot-Com Trial and Error." *Repertoire* 8(10) (2000): 18–19.

90. Ibid.

91. Cap Gemini Ernst & Young. *The New Road to IDN Profitability: Realizing the Opportunity in the Health Care Supply Chain.* Chicago: Cap Gemini Ernst & Young, 2001.

92. See Note Twelve.

93. Everard, Lynn. "The Supply Chain's Dirty Secret." *Repertoire* 9(5) (2001): 18–19.

Part V

Conclusion

12

. . . .

Conclusion

Lawton R. Burns and John R. Kimberly

Resources and Capabilities of Major Players

This book has devoted considerable attention to three major segments within the health care value chain: producers of health care products (manufacturers of pharmaceuticals, devices, and medical-surgical supplies), purchasers of those products (GPOs and wholesalers or distributors), and the providers that utilize them in institutional settings. The bulk of chapters have described some of the major players in these segments and their respective resources and capabilities. In a nutshell, manufacturers possess important capabilities in product innovation based on extensive investments in research and development, as well as capabilities in direct marketing to providers that utilize their products. Purchasers possess important capabilities in aggregated buying (for example, bargaining and negotiating over price) and physical distribution of large quantities of these products. Providers possess a near monopoly in the choice and use of these products for treatment, as well as a close proximity to the end user—the patient.[1]

Complexity in Value Chain Operation

The book has also devoted considerable attention to describing the complexity of the health care supply chain's operation—including flows of product, money, and information—and how this operation varies by type of product. We have offered various explanations for the observed complexity, including the lack of real-time information on point-of-service consumption of products, the resulting need to gather information on product use in other ways (for example, payment of tracing fees to distributors), the opportunity to earn profits at the expense of other supply chain players, and the desire by purchasers (intermediaries) to insinuate themselves more deeply into the value chain and more closely partner with both producers and providers.

Strategic and Competitive Issues Facing Major Players

The book has also analyzed the competitive and strategic issues confronting these three segments of the health care value chain. There are both commonalities and differences here. A major common thread among most value chain players has been the focus on mergers and acquisitions. Hospitals have horizontally integrated into systems and networks to deal with large managed care organizations (which are the product of mergers), GPOs have merged to focus greater buying volumes and bargaining demands on suppliers, wholesalers have merged to extract greater economies of scale from their warehousing activities and share some of the savings with their hospital customers, and producers have merged to develop broader product portfolios and deal with larger providers and purchasers.

There are also important strategic differences among the three players. Among producers, the major issues are continual product innovation, increasing market share, and developing close customer relationships. For diversified manufacturers, additional issues include how to bundle products to sell more goods from a large number of divisions and how to represent all of these divisions to the customer with a unified face. For purchasers, the major issue is to demonstrate the value they add to the supply chain in linking producers with providers, and thus avoid any attempt at disintermediation. A related issue is how to diversify out of their core function (group buying and physical distribution of product) and develop capabilities in the service arena. For providers, the key issue is the short-term focus on cost control.

Impact of E-Commerce on the Value Chain

Contrary to the stock market craze and hype of 1999–2000, the impact of e-commerce on health care appears to be more evolutionary than revolutionary. Unfortunately, this evolution will be slow. Some of the major players (for example, producers and GPOs) have developed their e-commerce strategies for primarily defensive reasons, and might not place a top priority on these efforts. Producers and purchasers have each developed large B2B exchanges that now confront one another and may have a difficult time attracting membership from the other side. Indeed, some of these exchanges now appear to be trying to coexist by listing themselves on each other's Web site, rather than developing a unified portal for electronic supply purchasing.[2] Providers appear to be limping into the B2B arena for a host of reasons, some of them financial, some of them cultural and professional. Their slow movement will retard the key development that producers are looking for: the availability of real-time data on point of use of their products that might enable demand planning.

Prospects for Extended Enterprise Models in the Health Care Value Chain

Finally, the book has investigated whether strategic alliances of the sort observed in the automobile industry are possible among the three segments of the health care value chain. We conclude that "extended enterprises" are not likely to emerge in health care in the near future for a host of reasons. The three key ingredients in such enterprises—dedicated asset investments in one's trading partners, effective knowledge management and information sharing, and trust—are all lacking. To be sure, some producers have occasionally developed national account managers and customer site representatives to more closely align with large GPOs and providers. However, providers are unable to collect and share critical information with upstream value chain players because they lack point-of-use data on product utilization and they underinvest in information technology. Moreover, there is a widespread lack of trust in supply chain players upstream and downstream and thus a reluctance to share information. This lack of trust is repeatedly exemplified by providers that purchase outside of GPO-negotiated contracts in search of better spot deals, by GPOs that engage in bargaining with producers over price in a "game of chicken" format, and by producers that engage in counter-detailing to providers when they lose GPO contracts.

Indeed, market structure conditions may not exist for extended enterprises to operate within health care. Unlike the "big three" auto manufacturers, health care providers are smaller and fragmented, even if you consider the number of systems and networks into which they have organized themselves. Health care producers are also fairly fragmented, particularly within pharmaceuticals and medical-surgical supplies. (Indeed, the most extensive consolidation in the value chain has occurred among the intervening purchasers—GPOs and distributors.) This means that, for any given pair of product buyers and sellers, there is very low economic penetration of one side into the other. As a result, the two parties with the greatest influence in the value chain suffer from a lack of industry leadership that might inculcate a vision of extended enterprise management to other value chain players. This, of course, presumes that they want to propound such a vision (see the following).

We might note here that the only previous effort to develop such an extended enterprise model in health care originated with an auto manufacturer (Chrysler) that not only had prior experience with the concept but had experienced large outlays as a payer for its employees' health care benefits. This effort focused on teaching total quality management practices to HMOs and providers, but did not extend to either producers or purchasers (intermediaries).[3] Chrysler's effort to extend the extended enterprise model to its health care suppliers began in 2000 with a lot of press but subsided in 2001 after its merger with Daimler and the firm's resulting financial trouble.

In addition to market structure, there are numerous agency problems within each of the three parties that inhibit the formation of trading relationships based on an extended enterprise model. These include the divergent incentives between producers and their sales representatives in the field, between product divisions and the coordinating units that seek to represent them to providers with a united face, between the GPOs and the IDN members they represent, and between the physicians and managers within an IDN.

Finally, extended enterprise efforts are blunted by the lack of aligned incentives across the three parties. As for-profit firms listed on Wall Street, producers are oriented toward growing sales, earnings, and market share. As largely nonprofit firms, hospital providers are oriented toward reducing today's costs and utilization levels to deal with managed care and lower increases in federal reimbursement rates, and perhaps toward standardization in some areas. As largely self-employed entrepreneurs, physician providers are oriented to their own practice preferences and matching products with patient needs and demands, much of which may run counter to hospital standardizing efforts. As intermediaries, purchasers (GPOs and wholesalers) must somehow seek to serve the interests of both sides by expanding producer market penetration via customized programs marketed to providers.

Some Recurring Themes that Inhibit a Value Chain Perspective

The Wharton study has identified a number of common themes across the three players that inhibit a shared value chain perspective. One recurring theme is the chicken-and-egg problem. For example, as discussed in Chapter Ten, it is unclear whether the success of an electronic supply chain rests more on aggregated buyers or aggregated suppliers. The development of rival B2B exchanges among both producers and purchasers suggests this issue has not yet been resolved. Another chicken-and-egg problem follows from the lack of consensus among providers regarding the value of e-commerce. As discussed in Chapter Eleven, the slow diffusion of B2B technology among providers reflects their tendency to delay adoption until there is some professional consensus. However, this consensus is unlikely to develop until providers see that their peers have innovated. Such problems have retarded the emergence of a clear technological platform for electronic commerce.

A related theme is the "game of chicken" played out among value chain participants. Producers and purchasers engage in bargaining showdowns to see which side will flinch at contract time. Producers that lose GPO contracts in a given year engage in counter-detailing at the IDN level to seek to regain some of the lost business. This exacerbates another game of chicken played out between IDNs and their GPO alliances: IDNs that dislike vendor contracts circumvent their own purchasing alliances and seek other producers. The result is the failure of standardization efforts, decreased GPO compliance, and the continued disorganization of buyers.

Perhaps the most important theme is the lack of a shared perspective regarding the importance of the health care value chain. As intermediaries, purchasers tend to place the highest emphasis on the value chain. GPOs and wholesalers have gone to great length to document their contribution to supply chain management and the need for greater efficiencies in procurement processes. Unfortunately for them, the other two parties (producers and providers) are less interested in the value chain. Their lack of interest stems from two different sets of reasons. Producers of branded products are most interested in innovation, research and development, and market share. Their Wall Street valuations, cost structures, and financial returns are more heavily shaped by product development than by product distribution. To the limited extent they focus on supply chains, their attention may focus more on upstream sourcing of their own supply inputs than on downstream distribution of finished products to providers. Moreover, producers regard GPOs and wholesalers as influencers, order takers, and information channels—but not customers. For their part, providers are most interested in reducing costs to satisfy managed care reimbursement constraints, improving quality to satisfy patients (for example, reduce medical errors) and attract physicians, and increasing utilization rates. Historically, there has been no clearly demonstrated path from supply chain management to the achievement of these goals. Materials managers within provider organizations have lacked the training and corporate-level position to make the case that such a path exists. The recent Novation and Arthur Andersen consulting report has tried to help them in this regard.[4]

What Will the Future Hold?

The development of a more widely shared value chain perspective and extended enterprise model in the health care value chain is not likely to soon develop. As noted in Chapter Eleven, the major stumbling block is the end customer—the hospital—and its supply purchasing and procurement activities. Major consulting firms are now targeting the hospital market with supply chain initiatives, with the result that supply chain management may become the next "new thing" in health care. If so, the effort will likely fail, as have prior hospital fads such as vertical integration, physician-hospital alliances, product line management, and restructuring and reengineering. A common problem with all of these efforts has been a top-down approach to organizational change without any concomitant change in how health care is delivered by local teams of providers.[5]

A fundamental improvement in the health care value chain will occur when hospitals employ point-of-use systems to capture product information and when these products have a unified numbering system (for example, UPNs). This will permit value chain players located upstream to analyze and forecast demand for their services and initiate cost efficiencies across the entire length of the chain. Providers will also be able to tie their burgeoning outcomes data to specific products utilized (for example, branded drugs or devices) in a manner that facilitates better product comparisons and cost-effectiveness analyses. Such comparisons may improve standardization efforts, resulting in appropriate targeting of supplies to patient segments and improved product development.

At least two developments are required to help turn this vision into reality. First, the federal government must require unique identifiers such as UPNs on medical supplies. The Medical Payment Advisory Commission (MedPAC) has discussed this possibility as part of its technology assessment activities, but has balked due to the disruptions this change would cause in Medicare coding and data collection. Such a change must be centrally imposed, given the lack of producer incentives to standardize product numbers and the lack of concerted provider will to demand them.

Second, there must be greater innovation and implementation of devices to capture data at the point of service. While a limited number of IDNs and major academic medical centers have invested in developing their own systems, most hospitals have not. Here, again, the impetus for change must come from outside the walls of provider organizations. This past year (2001), a coalition of Fortune 500 firms called the Leapfrog Group called on providers to adopt computerized physician order entry (CPOE) systems to reduce prescribing errors. Given their tight operating margins, providers are unlikely to widely adopt such systems without the financial support of these corporations or product vendors.

To be truly useful, such systems must be easily integrated into practitioner work flows. In this light, there are some subtle but important transformations already taking place. A small number of elite medical schools (Harvard, Stanford, and Duke, to name only the earliest cases) have signed agreements with the providers of personal digital assistants (PDAs), whereby each new medical student will be given a PDA at the beginning of school. This hardly seems radical on the surface. But two facets of this example are particularly noteworthy in their implications for the value chain. The most obvious is the fact that, unlike their predecessors, these students will go through their entire training experience digitally linked to a variety of data storage and retrieval entities and multiple information sources. Students will thus both provide data in digital form to various storage and retrieval entities, and receive information from a variety of sources. Having these linkages will become second nature to them—and perhaps as natural as wearing a white coat.

Moreover, the distributors of the PDAs in these arrangements with medical schools also have relationships with software manufacturers. These manufacturers have developed products that are designed to be both productivity enhancing and clinically useful. The software may, for example, enable them to send and retrieve diagnostic images instantaneously, thus enhancing productivity. It may also provide up-to-date information on drug interactions, thus helping them avoid medical errors. So, in the future, by consulting his or her PDA, a physician will both provide and get access to information instantaneously that will shape important decisions, singly and in the aggregate.[6]

It is not just the physician's world that will change as a consequence of the widespread use of the PDA. The roles of producers (medical suppliers) and insurers will also be affected by the access to data such a device provides, as will the organization of the entire value chain.

Nevertheless, the central role of physicians in the health care value chain (see Exhibit 1.1), physicians' near monopoly over key transactions (for example, drug prescribing, test and product ordering, and hospital admission), and the producers' view of them as key customers make them the key to health care transformations. As individual physicians embrace these new point-of-use systems that capture product data and incorporate them into their daily work flow, the health care value chain can become more electronically enabled to thereby facilitate demand planning by producers.

Changes such as these at the local-provider level will provide a more firm foundation for organization-wide and systemwide transformation. However, to be successful, these changes must not only be integrated into practitioner work flows but must also be accompanied by concomitant changes in other parts of the provider organization. These additional changes are legion. They include improved training and elevation of the materials manager role, increased salience of procurement in the top executive suite, technological investments in information technology to automate inventory and procurement functions, investments in process redesign to eliminate steps in these functions, and behavioral and cultural change interventions to break down professional resistance (for example, to standardization and utilization programs).

Moreover, to avoid the failure of prior organizational innovations (for example, integrated health care), the revamped health care value chain must find parties willing to pay for it. Technology firms have already shown a willingness to give handheld devices to physicians in hopes of building their software businesses. Producers of medical-surgical, device, and pharmaceutical products may be willing to help finance the needed investments in return for improved data on utilization of their products. Purchasers such as wholesalers may also assist in financing these investments as part of their continued effort to upgrade the information systems and provide value-adding services to their hospital customers. Finally, large corporations may need to help support these innovations if they wish to promote their vision of reduced medical errors for their employees.

Endnotes

1. There are two limitations to the claim that providers possess important capabilities in the choice and use of health care products. The first is the current shift toward consumerism and increasing patient requests for certain products (for example, prescription drugs). The second is the lack of an evidence base for the majority of medical practice, according to the Dartmouth Atlas (cf. DartmouthAtlas.org).
2. Hospital Materials Management. "E-Commerce Consolidation Continues with Deal Uniting Platforms of GHX, Neoforma." *Hospital Materials Management* (October 2001): 6.
3. Oswald, Kathy. "Making the Business Case for Quality Management." Presentation to the Wharton School, October 2000.
4. Lacy et al. *The Value of E-Commerce in the Healthcare Supply Chain.* Chicago: Arthur Andersen, 2001.
5. Burns, Lawton, and Mark V. Pauly. "Integrated Delivery Networks (IDNs): A Detour on the Road to Integrated Healthcare?" Paper prepared for Council on the Economic Impact of Health System Change, Washington D.C. (December 2001).
6. This scenario raises at least as many concerns as it portends positive changes, and these need to be fully acknowledged. Among the most significant are data security and the objectivity of the software developers. The privacy of individual records needs to be protected, and information content needs to be free from undue commercial influence. Assuming that these concerns can be satisfactorily addressed, one can imagine that the clinical dimension of the physician's world will change dramatically.

Index

• •